Praise for *The Inside Tract*

"*A fine, clear guide to the many ways our gut serves us.* The Inside Tract *shows us how we can easily use delicious food and science-tested supplements to keep our GI tract humming and ourselves healthy and happy.*"
—JAMES S. GORDON, MD, AUTHOR OF *UNSTUCK: YOUR GUIDE TO THE SEVEN-STAGE JOURNEY OUT OF DEPRESSION* AND FOUNDER AND DIRECTOR OF THE CENTER FOR MIND-BODY MEDICINE

"The Inside Tract *is full of wisdom and easy to understand, useful information. Highly recommended.*"
—BERNIE SIEGEL, MD, AUTHOR OF *FAITH, HOPE & HEALING* AND *101 EXERCISES FOR THE SOUL*

"*Kathie Swift, RD, and Gerard Mullin, MD, have put together the first comprehensive integrative approach to digestive health that centers around using 'food as medicine' to heal the gut. This book is an invaluable resource for clinicians and patients alike.*"
—DR. CYNTHIA GEYER, MEDICAL DIRECTOR, CANYON RANCH IN THE BERKSHIRES

"*If you're one of the millions who struggle with digestive distress, this is the balance of scientific grounding and practical tools you need to discover your unique lifestyle for healing.* The Inside Tract *provides a clear, custom path to wellness.*"
—ANNIE B. KAY, MS, RD, RYT, AUTHOR OF *EVERY BITE IS DIVINE* AND LEAD NUTRITIONIST AND REGISTERED YOGA THERAPIST, KRIPALU CENTER FOR YOGA AND HEALTH

Testimonials for Dr. Mullin

"Having Dr. Mullin as my gastroenterologist has truly been a godsend. His professionalism and knowledge is truly unique."

—TS

"I now look at my life in two parts: the time before Dr. Mullin, and the time after. He helped me progress from feeling as though I might be crazy to being someone with a real, manageable condition who was capable of living a fulfilling life. This condition isn't easy, but with Dr. Mullin's guidance and support, I'm able to take advantage of all life has to offer. Truly, I don't know where I would be without him."

—ER

"Finally, finally, finally . . . a doctor who listened to me! I have started to see the rewards of Dr. Mullin's treatment. I have even started working out at a gym—something for which I previously never had the energy. I am extremely grateful to Dr. Mullin and so very thankful that I have found such a committed, caring, and wise physician. I have hit the lottery indeed."

—LK

"I have been seeing Dr. Mullin since June and still I am not on any prescription medication! For someone who struggled through digestive distress for so many years, this is better than any magic or previously prescribed medication. Taking a natural remedy that I know does not have any known negative impact on my health is wonderful. I feel like I finally have a peace of mind."

—NT

THE
INSIDE
TRACT

THE
INSIDE
TRACT

YOUR GOOD GUT GUIDE TO
GREAT DIGESTIVE HEALTH

GERARD E. MULLIN, MD, AND
KATHIE MADONNA SWIFT, MS, RD, LDN

RODALE.

© 2011 by Gerard E. Mullin and Kathie Madonna Swift

Rodale books may be purchased for business or promotional use or for special sales. For information, please write to:
Special Markets Department, Rodale Inc., 733 Third Avenue, New York, NY 10017

Printed in the United States of America
Rodale Inc. makes every effort to use acid-free ♾, recycled paper ♻.

Illustrations by Paul Girard
Book design by Rachel Reiss

Library of Congress Cataloging-in-Publication Data

Mullin, Gerard E.
     The inside tract : your good gut guide to great digestive health / Gerard E. Mullin, Kathie Madonna Swift.
          p.   cm.
     Includes bibliographical references and index.
     ISBN 978–1–60529–264–9 paperback
     1. Digestion—Popular works.   2. Nutrition—Popular works.   3. Digestive organs—Diseases—Alternative treatment.   I. Swift, Kathie Madonna.   II. Title.
     RC801.M85   2011
616.3—dc22   2011003275

Distributed to the trade by Macmillan
          8   10   9   7   paperback

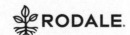

We inspire and enable people to improve their lives and the world around them.
www.rodalebooks.com

To the more than 60 million Americans who are known to suffer from digestive disorders.
To our loved ones for their unwavering support.
To those who mentored us over the years.
And to the beloved memory of our parents.

Contents

Foreword

by Andrew Weil, MD

Digestive disease afflicts 60 to 70 million Americans, according to the National Institutes of Health. However, the rising prevalence of just a few gut disorders calls into question the real scope and magnitude of the problem. For example, 42 million Americans experience heartburn weekly and 30 to 45 million suffer from irritable bowel syndrome. These are just two of the many disorders affecting the digestive system. The numbers don't quite add up!

For many years I have taught patients and physicians that optimum health and spontaneous healing can he achieved through dietary and lifestyle measures and the appropriate use of dietary supplements and natural remedies. Despite the evidence, we as a nation continue to promote the use of costly and potentially toxic prescription medications to treat chronic illness. The most common medications used to treat digestive disease, proton pump inhibitors, are among the best-selling drugs worldwide, but we are becoming increasingly aware that they produce myriad health problems and are far from a home run as therapy. I know there are better, safer, more cost-effective ways to address the rising tide of digestive disease in our population.

The Inside Tract is a groundbreaking book that will serve as an indispensable guide to the millions who suffer from digestive disorders. *The Inside Tract*'s message is simple, but profound: People with these problems can experience relief and healing through the use of a personalized nutrition plan, self-prescribed lifestyle modifications, and the judicious use of targeted natural remedies. Dr. Mullin and Kathie Swift have developed a unique profiling system for digestive illness to help individualize therapy—the Gastrointestinal Point System (GPS)—as well as a unique three-tiered nutrition program that eliminates provocative foods while incorporating ones that heal. They have also provided self-assessment tools to help readers navigate relevant lifestyle factors. Their belief in the power of food as medicine, in mind over matter, and in the benefits of nutraceuticals is supported by many case histories that highlight the successful resolution of chronic digestive illness using the system outlined in this book. In most of the cases, their integrative approach succeeded after a long history of conventional interventions failed.

The heart of this book reflects the very highest ideals of integrative medicine: that the disease can be addressed before it damages tissues and organs and requires drastic, costly intervention; that the body can heal itself if given a chance, that mind/body interactions are real and often very relevant to issues of health and illness, that all aspects of lifestyle must be considered when evaluating the onset of disease and its resolution, and that the doctor/patient relationship strongly influences the outcome of treatment. Mullin and Swift are deeply familiar with a wide range of therapeutic options other than drugs. In recommending therapies not commonly included in mainstream practice, they pay attention to the scientific evidence that supports them, always working from the principle that the greater the potential of a treatment to cause harm, the stricter the standards of evidence for efficacy it must be held to.

I am certain that the integrative transformation now taking place in medicine—a transformation of which this book is an important part—is a necessary prerequisite for building a functional, cost-effective healthcare system, one that emphasizes prevention and health promotion over disease management and that uses costly, technology-based interventions (including pharmaceutical drugs) only when they are truly indicated. We can manage common forms of illness with simpler, less expensive interventions. *The Inside Tract* beautifully illustrates this truth and reflects the principles and practices of integrative medicine.

I have devoted the past 32 years to developing, practicing, and teaching this system. In 1994, I established the University of Arizona Program in Integrative Medicine, now the Arizona Center for Integrative Medicine. Since its inception, the program has trained hundreds of physicians. Gerry Mullin, one of our graduates, recently developed and implemented a digestive disorders module for our fellowship training; it is now an integral part of our program. Gerry is also the editor of *Integrative Gastroenterology* in my Integrative Medicine Library series published by Oxford University Press. As the nation's most prominent integrative gastroenterologist he is pioneering and advancing the field. I have the utmost confidence in his approach to patients as exemplified in *The Inside Tract* and have referred and will continue to refer patients, colleagues and friends to him.

Every patient with digestive disease can benefit from the information and recommendations in this timely book.

Tucson, Arizona
March, 2011

Introduction

You aren't what you eat. You are what you absorb.

When it comes to food and health, most of us grew up listening to the conventional wisdom of our mothers and grandmothers. As children, when we refused to eat our peas, Grandma would look at us menacingly and say, "You are what you eat, you know," meaning that if we ate healthy, we'd live healthy lives and if we didn't, we wouldn't.

This advice is profoundly wise. The link between what you eat and how healthy (or unhealthy) you are cannot be denied. Human beings have known about the connection between food and well-being for millennia, and modern nutritional science has borne out the prudence of our ancestors regarding food in ways unimaginable to most people (including physicians) today.

Poor diet has been linked to chronic illnesses that are so prevalent in the modern world. Changing your diet and consuming the whole, real foods human beings evolved eating can slow and even reverse the progress of a vast array of chronic illnesses.

Despite this fact and the massive body of research regarding how important it is to eat well, we live in a culture that is inundated by products that aren't truly food. Inside your local grocery store, 70 percent of what you can buy isn't food. Put aside the aisles of chemical cleansers, paper towels, toilet paper, and magazines, and the great majority of the items that remain still aren't real foods. They might be better referred to as "ingestibles"—synthesized products you can ingest and which may give you some nutritive value but can't be called "food" in any formal sense.

We are having a cultural food crisis. We have what prominent food writer Michael Pollan calls "a national eating disorder," and it's one that threatens to destroy our very society. The magnitude of the problem really can't be understated. It's killing us.

America ranks last in longevity worldwide among industrialized nations[1] and was the leader in preventable deaths in a study of 19 countries.[2]

Despite the fact that we pay more for health care than any other nation in the world, we are far from healthy, and the foods most Americans eat are surely a factor in this.

But this book isn't about food (though we will talk extensively about how food affects your health and how it can be used as medicine), nor is it about the state of health care in America today (though we will talk about that, too!).

In this book, we are going to approach the whole problem of food and health from the other end of the food chain (from the "other side of the track," so to speak). We are going to look "inside" the problem and analyze one of the primary reasons Americans are so sick today. We are also going to teach you how you can overcome some of the illnesses you may be suffering from by treating yourself, not your illness; by eating what nourishes you, not what profits the food industry; by developing communities and connecting with people you care about; and by finding balance and meaning in your life.

To do this we are going to explore a simple yet profound truth. Here it is:

As astute as the expression "you are what you eat" is, in the end, it isn't quite accurate. The truth is, you aren't what you eat. You are what you absorb.

If you eat nothing but junk food, you're obviously not going to absorb the nutrients you need to live a healthy life. Junk in, junk out. Your health will most likely crumble sooner or later if you live this way.

Imagine what would happen if you started absorbing foods that nourished your body and soul. Imagine what it would be like if you could absorb the emotional stability and sense of peace that makes you feel whole instead of the stress that is making your life so overwhelming. Imagine how free you would feel if you could stop absorbing the toxins and unnecessary pharmaceuticals that are slowly poisoning your body and your life.

You can, but you need to clear up toxins (chemical and emotional) in your life in conjunction with changing what you put in your body if you want to enjoy good health.

The place where this absorption occurs is the place no one thinks to look. It's the place in your body that either makes you healthy or ill, but it's one most of us would prefer to ignore (and we usually do, until it's too late).

The interface between the outside world and the world within your body is not your heart or your brain; it's not your skin or your breath. It's your gut.

Your gut is your inside tract to health and wellness, and it is what this book is all about.

We will tell you more about exactly why your gut is the "inside tract" to health and wellness in the chapters that follow. We will also outline a complete treatment program tailored to your personal experience and needs. This program will allow you to heal your gut and thereby overcome many of the illnesses you may be suffering with. These include common

GERRY'S STORY

I (Gerard Mullin; aka Gerry) began my career as a healer well before I entered medical school. When I was young, my mother suffered from irritable bowel syndrome. I was in high school at the time, and together, she and I went from doctor to doctor looking for ways to treat the extraordinary pain that would keep her writhing in bed for days at a time.

At that time IBS was hardly on anyone's radar, so when my mother developed symptoms that didn't fit the paradigm most doctors had been trained to understand, they dismissed her out of hand, assuming she must be a hypochondriac. After each visit, we both came away disappointed and confused at hearing doctors say, "Mrs. Mullin, your symptoms are from hysteria. This is all in your head."

My mother was a courageous and intelligent woman. She knew her symptoms weren't "all in her head," and she knew there must be a way for her to heal. So she began researching complementary and alternative therapeutic approaches to treating her gut problems—reading books and magazines on natural healing, listening to radio shows on the subject. You name it, she did it.

Using the concepts she learned about how to treat her illness with a whole-foods diet, supplementation, prayerful meditation, and social support, she began to create a protocol for herself to overcome her illness.

To assist her, I shopped for groceries and cooked her meals, and I helped her procure and organize supplements. Her healing became a team effort, and it was in this way that my mom became my first mentor as a healer.

Six months after we began this treatment protocol, mom was a new person. Her friends and family were amazed.

You might say that I grew up around a holistic healing tradition. But what I didn't know then was that history would repeat itself and that I, too, would one day end up on my back looking for answers to an illness that doctors couldn't treat. I never would have imagined that through this experience I would discover the holistic healing program you will learn about in this book.

digestive ailments like gastroesophageal reflux disease (GERD), irritable bowel syndrome (IBS), and others, as well as illnesses that happen "outside the tract," including asthma, allergies, skin problems, myalgias, and more.

From Integrative Gastroenterologist to Autoimmune Patient

Inspired by the experience of my mother's illness and recovery, I decided to become a gastroenterologist. For 13 years I integrated the techniques I learned while helping my mom with the medical training I received at Johns Hopkins, the education I received while earning my master's degree in nutrition, and the dozens of holistic nutrition seminars I attended over the years.

Instead of the typical 10-minute visit you got with most doctors, I spent hours with my patients discussing different therapeutic options, explaining drug treatments that were available, and helping them analyze their diets and lifestyles to see what factors might have led to their gastrointestinal (GI) upset. My goal was to integrate any treatment that worked into a holistic approach designed to treat people, not diseases.

Then, one day in September of 2003, during an extremely stressful period of my life, I went from being a successful integrative GI specialist to being a patient in the hospital.

Without warning, I started having episodes of muscle twitching. The muscles in my arms and legs would buzz with strange tremors; it was unlike anything I'd ever experienced before. My gut instincts told me that my symptoms were stress related. I suspected that my magnesium levels were low—which often happens when people experience chronic stress—and that this was leading to my muscle twitching.

I began to work up the same kind of integrative analysis on myself that I typically did for my patients.

In the meantime, I spoke with doctors about the muscle twitches and asked their advice. Their prognoses were all different and more terrifying than my own.

One doctor suggested it may be ALS (Lou Gehrig's disease), a neurodegenerative disorder that affects nerve cells in the brain and spinal cord, ultimately resulting in total paralysis. Since motor function is always affected when ALS strikes, it was a possible explanation for my twitching.

Another doctor, a multiple sclerosis (MS) specialist, said it may be MS. Though the possibility of MS was remote, since the only symptom I had was these muscle twitches, she suggested I have a lumbar puncture (a procedure where spinal fluid is drained for later analysis) to rule out affliction with the disease.

My gut instinct was to wait for the results of my red blood cell mineral count and other integrative tests to see if low magnesium levels were the problem. I wanted to postpone the lumbar puncture for a few months and try to treat myself. But I trusted his expertise, and agreed to the lumbar puncture.

As soon as I saw the blood-tinged tube of spinal fluid in the doctor's hand, I knew I had made the wrong choice. The doctor performing the procedure entered the conus medullaris—the place where your spinal cord ends. One bad move here, and I could have been paralyzed for life.

Within hours of the procedure, excruciating pain radiated from the spot of the spinal tap down my back and through my legs. While I was writhing in pain, the doctor started testing my reflexes to make sure my spinal cord was not seriously injured. Thankfully, it wasn't, but I was in the worst pain I had experienced up to that point in my life. On a scale from 1 to 10, I was at a 10. I could hardly sit up in the hospital bed. I could barely walk.

He sent me home. So much for professional courtesy!

My brother Patrick picked me up from the hospital, and I asked him to call a neurosurgeon that we knew. When I explained what had happened, the doctor said, "What are you doing at home? You need to be in a hospital right now. I am going to have you admitted."

From Bad to Worse

When I got to the hospital, doctors recommended a blood patch (a procedure where blood is taken out of your arm and shot into the space around your spinal column) to close the leaking lumbar puncture and stop the headaches. When it works, this treatment can be extremely effective. When it doesn't, it can be catastrophic.

For a blood patch to work correctly, the blood has to be shot into a tube that runs around the spine. This is called the epidural space. If it is shot here, you are safe. However, if blood ends up in the subarachnoid space, where only spinal fluid is meant to be, your body sees this blood as an enemy and begins attacking it viciously. Antibodies are sent to wipe out these "foreign invaders." In short, you have an autoimmune response where the body mistakenly attacks its own cells.

That is what happened to me. And it resulted in one of the most difficult autoimmune disorders to treat—arachnoiditis.

Arachnoiditis is a pain disorder caused by inflammation of the spinal nerves running off the spinal cord and coursing through the arachnoid membranes (membranes normally meant to surround and protect the spine). This inflammatory reaction can be set off in many ways. Spinal surgery, which is bloody, is one possibility. Blood patches that go awry and botched spinal taps are less common causes, but they can cause it as well.

The cascading inflammatory response set off by arachnoiditis scars the tissues of the spine. In my case, I was left with constant, almost unbearable burning pain that coursed through my lower back and pulsed down my legs.

There's no known cure for arachnoiditis. In the worst cases it can cause paralysis, loss of bowel function, and loss of sexual function. Even those whose symptoms aren't quite so grim can expect a life of constant pain. It wasn't looking good for me at that stage.

But I didn't know any of that at the time.

What followed were dark days for me. Upon returning home, I had no idea why I was in so much pain. I was beginning to feel fed up with the doctors who had offered no explanations for the complications that I experienced. The pain soon became so unbearable that it was impossible to go to work, so I stayed home. I had a hard time walking. I was at my wit's end.

I realized that I was going to have to look for answers on my own and began typing my symptoms into an Internet search engine. Eventually Dr. J. Antonio Aldrete's Web site popped up, and when I saw the symptoms listed there and the causes of them, I knew I had arachnoiditis.

I sent Dr. Aldrete an e-mail asking whether or not he thought I might have the disease. His response came that afternoon, far faster than I expected. It was brief and to the point: *Yes, you could have it. Contact us immediately. Time is of the essence in treatment.* Needless to say, I called his office that day. Dr. Aldrete agreed to look at the films of my spine and talk to my doctor. He confirmed what I had begun to suspect: It was indeed arachnoiditis.

The treatment Dr. Aldrete recommended was an extremely aggressive dose of intravenous steroids. He has had some success using this method at the inception of the sickness. High-dose steroids can arrest the inflammatory response in some cases and slow the progress of the disease. The doses required are toxic and are usually only given to MS patients for severe disease. But Dr. Aldrete's success rate looked good, so I agreed to try the drugs.

The Medical Mishaps Mount

In response to the third cycle of high-dose corticosteroids, my cardiac rhythm destabilized into atrial fibrillation (a cardiac arrhythmia that involves the upper two chambers of the heart). This could have been complicated by a stroke, so I had to be rushed to a hospital to be shocked out of it.

A couple of months after this, my doctor suspected that I had a blood clot in my leg. I ended up being admitted to the hospital. There, I was treated with blood thinners that were ultimately unnecessary. I didn't have a clot, but I was given blood thinners nonetheless.

I was eventually put on yet another round of anti-inflammatory medications; these ate a hole in my gut and caused a peptic ulcer that bled heavily. I knew I was bleeding internally, but when I expressed this concern to the on-call doctor at the time, she told me, "You really need to stop trying to be your own doctor." It wasn't until I handed a commode filled with blood to a nurse on staff that anyone took me seriously. The doctor reacted in a panic and asked for my advice.

Luckily, an outstanding intensive care specialist, Dr. Roseanne Russo, and my former partner (who I trained as a fellow), Dr. Lisa Lih-Brody, were in the hospital that morning. They moved me into the intensive care unit within minutes and treated the huge peptic ulcer in my duodenum (the first part of the small intestine). My bleeding was so profuse that the attending anesthesiologist involved in my treatment told me that my blood was the color of Hawaiian Punch.

While in the intensive care unit, I was given penicillin, which I am extremely allergic to. My medical records indicate the allergy quite clearly, and I was wearing an allergy bracelet stating that I would have a reaction to the drug, but no one seemed to notice. It wasn't until I saw my skin turning red and my blood pressure bottoming out that I began to suspect what had happened.

Because my concerns were ignored, I had to hit the "CODE" button myself when I saw my blood pressure finally drop down to barely detectable levels. Doctors rushed in and put me on leg pressers to keep my blood pressure high enough to sustain life while they gave me high doses of blood pressure medication until the allergy rode itself out.

My immune system was so weakened at this point that I contracted pneumonia and was again assigned an antibiotic that I was allergic to; I then suffered from renal failure that improved once the antibiotic was discontinued. Again, I noticed what was going on, and again, my concerns were dismissed. I was actually told to "be quiet" when expressing my concerns by one of my ex-colleagues who was caring for me. It wasn't until I personally asked a nephrologist (a kidney specialist) to come in and have a look at me that the renal failure was confirmed and treated.

Although I was disturbed by this dark comedy of medical errors, it gave me the opportunity to witness firsthand how medicine, as a profession, has lost its way. Doctors don't listen to patients anymore or react to their health concerns. We ignore patients not only when they present with subtle symptoms, but even when they show up with the red flags of serious illness. This is the real tragedy of medical care today.

Even after I left the hospital, my struggles were far from over.

Upon being released, I was prescribed physical therapy. This is a ludicrous treatment for someone who has a spinal injury with arachnoiditis. In many cases, when people have a spinal injury and undergo physical therapy, their progress is reversed because the inflammation increases from being pushed too hard. That's what happened to me.

As my condition worsened, the hospital where I was working made it clear that I was on the verge of losing my job. So I kept at the physical therapy despite the fact that it caused me agonizing pain, and I began swallowing ever more powerful pain medications in the hope that I could make it back to work and salvage what was left of my professional life.

Overcoming the Incurable Disease

What I was doing clearly wasn't working. The pain medications gave me little relief and made my mind dull and fuzzy. The physical therapy worsened my condition instead of improving it. I had come to the end of the road with Western medicine; I had turned into another one of those "hard-to-treat" cases. I was almost certainly going to lose my job, and on top of everything, my mother was dying over 90 miles away and I very much wanted to be with her to help her with whatever she needed. Given my condition, I didn't think I would make it to see her until it was too late.

When it became completely clear to me that nothing I was doing was going to help me, I had a kind of revelation. I guess hitting that rock bottom spot of desperation was, in some ways, a blessing. It suddenly occurred to me that I had been overly reliant on a system that emphasizes invasive tests and magic bullet medications. Conventional Western medicine had spun its web and trapped me as it had trapped so many others.

I knew I had to finally take charge of my life and my treatment before it was too late. I decided I was going to be my own doctor for a change and concentrate on healing myself.

The first thing I did was let go of my job. I thought, *If I lose my job, so be it. I'm just going to get better and figure out what I will do with my life from there.*

With that resolution in place, I watched an old, reliable, inspiring movie—*Rocky*. I always loved it when Rocky's trainer, Mickey, came on the screen and said, "Can't? There ain't no such thing as can't." It gave me the motivation to keep going, despite the odds.

Over the next few weeks, I put my laptop on my knees while lying in bed and began sifting through thousands of scientific and medical journals looking for alternative ways I could treat myself. It was the same path my mother had walked all those years ago.

Slowly I began to put together pieces of a treatment protocol for myself. I found new ways to get pain relief without being on those junky narcotics. For example, I learned that a derivative of cough syrup, dextromethorphan, sits on the same nerve receptors as narcotic painkillers yet doesn't have as many side effects. I used that until I could find other solutions.

I started looking for nutraceutical supplementation that would modulate pain just like the dextromethorphan did. I finally found an all-natural substitute so I could get off the drugs entirely.

I also started discussing treatment options with respected colleagues who took a more integrative approach to care. People like John McCorrie (a master herbalist in Nottinghamshire, England), Dr. Russel Portnoy (a leading integrative pain specialist), and Dr. Fred Smith (an integrative primary care physician).

I began to understand and treat my condition as a self-perpetuating chronic inflammatory response. I iced my back and took supplements that helped reduce inflammation.

Within a matter of weeks, my pain began to diminish.

The real shift in my condition occurred when I went back to the whole-foods diet I had been eating since my mother discovered the power of food as medicine when she was sick. You see, I had been eating a "special diet" prescribed for my peptic ulcer. This consisted of mashed potatoes, gelatin dessert, and a bunch of other processed, tasteless, unhealthy foods. It is unfortunate how little many doctors know about nutrition. It isn't addressed sufficiently in medical school—a lecture here and there is all most physicians-in-training get about the value of nutrition in health.

When I went back to my whole-foods diet, the difference was like that between day and night. My pain diminished even more rapidly. I began to feel more energetic. I could get up and move around more freely and for longer periods of time. In short, I was getting better.

About 6 weeks after I began treating myself, it became clear that my mother would not make it. She was admitted to a hospital in Manhattan, but rather than being stuck at home, I was now well enough to get in the car and make the drive to see her.

When I got there, I shared with her my renewed beliefs in an integrative, holistic approach to treating illness. I told her I had decided to pursue a PhD in nutrition and continue the work we had begun together so many years before. She never scolded me or said, "I told you so." She just looked at me and said, "Well, I think it's about time."

A few weeks later, my mother passed away at the ripe old age of 82. The length and quality of her life were her final testament to the power of integrative medicine. People who are as sick as my mother typically don't live to see 82. Her cardiologist was baffled that she made it as long as she did, and Mehmet Oz—best known as Dr. Oz—who was my mother's cardiac surgeon, was impressed that she was able to sustain such a high quality of life for so many years using integrative therapies she had researched herself.

It was a blessing that I was there to be with her when she went—a blessing that was a direct outcome of the lessons she taught me about health and healing when I was a child. If I hadn't gone back to my roots and embraced the integrative approach she introduced me to all those years ago, I may not have made it to the hospital in time to share her last moments.

After my mom died, I continued to refine my treatment protocol. I kept taking the supplements that Dr. Loren Marks (a colleague, friend, and board-certified nutritionist from New York City) and I configured, stayed on my whole-foods diet, and I got better and better.

By the spring of 2005, I had started to feel like my old self again in many ways. I was on the road to recovery.

My Journey Back to Johns Hopkins

It was about this time that Dr. Tony Kalloo called me from the gastroen-terology department at Johns Hopkins and offered me a job. He knew what had happened to me at my previous place of employment, understood the history and complexity of my illness, and wanted to help me salvage what was left of my professional life. Tony and Johns Hopkins gave me an opportunity no one else was willing to at the time, and I will be forever grateful to them for it. Tony started the newsletter *Inside Tract* shortly after becoming director of Gastroenterology and Hepatology at Johns Hopkins in 2005. Because of his heroic efforts I named this book in his honor.

Tony hired me for a desk job. Even though I was getting better, neither of us really expected that I would be walking the halls of a hospital or actively treating patients again. We both turned out to be wrong.

As long as I continued on the integrative, holistic treatment program I had developed for myself, my condition continued to improve. In fact, it improved enough that shortly after being hired at Johns Hopkins, I was able to start being a doctor again—I would not be relegated to a desk job forever.

Today, if you look at me, you would never know that only a few years ago I had been so sick that I was bedridden from the pain. I am now an associate professor at Johns Hopkins University. I'm also editing the first textbook on integrative gastroenterology for physicians (for Dr. Andrew Weil), co-editing the first gastrointestinal nutrition pocket guide for the American Dietetic Association, and co-editing the first gastrointestinal and liver disease desk reference for CRC Press.

As long as I stick to my regimen of proper eating, stress reduction, life-style maintenance, and supplementation, I keep my symptoms at bay. Dr. Aldrete himself considers my recovery miraculous. He says he has never seen a case like mine. In fact, at his request, I have coauthored a chapter on nutrition and diet for the second edition of his authoritative textbook on arachnoiditis for physicians, and I have addressed an inter-national conference on the role of nutrition in treating this disease.

Take a few moments to consider the approach I took to heal myself. There were four essential ingredients to it.

1. **Whole-foods diet.** I stick to a primarily vegetarian, whole-foods diet that includes lots of vegetables full of phytonutrients, plenty of fiber, whole grains, little gluten or dairy, and wild cold-water

fish that are full of omega-3 fats. It wasn't until I got back to this core diet that my condition really began to turn around.

2. **Nutritional supplementation.** Despite the fact that scientific studies support the use of nutritional supplementation, many doctors are still skeptical of the value of supplements. For me, supplements were absolutely essential in my healing. I feel they are essential for others as well and recommend them regularly to my patients.

3. **Detoxification.** I always include freshly prepared vegetables (a combination of root and leafy vegetables) to help optimize my body's detoxification abilities.

4. **Lifestyle changes.** When I finally gave up my stressful job and took care of myself instead of worrying about the needs of profit-driven workplaces, I was able to overcome my condition. Stress kills. Relaxation is essential. Exercise is important, too. If you don't look carefully at the larger aspects of your lifestyle and analyze how your psychological and spiritual needs are involved in your health, it is much more difficult to heal.

The steps that I took to heal myself are the essence of the treatment approach you will find in Part III of this book. There, Kathie and I are going to teach you techniques that she and I have used for decades to successfully treat patients.

These tools are especially effective in treating digestive disorders. By using these techniques to heal your gut and treat inflammation in your body, you can overcome the debilitating symptoms you have been struggling with for so long.

However, the techniques you will learn aren't limited to treating gut conditions. After all, my condition did not technically begin in my gut. Many other health conditions can be handled the same way. By treating your inside tract and reducing inflammation throughout your body, you set the stage for a lifetime of wellness.

Your gut knows more than you think it does. You should listen to its intuition and wisdom. I wish I had listened to my own gut all those years ago when it told me to treat the muscle twitches I was experiencing (the ones that set off the cascade of medical mishaps that eventually led to arachnoiditis) using the holistic approach I have been using for decades. If I had, it's pretty likely that I would never have gone through my horrific health nightmare. You see, my red blood cell mineral count came back just weeks after I had that fateful lumbar puncture. It turned out that my magnesium levels *were* low, just as I suspected. Once my magnesium levels were replenished, the twitches went away!

Yet if I hadn't gone through that experience, I wouldn't know what I know today. I wouldn't be able to fully apply the holistic, empathetic model I now use to treat my patients if I hadn't used my own health crisis to refine my healing practices. I wouldn't be part of a movement that is actively trying to change the way medicine is practiced in this country.

I may not have met my coauthor, Kathie Swift.

And we may not have written this book.

For me, that would be a tragedy. This program is something I am proud to share. I hope each of you chooses to use it to develop a new relationship with your gut, overcome your digestive disease, and live a vitally healthy life for many years to come.

Why a GI Specialist and a Nutritionist Teamed Up to Write a Book on Gut Health

Kathie Swift and I came together to write this book because we wanted to put the tools we use to heal digestive disorders (whether they are the core cause of your health problems or the underlying factor in another illness) into the hands of people like you, who need them.

As a GI specialist who focuses on holistic and alternative methods for healing the gut, I bring to this book nearly two decades of knowledge in the science and treatment of the gut. I also bring my personal experience in developing a treatment protocol that I used to overcome my "incurable" illness.

I also happen to understand just about every diagnosable digestive disorder there is, the standard protocols used to treat these disorders in conventional Western medicine, what kind of response and treatment you can expect from your doctor (since I am one), and what kind of alternatives you have in terms of treating and healing your gut.

Kathie has an exhaustive background in integrative medical nutrition therapy. She worked as the director of nutrition at Canyon Ranch for years, and during her tenure there she initiated a revolution in the way they treat people by using food and nutritional therapies as medicine. She is the curriculum designer of the Food As Medicine professional training program held and sponsored every year by the Center for Mind-Body Medicine.

This is where leaders in the field of nutritional therapy gather to disseminate information about how to integrate dietary practices into a clinical setting. She served as the inaugural chair of the American Dietetic Association's Dietitians in Integrative and Functional Medicine, a dietetic practice group leading change in nutrition care. Kathie also helped her long-time friend and colleague, Dr. Mark Hyman, create the UltraWellness Center, a clinic for individuals suffering from chronic, complex conditions. She started the first holistic Digestive Healthy Living Program at Kripalu Center for Yoga and Health and helps workshop participants heal using whole foods, supplementation, and lifestyle changes. The nutritional therapy protocols she has developed and the fact that she is at the very hub of an ongoing revolution in the way food is used to help people heal make her one of the most unique dietitians practicing in America today.

In teaming up with one another, what we offer you is the first completely comprehensive self-help program that will allow you to heal your digestive disorders, optimize your health, understand what to expect if you *do* end up in a medical setting (what tests you might anticipate, for example), and reconnect with your gut—your inside tract to health and well-being— in a fundamentally new and different way.

How to Use This Book

In Part I, we review what digestive disorders are, how many people have them, the kinds of digestive disorders that exist, and why the epidemic of digestive disease in this country is a reflection of the imbalances in our society. With that information in place, we then take you on a guided tour of your inside tract.

In Part II, we give you a detailed explanation of the dietary and lifestyle changes previously outlined that form the core of this program. We review some of the scientific literature that tells us how making these changes will help you heal, and we review many of the physiological mechanisms triggered that create and support a move toward greater health. Along the way you will read stories about miraculous recoveries our patients have made using many of the same techniques presented in this book.

Part III is really the guts of the book, if you will. Here we move from the theoretical to the practical and offer you a step-by-step way to integrate all of the dietary and lifestyle changes recommended in Part II over a period of 2 or more weeks. We include real-life case stories to show how the program works, simple checklists you can use to follow the program, a complete set of gut-healing meal plans (with recipes in the Appendix), and our GPS self-assessment tool that will place you on one of three tracks to healing your digestive system.

Track 1 is designed for people with periodic minor digestive symptoms or those who simply want to maintain optimal health. In it you will find a delicious meal plan as well as whole food recipes to help you live a long and healthy life.

Track 2 is for people who have an established digestive disease requiring medical intervention, such as GERD, nonulcer dyspepsia, or IBS with moderate symptoms. People who fall into this category are those whose disease may end up progressing if they don't take action now. If you follow the steps outlined in this section, you will go on an elimination diet that will help you heal your gut.

People with digestive disorders with severe symptoms will most likely end up on Track 3. This is where we give a full program for improving even the worst cases of Crohn's disease and ulcerative colitis, as well as other challenging GI conditions. Stricter dietary strategies are outlined in part of this track.

You don't need to worry about which track to go on right now. The GPS quiz on page 161 of Part III will give you all the information you need to know. Just read Parts I and II, take the quiz, and follow your path to health.

We will be there with you every step of the way. We help you see how far along you are in recovery, tell you when it might be okay for you to switch from one track to the next, and explain *how to* employ the techniques we prescribe.

You will come away from this book with an understanding of many of the natural tools currently available to help you heal your gut.

We believe that integrative medicine—medicine that includes the best of every healing tradition in the world—is the future of health care, and we know that many patients see this as the future of health care as well. Truly integrative medicine doesn't preclude any possibilities. In some cases, all that's needed is a nourishing diet that supports healing. In other cases, medications are called for. Surgery can even be helpful for some.

The problem with the present model of medicine is not that it has developed drugs and surgical interventions to help heal people. The problem is that these have become the *only* tools we use—even when better, scientifically sound, less-intrusive options exist. Hippocrates, the founder of Western medicine, said: "Leave your drugs in the chemist's pot if you can heal your patient with food." The way medicine is practiced in the West today is a far cry from Hippocrates' vision. Today, patients are given prescriptions without first being given the option of altering their diets and lifestyles, even when food, relaxation, or supplements would work just as well.

Sometimes, even if you make all of the right choices, surgeries and medications are still necessary. If you try going on Tracks 1 and 2 and you can't find a solution to your digestive disorder, it may be time to see a physician or a GI specialist and look for some answers. Track 3 should only be attempted under medical supervision. If this is the case for you, you will need to educate yourself about what some of these interventions entail and what the potential side effects may be. We hope this information helps you take the reins and guide the direction of your treatment to health and a better quality of life!

The earliest medical traditions in the world thought of the gut as the center of health and wellness, and they understood that to be vitally healthy you must first treat your gut properly. How strange it is that we live in a world that has become so disconnected from this simple truth. How odd that conventional medicine has spent centuries researching the heart, the brain, and every other organ in the human body and yet still has such a hard time understanding that what we eat and how we treat the gut determines much about how healthy we are.

We are living in a world out of balance. The way back to balance is through the gut. Follow your gut instincts—listen to what it tells you about the foods you eat, the medications you take, the stress you endure, the life you live—and it becomes easy to see through the illusions under which we are laboring today. Your body has inherent wisdom that no doctor anywhere on the planet can ever surpass. Listen to your gut—that seat of wisdom—and it will lead you back to a healthy and vitally engaged life. It truly *is* your inside tract to health and wellness.

Welcome to the journey.

PART I

The Gastrointestinal Superhighway

CHAPTER 1

The Gut: Your "Inside Tract" to Health and Wellness

Everyone has a doctor in him or her; we just have to help it in its work. The natural healing force within each one of us is the greatest force in getting well.

—Hippocrates

This book is about your gut.

No, we aren't talking about those extra inches around your middle. We're talking about your alimentary canal, your gastrointestinal (GI) tract, your inner core of life, your inside tract to health and well-being.

We know it's a hard sell. Most people have an almost overwhelming aversion to contemplating their gut—one that borders on absurdity, when you stop to think about it.

After all, we revere the hard work our hearts do for us, and our culture feeds us endless rhetoric on how important it is to protect your heart with diet, exercise, and a healthy lifestyle. We love our hearts. There is something downright romantic about the pump of life—that muscle that beats 72 times per minute and will contract approximately 2.5 billion times before it pumps its last pump and finally stops speeding our blood through their vessels. What a lovely and refined organ! What a powerhouse! What a masterful example of evolution!

And the brain? We have a nearly mystical appreciation for the human brain. We worship those 2 pounds of custardlike gray matter that resides between our ears more than we do any other system in the human body. Admittedly, it is impressive and more than a bit mysterious. Despite centuries of scientific analysis, the inner workings of this seat of human cognition and consciousness are still not particularly well understood. Indeed, the brain is a marvel of creation—one that most likely holds some of the most profound secrets about what it means to be human.

If you're like most people, you would probably be apt to ponder the inner workings of many organs and bodily systems before you would think about your gut. You may look out for your skin by staying out of the sun, contemplate the mechanisms by which your reproductive system works, or be held in awe of the complexity of your eyes, ears, nose, or tongue.

You know that the health of these various parts and systems determines much about your quality of life, and you are likely vigilant in caring for them. You may visit eye doctors and dentists annually and carefully consider the latest dietary information the media feeds you regarding heart health, but few people put that kind of energy into their gastrointestinal tract, much less become intimate with the way it functions and the impact it has on their overall health and well-being.

The result is that your inside tract often goes ignored—in some cases, until it's too late.

Perhaps we ignore the gut because its job is so gritty. Or maybe it's because we are in constant contact with it on a daily basis, so we forget it's even there—like that unrecognized employee at the office who's a real workhorse but is taken for granted. Your days revolve around your gut. You eat during the day to satisfy its hunger. You go to the bathroom to excrete the waste it creates. It's the center of your world in many ways. But it's so easy to simply let it slip one's mind.

It could also be that our society has drawn us away from the gut. People these days turn up their noses at the idea of gut instinct. We eat a Standard American Diet—SAD—that puts the gut in constant peril. (You'll learn more about this in Chapter 4.) We are practically encouraged to beat up the gut with excess antibiotics, toxic chemicals, stress, lack of exercise, and any number of other poor lifestyle choices our world makes it all too easy to embrace and very difficult to avoid. Maybe we just can't face how much we torture the poor gut.

Whatever the case, most people tend to ignore GI function. And we are all suffering because of this ignorance.

As we will explain a little later in this chapter, digestive disease has reached epidemic proportions in our society. A minimum of 60 to 70 million people suffer from some kind of digestive disease, and research presented later in this chapter suggests that even more are suffering. Seventy percent of Americans either have a digestive disease or will suffer with digestive symptoms over their lifetime. According to a study produced in 2004 by the American Gastroenterology Association, the estimated cost of digestive diseases was $141.8 billion. Digestive disease costs in 2004 accounted for 10 percent of all health care spending in the United States ($1.9 trillion, 16 percent of its gross domestic product).

This figure will not come as a shock to you if you are one of the 60 to 70 million Americans who suffer with digestive disorders. But did you know that unhealthy gut function has been linked to a multitude of other diseases and chronic health conditions as well?

What's more, an unhealthy gut has been linked to a plethora of systemic symptoms including headaches, skin conditions, joint and muscle pain, allergies, asthma, menstrual pain and irregularities, and more. Even mental illnesses like depression have been linked to gut dysfunction.

Is it possible that a part of us that's so often ignored by our culture could be the very seat of health and disease prevention? Is there *really* a connection between gut health and our day-to-day lives? If there is, how can we get back in touch with this inside tract to health and well-being so we can thrive once more?

In this book, we will revolutionize the way you understand health and well-being. The simple truth is this: Your gut is at the center of your being in every way imaginable. Heal your gut and you will be on the superhighway to health.

The Inner Tube of Life

The average adult human is, in essence, a 30-foot-long tube that starts at the mouth and ends at the anus. The inner lining of this tube—the gut—is your interface between the outside world and the world within.

Perhaps most importantly, your gut is the place in your body where food is broken down into its constituent elements so it can be processed and turned into the vitamins, minerals, and energy you use to live every single day of your life.

On the surface, this sounds pretty mundane. Not many people are awed by the idea that their gut digests food. You eat, it goes into your stomach, a little acid is poured on it, you get the nourishment you need, and the rest goes into the toilet. That's the end of the story, right? What's so special about this?

What's funny (and sad) is that we have become so disconnected from our inside tract that most of us believe this is essentially all that happens when we eat food. We've lost touch with the wondrous transformation that occurs when other living beings (plants and animals) that were nourished by the sun and the earth give their lives to provide us with the energy we need to live.

Consider that human beings eat a more varied diet than virtually any other species on the planet. Over tens of thousands of years, the human digestive system evolved so that it could consume millions of different species. We go around eating pretty much anything we want to all day long, and we don't even have to think too much about it. (Or at least we don't *think* we have to! Later on you'll learn why being attentive to what you eat should be one of your biggest priorities.)

Besides breaking down food into its constituent elements and then using those vitamins and minerals to fuel your body, your gut also acts as the first line of defense against microbes and intrusive invaders: viruses and bacteria that make you ill. Seventy percent of your protective immune system cells and antibodies live in your gastrointestinal (GI) tract, and they work hard every day to keep out foreign cells that would leach out your life force.

To accomplish these tasks, your GI tract supports an entire ecosystem of its own. Trillions of bacteria live inside your gut. Most counts suggest that there are about 500 different species of bacteria living in there and that the average healthy adult carries 5 to 8 pounds of "flora" inside them at all times. The total number of bacteria in your gut exceeds the number of cells in the rest of your body by a factor of 10. In a strange way, we are more bacteria than human—more bug than human. An entire universe of beings lives inside us. This "microflora" is like an organ within an organ—an undiscovered country of organisms that live in harmony with us.

Under normal, healthy conditions, these bacteria are "friendly" helpers that assist us in the task of living. They have a number of important jobs that we will discuss in detail later in this book, but one of their main functions is to help you digest and process the foods you eat. Chewing, stomach acid, and even enzymes by themselves don't do the trick; we need our little symbiotic friends to helps us transform our victuals into the vital substances needed for our bodies.

Your gut provides a safe shelter for these "friendly" bacteria. However, the sanctity of their home is constantly being challenged by pathogens, aka "bad" bacteria that would very much like to take up residence there. In this war for space, the army that's getting fed the best typically triumphs. When you eat too many poor-quality foods that are filled with sugar and low in fiber (foods the "bad" bugs thrive on), take too many antibiotics, or don't get enough exercise, you set the stage for the microbial terrain of your gut to shift in unhealthy ways. The "bad" bugs overtake the "good" bugs, and the results can be harmful to your health.

But this is not the only thing that can go wrong in the gut.

In addition to supporting this ecosystem of friendly bugs, your gut also has a brain of its own that it uses to take care of the digestive functions in your body. This enteric nervous system (ENS) has garnered much attention in recent years, particularly due to the work of Dr. Michael Gershon, an internationally renowned neuroscientist who coined the term "the second brain" for the ENS. Yet most people still aren't aware of the miraculous work the gut-mind performs.[1]

Half of all the nerve cells in your body actually reside in your gut. There are more nerve cells in your bowel than in your spine. A lot of people are pretty amazed by this, because most of us think of the brain as Grand Central Station for our bodies. Maybe we live a little too much in our heads and need to get back to the center of our being—the gut.

Neurotransmitters (chemicals that allow neurons to communicate with one another) are also found en masse in your gut. Your gut has as many neurotransmitters as your brain, and every class of neurotransmitter in your brain can also be found in your gut.

YOUR SECOND BRAIN

You've had "gut instincts" and "gut feelings," but what you may not realize is that your gut literally has a mind of its own—the enteric nervous system (ENS). The word *enteric* means "of or having to do with the small intestine," which is precisely where this second nervous system is located.

Except for your brain, your gut is the only system in your body that has its own dedicated nervous system. In fact, your ENS is highly integrated into your central nervous system, and it interacts with it constantly. If you're afraid, your gut-brain knows it and your digestion is altered. Likewise, if you eat something that "doesn't sit well with you," it may put you in a bad mood.

German psychologist Gerd Gigerenzer called the enteric nervous system the "intelligence of the unconscious." So the next time your gut tells you something, listen to it. It knows more than you think.

Your gut-brain, or "second brain," commands the functions of digestion independent of your actual brain. This is absolutely amazing when you think about it. In grade school, most of us were taught that the brain controls all the functions of the body—like a commander overseeing its troops, the brain is thought to tell every other cell in the body what to do. This turns out not to be the case. The ENS can function autonomously from the brain. And yet, it is connected to it. Your brain and your gut are actually in constant communication through the vagus nerve. This nerve starts in your brain stem, runs through your neck and chest, and ends in your abdomen. It's a highway of information that connects your gut-brain to your brain, ensuring that both are in constant communication.

Little wonder then that stress, anger, anxiety, depression, and other negative emotions have a profound impact on gut health. When you perceive something as stressful, your brain tells your gut about it, and it usually doesn't react so well.

By the same token, your ENS can perceive stressful events without the help of your brain. You know those butterflies you experience when you get nervous? When your gut gets stressed-out, it tells your brain about it, too. Again, the results usually aren't so great.

These are but a *few* of the ways the gut acts as your interface between the outside world and the world within. (You will learn more about digestive biology throughout this book. In Chapter 2, we will give you a complete anatomical overview of the gut; we'll review gut flora, the gut–immune system, the ENS, and the rest of the digestive system in more detail.) What you may be unaware of is that you sense the world with your gut as much as you do with your brain. In fact, your inside tract is exquisitely sensitive to everything you absorb in your environment, from the foods you eat to the stress you experience to the toxins you ingest. Our gut function and our gut feelings are absolutely essential to healing ourselves and our world.

The sad and ironic reality is that, as a society, we are out of touch with the importance of maintaining good gut health, and we believe that it is okay to eat junk while taking acid blockers to try and maintain optimal digestive health and well-being. The result is an epidemic of gut-related diseases that are destroying the health of our society and wreaking havoc for many of us. Despite the fact that we live in a wonderland of medical miracles, we have lost touch with some simple truths about health and wellness that humanity has been aware of for millennia.

We need to get back on track.

Ancient Secrets to Health: The Importance of the Gut in Ayurveda and Traditional Chinese Medicine

The idea that the human digestive system is the key to balanced health and vitality has been the basis of Eastern civilization healing practices for centuries. Let's consider a couple of examples.

Ayurvedic medicine is a Hindu system of health care that is native to the Indian subcontinent and has been practiced since approximately 2000 BCE. The term *Ayurveda* translates to "the wisdom and science of life." In this system, disease is considered to be the absence of vibrant health, which constitutes a major difference with the way medicine is practiced in the West today.

People who practice the Ayurvedic tradition believe that illness commences with a breakdown of the spirit and evolves in definable stages, beginning with improper digestion and toxin elimination.

The *Sushruta Samhita*,[2] a comprehensive guide to Ayurvedic medicine that dates to the 3rd or 4th century AD, defined health as follows:

> A person whose basic emotional and physical tendencies are in
>   balance,
> Whose digestive power is balanced,
> Whose bodily tissues, elimination functions, and activities are
>   in balance,
> And whose mind, senses, and souls are filled with vitality,
> That person is said to be healthy.

It goes on to say that the Ayurvedic secret to a long, happy, and vital life is predicated upon balanced energetic, metabolic, and protective forces; *strong digestion*; optimal cellular, tissue, and organ function; efficient elimination; and clear senses, a joyful mind, and transpersonal connection.

Digestive Fire

In Ayurvedic medicine, digestive fire (called *agni*) is required to process our food correctly, or else toxins (called *malas*) are disseminated and we begin down the road that leads to illness and disease.

However, the principle of digestive fire energizing our life force is not unique to Ayurveda. Traditional Chinese Medicine (TCM) was the first formalized system of health and healing in modern civilization, and it has similar things to say about the importance of digestion and your inside tract.

In TCM, all life occurs within a circle of nature, with all things in this matrix interconnected and mutually dependent upon each other. Human beings represent a microcosm of nature and are considered the juncture between heaven and earth. Health and vitality are predicated upon spiritual connection, balanced living, a plant-based diet, *proper digestion,* and peace of mind. The free and unimpeded flow of energy, or *chi,* is the essence of health and well-being. A blockage in the flow of chi through energy channels called meridians is the root cause of illness, and loss of adaptability is the beginning of disease.

TCM suggests that the foods we eat are not merely nutrients, but rather are vehicles for this life force to be dispersed to our bodies in either a healthy or unhealthy manner as is determined by the outcome of digestion. When the digestive fire is too weak or too strong, the resulting energy imbalances create disharmony and illness.

The major source of chi in the human body is thought to be centered around the digestive tract in a ball of energy called the *don tien.* This virtual force field of energy circling our digestive tract is essential to health and well-being.

Practitioners of TCM believe that food contains the energy we need to live, that this energy is extracted in the gut from the foods we eat, that the gut is thus the home of our life energy, and that our chi flows out from this don tien to the rest of the body, nourishing the mind, body, and spirit.

Here are a few of the basic principles of TCM:

- Disease is not considered to be the existence of a particular disorder, but the absence of vital health.
- Human beings are more than their bodies; health and illness go beyond the body to include the mind and the soul.
- A sound mind, peace, wholeness, and harmony are critical if you wish to achieve an experience of vital health.
- Proper digestion of a healthy, vegetable-based diet is the key to a life filled with vibrant health and free of disease, stress, and toxins.

The gut is the place where health or illness is born; it is the holding tank for our life energy, and treating it well as TCM and Ayurveda principles suggest is the first step toward a healthy life.

In contrast, in the West, we have embraced a concept called reductionism. This concept divides people into parts instead of understanding them as whole human beings.

Reductionism has taken us away from the more holistic perspective that ancient forms of healing (such as Ayurveda and TCM) embraced centuries ago and still use to treat people today. Systems like these are extremely effective at providing a method of preventive care that keeps people healthy, as well as a system for coping with chronic illness.

Despite the progress we have made in medicine in the West, the shift away from a holistic understanding of human health has proven costly. Both Ayurveda and TCM emphasize that gut function influences health and well being. We live in a world where obesity has become the number one health problem. The health of your gut strongly correlates with the size of your waist. When the little symbiotic bacteria we previously discussed are out of balance or you eat a diet that sends the wrong messages to your genes, you set the stage for weight gain and immune dysregulation.

Our poor digestive health is a symbol of how far out of balance our society actually is.

The Epidemic of Digestive Diseases: A Society Out of Balance

The word *epidemic* is thrown around so much these days that it's hard to know what it means anymore. We have an obesity epidemic, a diabetes epidemic, an overall chronic illness epidemic, an autoimmune disease epidemic, an epidemic of mental disorders—the list just seems to go on and on. But what does this actually mean? Can we really have so many epidemics at one time? If so, why are they all happening concurrently? Could they be related? How?

Reviewing a few statistics on digestive disease will make it easy to see why this problem is, in fact, an epidemic.

The National Institute of Diabetes and Digestive and Kidney Diseases (NIDDK), which is the major national agency dedicated to gastroenterological disorders, states that 60 to 70 million Americans are affected by a digestive disease.[3] Not only are these statistics wildly out of date (they come from an interview survey done by the National Center for Health in 1996), they also fail to take into consideration a number of factors, which means the problem may actually be even worse than it sounds. Recent studies suggest that 7 percent of Americans (21 million people) have heartburn at least once a day, 14 percent (42 million people) experience it once a week, 21 percent (about 60 million people) report having acid regurgitation once a month, and over 50 percent (about 150 million people) encounter it annually. These numbers continue to increase as we become fatter as a nation.[4] The NIDDK's estimate of the number of people suffering from digestive diseases annually is accounted for by this one malady alone. It is, therefore, rational to conclude that the actual number of sufferers is a great deal higher than government estimates would indicate.

There is also excellent reason to believe that many of the other chronic illnesses our society suffers from originate (at least partially) from GI imbalances. Chronic conditions such as allergies, arthritis, chronic fatigue, depression, menstrual irregularities, migraines, neurological disorders, osteoporosis, PMS, skin conditions, and other symptoms may be related to undiagnosed digestive disease, such as celiac disease.

Even if we consider only the most conservative of these statistics, it's clear that we have a digestive disease epidemic on our hands. Today (15 years after the NIDDK data was produced), doctors know that more people than ever before are currently seeking a physician's care for digestive diseases. An increase of this magnitude cannot be explained by better reporting; it is not something we should "expect."[5] The digestive disease problem in this country is an epidemic.

We live in a society that's out of balance. We eat a diet filled with chemicals that aren't fit for flies (and even flies won't eat them). We experience chronic stress at record levels. We work more than any other nation in the world. We are disconnected from our communities. We exercise less than we ever have. Often times, the only solutions our doctors offer us are more pharmaceuticals and intrusive procedures—"magic bullet" medicine—even though complementary and alternative therapies are far safer, have a growing track record of success, and don't pose nearly the health risks.

To reverse this trend, we have to get in touch with our gut instincts once more and return to the very soul of medicine.

In fact, 50 percent of people who seek care from gastroenterologists pursue some form of "alternative" therapy at the same time. One might wonder how many of them tell their physicians about this choice. National statistics state that 72 percent of them *don't* tell their doctors because they are afraid of being criticized. What a shame!

The disconnect between you and your gut and our society's deviation away from pursuing dietary and lifestyle changes as frontline therapies are at the very core of the health crisis we are facing as a nation. Treating the gut is the beginning of healing. The epidemic of digestive disorders in this country, as well as all of the other associated symptoms that can come up when the gut is out of balance, bear out the reality that we need to start by treating the gut. We have to learn to embrace some of what ancient cultures like India and China began sharing with humanity millennia ago.

Treat the gut and you treat the illness. Heal the gut and you heal yourself. Maintain balance in the gut and you balance your body, mind, and spirit—and vice versa. Ignore your gut and the balance of your health is compromised. Your body spirals down into illness in a relatively definable set of stages, just as Ayurvedic practitioners have known for centuries.

Accordingly, this devolution of health often shows up in the gut first. Over the course of this book, we will describe why this happens and provide you with concrete steps you can take to reverse this trend and overcome your digestive illness. But to use this program effectively, you need to have a better grasp of the territory we are exploring. So in the next chapter we will take you on a guided tour of your inside tract and reveal its wondrous anatomy in detail.

CHAPTER 2

Taking a Ride on the Tube: A Guided Tour of Your Gut

Your gut is a bit like the metro station in and around London, England—which, incidentally, is also referred to as "The Tube." It is a complex array of organs (stations) that are all connected by your gastrointestinal (GI) tract (the tube or railway itself). The primary job of this railway is to transport food from station to station so it can be broken down into its component parts, absorbed by your body, and eventually transformed into the building blocks that make up your body.

The railway itself is immense. Your GI tract is one of the largest systems in your body. It is a staggering 30 feet long from end to end. If removed from your body and stretched to its full length, it would be the height of a telephone pole.

It is also unique in that it is, strictly speaking, "outside the body." It is a long, continuous tube that stretches from your mouth to your anus, and it is constantly in contact with and communicating with the outside world. Aside from air, visual data, and a few other things, everything you "ingest" has to take a long trip on this inner railway.

In this chapter, we want to take you on that same trip. We are going to look at your gut from a food's-eye perspective and take you on a fantastic voyage through your gut. Along the way we will talk about what digestion is and how it works, we will stop and investigate each of the major stations along the railway, and we will look at what happens when the railway breaks and the train goes off course.

Welcome to your guided tour of the inside tract.

Digestion: Transforming Food into Life

Eating is an intricate, dynamic event.

The process of digestion is a complex and highly coordinated effort that involves the body's entire nervous system. Digestion begins before food ever enters your mouth, and it goes on long after you have chewed and swallowed. In fact, there are four phases of digestion. Using our train metaphor, if food is the train, your GI tract is the railway, and the organs connected to your GI tract are the stations, then the phases of digestion are synchronized according to a schedule that governs when food (the train) will move from one station to the next.

Preparing for the Journey of Digestion: The Cephalic Phase

The first phase of digestion affects your gut but is not driven by it. The cephalic phase is actually "all in your head." That doesn't exactly mean that your brain digests your food, but your brain *is* intimately involved in the process. The sight, sound, smell, or even just the thought of food elicits signals from your brain; those signals are transmitted down your central nervous system via the vagus nerve (more about this important nerve momentarily). These signals drive your digestive processes and prepare the way for food to enter your inside tract. In essence, the cephalic phase of digestion gets the track ready before the train enters the tunnel. And it does an amazingly efficient job. You may secrete as much as 40 percent of the hydrochloric acid and digestive enzymes needed to break down the foods you eat *before* you consume a single ounce of food! Even insulin secretion has been shown to occur in response to tasting sucrose or saccharin without consuming any sweets.[1]

In high school biology class, you probably learned that digestion starts before you begin eating, but it's unlikely that you've given much thought to that fact since then. Despite the fact that most of us ignore or are simply unaware of this part of the digestive process, it is extraordinarily important, and understanding the cephalic phase of digestion is essential if you want to heal your inside tract.

To begin to appreciate just how important your brain is to digestion, you must first understand a little bit about your nervous system and the parts of it that are related to digestion and gut function. You may also remember from high school biology class that there are several different branches or pieces of your nervous system. We want to focus on just one branch of it: the autonomic nervous system and its intimate relationship to digestion and gut function.

The autonomic nervous system is divided into three subsystems: the sympathetic, parasympathetic, and enteric nervous systems, each of which plays a critical role in gut health. The parasympathetic nervous system governs digestion (among other "vegetative" processes, such as relaxation). The sympathetic nervous system governs your fight-or-flight response, which, when activated, inhibits digestion (more on this in a moment). And your enteric nervous system is the part of your neurobiology that resides in your gut—your second brain. (See "Your Second Brain" on page 23 for more information.)

⊶ KEY POINT: What happens during cephalic digestion depends on your state of mind.

Let's say you've been having a great day. You just learned that you got a promotion, you won a gift certificate to your favorite spa, and the kids are happily playing together in the backyard. You feel as relaxed and centered as you've felt in weeks. Slowly, you notice that familiar sensation of hunger creeping up on you. The thought of food triggers impulses in your brain that then flow nicely down your vagus nerve—a long nerve that starts in your medulla oblongata (the lower part of your brain stem) and wanders through your neck and chest and into your abdomen. This nerve mediates the parasympathetic nervous response. It only functions properly when you're relaxed. So on this particular day, in your happy, peaceful state of mind, it is operating at peak performance. It's telling your gut to secrete optimal levels of digestive juices and promoting the healthy movements required for proper digestion.

Now let's look at another example. Imagine that, instead of feeling happy and peaceful, you're really grumpy and stressed-out. You've been missing deadlines at work and you know your clients are getting frustrated with you. You just had a fight with your spouse. Your best friend was recently diagnosed with breast cancer. In this anxious frame of mind, you start to feel hungry. But this time your parasympathetic nervous system isn't activated, so those signals can't flow down your vagus nerve properly. Instead, your *sympathetic* nervous system is activated. In this frame of mind, with this part of your nervous system activated, your digestive train is going to get derailed before it even has a chance to start down the track.

Under stress, a set of biochemicals (adrenaline, noradrenaline, and cortisol, among others) is produced that put the body in a crisis/response mode. This response is designed to help your body react properly to a life-threatening emergency. To facilitate this, the system diverts much of its resources to lifesaving functions (like circulation) and inhibits biological processes that aren't immediately necessary at moments when your life is truly in danger (like digestion).

In states of acute stress, there are times your gastrointestinal motility (the movement of your digestive tract) is temporarily frozen. It's like a train getting stuck on the tracks. In some cases, food is actually evacuated from the tract under conditions of severe alarm. If you've ever felt like you had to vomit or defecate when you were extremely stressed-out, this is why.

Consider how adaptive these responses are in certain circumstances. If you are running for your life, your stress response is precisely what you'd want and need your body to do. Forget about digestion. Let's pump blood down into those legs so you can run, or so you can fight if you're caught. Frankly, we wouldn't have survived long without this system in place.

The problem with stress, as we all know, is that most of us *aren't* running for our lives when we get stressed-out. Stress happens in response to a real or a perceived threat. So anytime you think you're in danger, your sympathetic nervous system is triggered and digestion slows or shuts down.

Think about how often each day that happens to the average modern human. You're stuck in traffic and late for work, and you start to get stressed. Then you walk into the office and you get a call from school letting you know that your child is sick. Phone calls, appointments, deadlines, projects—work, work, work—coffee, coffee, coffee—rush, rush, rush—and all day long you get ever more stressed-out. Then you go home, cook dinner for the kids (who are vying for your attention and fighting with each other), and the stress continues to build until you go to bed.

If this or a similar scenario describes your life, it means you suffer from chronic stress, and that carries many digestive consequences of its own. One telling example of how your gut reacts to chronic stress has to do with your upper digestive sphincters (the pylorus and lower esophageal sphincters). These important passages in your GI tract remain open under stress. When this happens, food and digestive enzymes can travel the wrong way in your tract, resulting in gastroesophageal reflux. This is one of the ways stress causes heartburn and other stomach problems.

The detrimental effects that a poor frame of mind can have on digestive function and the emerging role that these effects have in digestive disease are only now beginning to be fully understood. What we do know is that the journey to healthy digestion starts well before you bring your fork to your lips. It begins with your frame of mind during the cephalic phase of digestion. Your mood and your gut function are intimately tied together. Your mind can either prepare you for healthy digestion or derail the process. Eating when you are in a bad mood, under stress, multitasking, or otherwise distracted drastically impedes the digestive process.

Does that mean you should only eat when you are in a centered, peaceful place? Well, that may not be fully realistic. But there are many things you can do to improve your frame of mind and prepare yourself for excellent digestion. Mindful eating is one of the most important techniques you can use, and in Chapter 4 we will show you how to eat more mindfully. Throughout this book we will look at this and other stress-reducing lifestyle modifications you can make to improve your digestion.

The good news is that you do have some control over how tense or relaxed you feel, and you can learn specific techniques that will help you set the stage for excellent digestion. Stress is a major, largely unrecognized threat to the health of your inside tract. Learning to manage this threat with relaxation techniques and mindful eating practices can have profound effects.

Digestion can be a "sensational" experience if you learn how to make it one. But for now, let's resume our journey through the GI tract. Now that we have prepared for the journey of digestion, let's enter the tube and see what we find there.

Your Mouth: The First Stop on the Line

Imagine you were on a train taking a journey through your inside tract, and the very first stop on the line was your mouth. There, teeth are delightfully chewing away in a sea of saliva that begins the process of transforming food into life. The train ride continues and the food takes a plunge into your stomach for the next adventure!

The train ride is smooth if the food is chewed into a pasty texture, which leads us to a question: Have you ever timed yourself when eating? How long does it take you to finish a meal? Is it 10 minutes? Maybe only 5? If you are one of the millions of people who gulp down their food in these brief time frames, you are shortcutting one of the first and most important steps in digestion: chewing.

Once food is ingested, it needs to be ground into tiny bits and mixed with salivary enzymes so they can begin breaking down the starches, fats, and proteins into a soft substance called chyme. This is done simply by

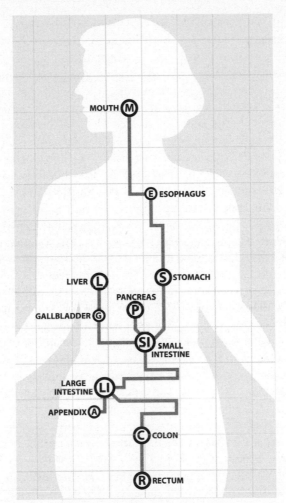

Metro station—whole GI system

chewing your food. But if you lead such a hectic life that meals are cut down to a fraction of what they should be and this important part of digestion is overlooked, you're going to make your gut very unhappy.

You can't swallow your food whole and expect to digest it well. When you don't take the time to sufficiently grind up your food, the particles are too big to be properly digested. This much is obvious to most people.

But what you may be unaware of is that important digestive enzymes are found in your saliva and are only properly integrated into the foods you eat when you chew enough. For example, one of the enzymes that your

LUCY'S STORY

At 47, Lucy was referred to me, Gerry, by her primary care doctor for ongoing digestive health issues. On the surface, you wouldn't have known she was ill—Lucy appeared physically fit and led a travel-oriented and energy-demanding lifestyle. But under the surface, illness was lurking.

Her history of health problems began in her midtwenties with an autoimmune thyroid disease. She had successfully managed the condition for years, but over time, life's challenges and stressors began to take their toll on her body. Eventually this showed up as a functional digestive illness. That's when she came to see me.

Our first visit lasted more than 2 hours. I heard how she worked hard raising children and traveling with her business. She sounded exhausted and overwhelmed. It was clear to me that Lucy never had time for herself and always put everyone else's needs in front of her own.

After listening to her story, we did some testing and my initial concerns about her health were confirmed: Lucy's body was chronically stuck in fight-or-flight mode and her "energy reserves" were running low. She had both clinical and biochemical evidence of adrenal insufficiency. This disorder occurs when your body produces insufficient amounts of cortisol and aldosterone—stress hormones that are produced by the adrenal glands.

The prescription I used to help Lucy heal her inside tract was simple: I asked her to recognize that her present state of unwellness was a consequence of her stress levels. What Lucy needed was scheduled downtime where she could hang a "Do Not Disturb" sign on her virtual door and relax. She needed a way of telling the universe that she was taking an hour or two for herself.

In addition, I suggested that she begin taking her meals in a relaxed, calming environment where she could incorporate mindfulness into her eating habits. Lucy already ate a healthy diet. In her case, the missing link was the vital connection between her state of mind and her digestion. She didn't need to change what she ate; she needed to change how she ate. This turned out to be one of the most important steps in Lucy's long-term recovery. Like many of my patients, she made strides by making one simple adjustment: eating mindfully in a calm, stress-free environment.

saliva contains is called alpha-amylase. This enzyme is responsible for breaking down starches into smaller molecules that the cells in your body can use for energy. When your food is not chewed properly, the alpha-amylase in your saliva does not have the opportunity to break down these starches. This could lead to symptoms of carbohydrate maldigestion and malabsorption, in some cases. Similarly, lingual lipase (another important digestive enzyme) is secreted by glands located under your tongue; it begins the process of digesting the fat content of food. If you don't chew enough, the fats you eat may not be properly digested as well.

All of this maldigestion of food in the mouth can interfere with the process all the way down the tract. Food particles that are too large end up in your intestines, where they become a breeding ground for bad bacteria. Such bacteria in excessive quantities in the small intestine can have a wide variety of negative health effects, but the most immediate and obvious symptoms are gas, bloating, and indigestion. If you experience any of these after a meal, it's a sign that you may not be chewing enough.

Besides the potential for bacterial overgrowth, you should also know that not all of the nutrients in your food get released when you underchew. That means you deprive yourself of the very nourishment you were trying to get when you put the food in your mouth in the first place.

Put simply, chewing is essential to good digestion. It will bring out more of the flavors in the foods you eat and slow down your pace at the plate. So take the time to put down your fork and simply chew. Savoring one bite at a time.

The Esophageal Phase: Moving on Down the Tract

Having passed through the mouth, the next stop on the tract is the esophagus. The esophagus is a muscular tube about 9½ inches long that is lined with soft, moist, pink tissue called mucosa. This mucosa, which looks very much like the inside of your cheek, lines not only your esophagus but also most of your digestive tract, and it allows for the easy movement of food through your entire gut. It also helps protect your inside tract from the acids and enzymes that are necessary for converting food into molecules.

Normally, food is propelled down your esophagus and through the rest of your GI tract by a set of rhythmic, wavelike muscular contractions called peristalsis. After you have swallowed, these involuntary movements are responsible for getting your food where it needs to go. Unfortunately, the process of peristalsis can be impeded or even reversed by any number of factors, such as strees, infections, environmental influences. Gut disorders like small intestinal bacterial overgrowth (SIBO), gastroesophageal reflux disease (GERD), and irritable bowel syndrome (IBS) can be associated with and worsened by problems with intestinal movement (also known as motility). When your food comes back up through your esophagus, it is generally not a good thing. It's called reflux, and it's an experience far too many Americans are far too familiar with.

Assuming you do not suffer from one of these disorders and peristalsis is working normally for you, chyme will travel down your esophagus and encounter a gateway called the lower esophageal sphincter (also called the cardiac sphincter). This gateway opens to let the food you have eaten pass into your stomach for further processing. Once the journey down the esophagus has been safely completed, food enters your stomach—the major powerhouse of the digestive process.

The Gastric Phase of Digestion: Entering the Body's Blender

When you mention the word *digestion,* most people immediately think of the stomach. While this is misguided to some extent, this idea prevails for good reason—the stomach *is* the place where the physical disassembly of food, which began in your mouth, is completed. By the time food passes from your stomach into your small intestine, it no longer resembles anything most of us would call food.

On landing in the stomach during a tour of the inside tract, you would find this muscular, elastic, pear-shaped bag to be something of a roller coaster ride. Lying crosswise in the abdominal cavity beneath the diaphragm, the stomach has the ability to change size and shape according to its present position in the body and the amount of food inside it. It's normally about 12 inches long and 6 inches across at its widest point. It can hold around 1 quart of food, but it will hold much more than that if forced to. And it secretes gastric acid powerful enough to burn you if you touched it and digestive enzymes so strong that they can rip apart proteins and fats. These chemicals are mixed with your food as peristaltic contractions thrust the food from side to side, banging it against your stomach walls. A ride in there would be like floating on a boat in an acid storm.

The stomach is responsible for three tasks.

1. Storing all swallowed food and liquid.
2. Mixing up food, liquid, and the digestive juices the stomach produces.
3. Emptying its contents slowly into the small intestine.

From the time a meal is finished, it usually takes your stomach about 4 hours to complete all of this. However, a number of factors determine the duration and completeness of the gastric phase of digestion.

First, the quantity of food ingested plays a crucial role in determining the outcome of digestion. The idea of "eating until you are full" is a relatively modern invention of Western culture. Ayurvedic medicine, on the other hand, suggests that you only eat until you are about two-thirds full. Okinawans follow a principle known as *hari hachi bu,* which means "eat until you are 80 percent full." These are both good rules of thumb, and they turn out to be scientifically supportable as well: Your stomach mixes and grinds food best when there is plenty of space for it to do its job. Think about it this way: When you make a smoothie, does your blender work most efficiently when you leave some space at the top or when you fill it to the brim? Obviously, foods are broken down much more easily when there is space at the top for them to move around. The same is true of your stomach. When you don't leave enough space to allow your stomach to do its job properly, you risk having undigested food particles travel into your small intestine. This is not a good thing, as we have already discussed. Furthermore, when you overeat or eat too fast, you risk building up pressure in your stomach. This pressure can force the lower esophageal sphincter to open, and you end up with reflux and the uncomfortable sensation of heartburn and chest pain. Much of this can be solved simply by eating an amount of food that gently satisfies you, but not to the point of fullness. Overeating places a strain on your digestive system.

The second factor that has an impact on the speed and quality of digestion in your stomach is the composition of the foods you eat—mainly their fat and protein content—and the degree of muscle action in the stomach. High protein and high fat foods take a longer time to traverse the digestive highway.

Finally, the acidity of the stomach plays an important role in the efficiency of digestion. Digestive enzymes in the stomach function optimally in highly acidic conditions. Slower digestion can be the result of too little stomach acid, when taking acid blocking medications, such as proton pump inhibitors (PPIs). Researchers have recently shown that stomach emptying is slower when proton pump inhibitors neutralize the stomach's pH.[2]

Why is all of this important? Because an inordinate delay in the clearing of food particles from the upper digestive system can lead to problems similar to those caused by underchewing. Such a delay establishes a breeding

DISORDERS ASSOCIATED WITH
SMALL INTESTINAL BACTERIAL OVERGROWTH

✓ Chronic diarrhea
✓ Chronic fatigue syndrome
✓ Cirrhosis of the liver
✓ Hypothyroidism
✓ Irritable bowel syndrome
✓ Fibromyalgia
✓ Migraine headaches
✓ Rosacea
✓ Restless leg syndrome
✓ Rheumatoid arthritis

ground for bad bugs in the small intestine. This may lead to SIBO, which has been linked to IBS and other conditions (see page 52 for more information).

Once the food in your stomach has been completely broken down, the pyloric sphincter at the bottom of your stomach opens and the digested mass passes through this gateway and into your small intestine (also known as the duodenum). As you will see, the intestines are a strange, wandering world filled with beautiful flora and special tentacles that capture fats, nutrients, and proteins so they can be assimilated and used to build your cells and sustain your biochemistry. It is the place where nontubular organs involved in digestion meet and contribute to the process. It is the central meeting place for the entire digestive process.

Intestinal Phase of Digestion: The Metro Station of the Digestive System

Upon entering the small intestine, we see a world that is very different from those we have encountered so far. Up to this point in the journey, every phase of digestion and every organ we have traveled through has simply been preparing us for the ultimate absorption of nourishment into our bodies. Little has actually been absorbed, and most of the organs we have passed through have had only one or two jobs to do. The small intestine is an entirely different matter. It's a bustling metro station where all of the different organs involved in digestion finally meet and dozens of tasks are undertaken so that digestion can be completed. Here are a few of the important jobs your small intestine does for you.

- Breaks food down into molecules you can absorb
- Differentiates molecules you can absorb from nondigestible food particles and pathogens, and shunts each into its correct place

---

Digestive Helpers: The Pancreas and Gallbladder

Because they are so important to digestion, and because they can both be affected by illness, it's worth taking a moment to look at these digestive helpers in a little more detail.

The pancreas is a small organ that weighs about 80 grams and is the shape of an inverted smoker's pipe. One reason it's so important is that it releases insulin, the hormone that helps sugar get into our cells. Stable insulin levels are essential to good health. Imbalanced insulin levels are the chief cause of type 2 diabetes and contribute to a variety of other health problems as well.

Pancreatic cancer has seen much press recently and is a growing concern both among physicians and the public. It is rapidly fatal in adults, with less than 5 percent of patients surviving for 5 years or more after being diagnosed. Interestingly, recent research has shown that drinking sugary sodas significantly increases the risk of pancreatic cancer.[3]

There's a simple solution that will help stabilize your insulin levels and limit your risk of pancreatic cancer: Reduce your sugar intake, especially from soda, and eat dark greens daily. These are rich in folate, which has recently been shown to reduce the risk of developing pancreatic cancer.

Your gallbladder is even smaller than your pancreas, and it lies between your liver and your small intestine. Its only job is to store bile between meals and send it into the small intestine during digestion.

Many patients ask if they can still digest fats after they have their gallbladder removed (a surgery called a cholecystectomy, most commonly necessitated by gallstones). Since the gallbladder simply stores bile (it does not produce it), in its absence the liver cannot simulate the surge of bile that was once released when the gallbladder was intact. So though you *can* consume fats without a gallbladder, we advise you to eat more frequent meals and spread out your fat intake throughout the day.

If you still have your gallbladder, you can reduce your risk of gallstones by eating meals that are high in fiber.

- Houses much of your immune system
- Absorbs nutrients, fats, and proteins that are then reconstituted into the cells that make up your whole body

The tactics, techniques, and tools employed to achieve these objectives are quite incredible.

The journey begins when chyme passes from the stomach into the small intestine. At this stage, digestive enzymes and caustic chemicals are released from several different places to complete the process of digestion. The walls of the small intestine itself release a few enzymes, including lactase, the enzyme that breaks down the lactose in milk. The pancreas also enters the game at this stage, releasing a fluid that contains a wide array of enzymes designed to break down carbo-hydrates, fats, and proteins. Bile, released by the liver and stored in the gallbladder between meals, is squirted into the mix to emulsify the fats in the foods we eat in much the same way that your dish deter-gent cleans grease off a frying pan. (For more on the pancreas and gallbladder, see "Digestive Helpers: The Pancreas and Gallbladder" on page 41.)

Once chyme has been mixed with these powerful chemicals, much of it is ready for absorption into the body. The rest will be transported further down your digestive tract, where it will feed your gut flora and ultimately be excreted from your body. We will discuss this process in more detail in a moment. For now, let's focus on how molecular absorption by the small intestine takes place.

The average human small intestine is about 22 feet long. This is incred-ible enough, when you consider that the average adult is less than 6 feet tall. Stretched end to end, the small intestine would be nearly four times as tall as you are. But its surface area is even more incredible: If you pulled it taut, it would be the size of a doubles tennis court. This increased surface area is possible because the small intestine is corrugated—shaped into a multitude of fingerlike projections.

Each of these fingerlike projections is covered with tiny villi—minuscule tentacles that further increase the surface area of the intestine.

Villi grab molecules from your digested food and feed them toward the surface of the small intestine, which is only one cell layer thick. This sur-face is like an internal skin, but it has about 150 times the surface area of your outer skin, and its job is much more sophisticated. It has to figure out

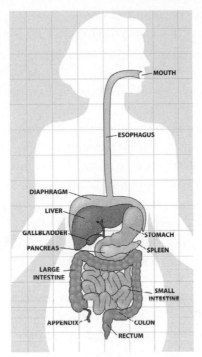

A cross-sectional view of the digestive tract

how to keep pathogenic organisms and damaging molecules out of your body while letting in the nutrients, phytonutrients, and other food components that you need in order to survive. One of the mechanisms the small intestine uses to differentiate between lethal enemies and nourishing friends is your gut–immune system. It's critical that you have a basic understanding of how the gut–immune system works if you want to get the most out of this book, overcome your digestive disorders, and remain healthy. So let's take a minor detour and look more carefully at your digestive defense system.

Homeland Security: Ensuring a Safe Digestive Journey

The gut–immune system is like a highly trained homeland security team. Its job is to defend you against lethal microbes and other unhealthy insults that are constantly bombarding you. This special force contains the largest number of immune cells in your body. Approximately 70 percent of your immune system is located immediately beneath the surface of your gut lining. It may surprise you to realize that more of your immune system is localized in your gut than in any other organ in your body, but when you consider it carefully, it makes sense: The gut comes in contact with far more molecules and foreign organisms than any other organ does.

Like a crack military team protecting a border in war-torn territory, the gut–immune system is responsible for seeking out threats and eliminating them while allowing friendly elements to travel across its lines.

When this force is functioning optimally, the gut–immune system achieves its objectives without fail. Over the course of your life, it successfully sorts through hundreds of billions of molecules, microbes, and toxins, allowing important nutrients, phytonutrients, proteins, and fats into your body while keeping invaders at bay or destroying them completely. Your health is dependent on this homeland security team.

However, there are times when your gut–immune system simply gets overwhelmed. This can happen for a number of reasons, including:

- Eating too many processed foods that are high in sugar and unhealthy fats
- Eating a diet that is low in fiber and nutrients
- Exposure to food allergens or other offensive dietary compounds
- Constant exposure to environmental toxins
- Excessive or chronic stress
- Lack of exercise or excessive exercise
- Infections viral, bacterial, fungal
- Foodborne illnesses from bacteria
- Endotoxins produced by yeast, bacteria, etc.
- Imbalances in other systems in the body

When the total load of stressors becomes too great, many problems can occur that affect your gut–immune system. For example, you may develop a leak in the epithelial barrier in your gut, and semidigested food particles and bacterial toxins may cross into your immune system and set off an allergic or inflammatory response—a great recipe for chronic illness.

Supporting your gut–immune system and helping it function optimally is one of the best ways to overcome digestive disorders and protect your long-term health. In recent years, medical science has established that one of the most important factors in supporting a healthy, balanced immune system is good nutrition. You need to nourish your homeland defense team well if you want it to do its job well. Here are some tips to help you do that.

- ☐ **Provide your "inner skin" the nutritional support it needs.** Increase your intake of choline (egg yolks), vitamin A (dark greens; yellow, green, and orange vegetables; fruits; and egg yolk), vitamin C (citrus fruits), zinc (pumpkin seeds, clams, lean chicken, and some fish), and fiber (found in all fruits, vegetables, beans, whole grains, nuts, and seeds).

- ☐ **Consume adequate protein.** Glutamine is a nonessential amino acid that is the preferred fuel for the lining of your gut. It comes from the protein you eat. Healthy sources include, fish, lean poultry and meat, eggs and dairy products, beans, nuts, seeds, cabbage, spinach, and parsley.

- ☐ **Maintain an optimal acidic environment in your stomach.** The digestive enzymes and acid in your stomach can destroy some bacteria and viruses that you ingest in food well before your gut–immune system has to deal with them. Inappropriate use of PPIs inhibits this process.

- ☐ **Balance your fats.** Clinical studies have shown that maintaining a healthy balance between omega-3 and omega-6 fatty acids is one way to support balance in your immune and inflammation response systems. Focus on foods with healthy fats, such as wild cold-water fish (sardines, anchovies, salmon), avocados, extra-virgin olive oil, olives, nuts, and seeds.

- ☐ **Avoid food allergens and intolerances.** If you have digestive symptoms whose source you cannot track, foods such as wheat, dairy, corn, or others may be overactivating your gut–immune system. A food elimination diet followed by a food challenge in which you systematically reintroduce the eliminated foods and monitor for effects can be most helpful in identifying food culprits.

- ☐ **Reduce your toxic load.** Choosing organic foods as often as possible is one way to minimize your intake of the toxins and unhealthy chemicals that can inhibit your immune system's ability to protect your health.

- ☐ **Maintain a healthy weight.** Recent research has shown us that fat is much more than a storage depot for excess calories. Certain fat cells in the body actually send inflammatory messengers (cytokines) throughout your body, leading to an overactive immune response. You can reduce the inflammatory burden on your body by achieving and maintaining a healthy body weight.

☐ **Reduce stress.** Stress increases your inflammatory response and contributes to an immune system out of balance. Studies have shown beyond the shadow of a doubt that excess stress has an impact not only on gut–immune function but also on the gut itself. Practicing mindfulness and integrating relaxation into your daily life will be soothing to your system.

☐ **Get enough good-quality sleep.** Sleep is the time when your body rests and repairs itself. When you don't get enough sleep, you weaken your entire system. Let your body recover by getting 7 to 9 hours of restorative sleep each night.

If your gut–immune system is working optimally, only molecules that your body can use are absorbed through your intestine, transported into your bloodstream, and eventually processed into all of the cells and chemicals you need to make your biology function. What is left is then transported further down the tract toward your large intestine, where it encounters a very interesting group of bacteria known as your gut flora.

THE LARGE INTESTINE AND FRIENDLY FLORA: ONE LAST STOP BEFORE LEAVING THE BODY

After food has passed through your small intestine, what is left can hardly be called food—at least not human food. In the final part of the intestinal phase of digestion, which occurs in the large intestine, no "digestion" as such takes place. But that doesn't mean that the compounds that pass into your large intestine aren't consumed. They are—just not by you. What is fed here are friendly organisms that live inside you—your gut flora. We introduced you to these wonderful bacteria in the previous chapter, but here we'd like to expand your understanding of these fascinating critters in hopes that it will initiate a more intimate relationship between you and these beneficial bugs.

Until recent times, the gut flora was largely ignored by science and medicine. Today we know these beneficial bacteria are helpers that are crucial to our health. Your flora performs so many functions that some now refer to these bacteria as "the lost organ."[4]

The average adult gut contains approximately 5 pounds of bacteria. It has been estimated that about 500 different species make up this flora, perhaps even more. The bacterial DNA in your body outnumbers your human DNA by a factor of 100. Some of these microbes are pathogens, or potential pathogens, under conditions of poor health. But fortunately, the vast majority of them are symbiotes—creatures that live inside you for the mutual benefit of the host (you) and the organism (the bacteria). You provide them with shelter and the nourishment they require, and they provide you with a number of benefits, which we will get to in a moment. When you are healthy, the vast majority of your flora is contained in your large intestine. When bugs move into your small intestine, this is called small intestinal bacterial overgrowth (SIBO), and as we have already mentioned, it is a leading cause of digestive problems for many.

After you have digested your food, the undigestible remains arrive in your large intestine, and your flora begin their meal. They ferment carbohydrates the human body is otherwise unable to process. In doing so, they produce biotin, vitamin K, and other essential nutrients. This fermentation also produces short-chain fatty acids that increase the gut's absorption of water, regrow gut cells in the colon, and may provide defenses against colon cancer and inflammatory bowel disease.[5] But this is only the beginning of what these beneficial flora are responsible for. They also:

- Help train the immune system to differentiate friend from foe
- Rebalance the immune system when it gets off-kilter
- Reduce gut inflammation
- Limit the amount of pathogenic microbes in the gut
- Stimulate and improve metabolic function
- Help prevent allergies
- Reduce gas production in the gut
- Prevent tumor growth and have antitumor properties

While you *can* survive without these wonderful little helpers, you wouldn't want to try it if you didn't have to. They are so beneficial that living without them very quickly leads to illness. When too many bad bacteria take over in the gut and run out the good guys, or when too much bacteria grows in the wrong place in your gut, you can develop a host of digestive illnesses.

Like much of the rest of your inside tract, the bugs are exquisitely sensitive to your diet and your environment. That means you have a great deal of control over the type and amount of bugs that grow in your gut. If you eat foods that are full of sugar, drink too much alcohol, and eat too little fiber (all behaviors that the bad bugs love), you will end up in a state where the bad bugs outweigh the good bugs. This is called dysbiosis, and it's not a condition in which you want to find yourself. On the other hand, if you reduce the amount of sugar you consume and increase the amount of fiber you eat (good bugs really *love* fiber), you make your good bugs healthy again and you regain a better balance of flora in your gut.

Another way to significantly increase the amount of beneficial bacteria in your large intestine is to take them as a supplement. When they are administered this way they are called probiotics, and they are an excellent therapeutic intervention and preventive strategy for digestive illness. They are an essential part of this program, and we will teach you in Chapter 6 how to use them to get back on track.

Aside from housing your flora, your large intestine actually does very little. Over the course of about 32 hours, while your beneficial bacteria are munching away, the large intestine passively absorbs the vitamins they produce and soaks up water from the mass that passes through it. Eventually, excretion takes place.

The Voyage Ends, but the Journey Begins: Moving from Illness to Health

This concludes our fantastic voyage through the gut. As you exit the train, please make sure you take the information you have learned in this chapter with you. It sets the stage for the rest of this book. Needless to say, there are endless ways your gut can get off track. If any of the steps along the path to digestion are inefficient or incomplete, if you eat the wrong kinds of foods or are exposed to too many toxins, if you eat too quickly or don't chew enough, if you have too few good bugs in your gut or too many bad ones, if the bugs you do have grow in the wrong place, if your gut–immune system is imbalanced or overactive, if you have a genetic predisposition for digestive illness, or if any one of a dozen other mishaps occur, you will likely find yourself trying to manage and cope with a digestive illness. How this manifests and what you can expect to experience when you develop such an illness is what we will be exploring next.

CHAPTER 3

WHEN YOU GET "OFF TRACT": DIGESTIVE DISEASE AND YOU

In this chapter, we'll review some of the data on a few of the most prominent digestive disorders and take a brief look at some of the many ways digestive ill health may manifest itself in your whole body. This will not only give you a sense of how prevalent gut dysfunction is, but will also help you better understand your own illness.

The seven most prevalent digestive disorders in Western countries are:

1. Gastroesophageal reflux disease (GERD) (30 to 60 million)
2. Irritable bowel syndrome (IBS) (30 to 45 million)
3. Gallstone disease (20 to 25 million)
4. Diverticular disease (2.2 to 40 million)
5. Celiac disease (gluten enteropathy) (estimated at 3 million but may be a great deal higher)
6. Inflammatory bowel disease (IBD) (700,000 to 900,000)
7. Colorectal cancer (approximately 255,640)

Let's briefly review the prevalence rates and the kinds of symptoms one may experience with each of these conditions. We will also look at some of the extraintestinal manifestations of digestive disorders.

Gastroesophageal Reflux Disease: Heartburn Gone Rogue

Gastroesophageal reflux disease has gotten a huge amount of press in recent years, and the incidence of GERD has skyrocketed over the last three decades. Thirty years ago, GERD was hardly recognized. You either had heartburn or chronic heartburn, and you were treated as such. The appearance of

GERD as a diagnosis has complicated the picture, so let's take a moment to tease this apart a bit.

Heartburn occurs when stomach acid creeps up into your esophagus. This is called reflux. When your gut is functioning normally, a valve called the lower esophageal sphincter (LES), which is located between your stomach and your esophagus, opens briefly to let food into your stomach or gas out of it. Otherwise it remains tightly closed, and your stomach acid is kept where it is supposed to be. However, in some cases the LES opens too often or doesn't close tightly enough. This is one cause of acid reflux.

Another common reason reflux occurs involves a failure of gut motility (sometimes referred to as disordered peristalsis) to sweep acid and digestive enzymes away from the esophagus. In either case, what you experience is that old familiar burning sensation in your esophagus as stomach acid creeps into it. When you are under anxiety, stress, and depression, the esophagus can become hypersensitive and minor irritation from GERD can cause severe pain.

GERD is usually experienced as heartburn, but some people have silent GERD, which is reflux without heartburn. Still others may experience a host of symptoms that manifest themselves in conjunction with GERD, including:

- Asthma
- Bad breath
- Belching
- Chronic cough
- Chronic sore throat
- Difficulty or pain when swallowing
- Erosion of tooth enamel
- Hoarseness
- Inflammation of the gums
- Postnasal drip
- Sleep disorders
- Sour taste in the mouth
- Water brash (sudden excess saliva)

We now know that 14 percent of Americans suffer from heartburn once a week, 21 percent suffer monthly, and 50 percent experience it yearly. It's actually quite frightening, when you consider the profound health complications that can come with GERD. These include:

- Barrett's esophagus (changes in esophageal cells that are precancerous, in some cases)
- Dysphagia (difficulty swallowing)
- Esophagitis (irritation and inflammation of the esophagus)
- Esophageal cancer

That doesn't mean you should panic. Even if you have daily heartburn, it doesn't automatically mean you will end up with esophageal cancer. What's more, the reason your LES isn't functioning properly or your gut motility is impaired most likely has to do with what you eat and how you live. That means that changing your diet and lifestyle can help you preclude and even reverse the symptoms of GERD.

A dysfunctional LES or disordered peristalsis may be caused by several factors.

- Certain medications (including calcium channel blockers)
- Eating foods that relax the LES (usually tomatoes, citrus fruits, garlic, onions, chocolate, caffeine, alcohol, and peppermint, though this is highly individualized)
- Foods high in fat and oil (especially excess animal fats)
- Obesity (which also puts pressure on the stomach)
- Overeating (which puts pressure on the stomach)
- Smoking (which relaxes the LES while increasing acid production)
- Stress (which increases acid production in the stomach, affects motility, and lowers your pain threshold)

As you may be able to intuit from the list above, the causes of GERD are extremely individualized, and thus treatment should be customized to the root cause or causes. This is particularly true when it comes to dietary factors that lead to GERD. It's not as though everyone who eats a tangerine or has a cup of peppermint tea will automatically have heartburn. These are simply a few examples of possible causes. The key is to find out what is setting off *your* symptoms and eliminate the sources of the problem for you. In many cases, when you treat the causes of GERD, the problem resolves itself. We will teach you more about how to do this in Part III.

Irritable Bowel Syndrome: It's Not All in Your Head!

Unlike many other digestive diseases, irritable bowel syndrome is a functional disorder. What this means is that the problem is due to the way the organ (in this case, the gut) works, not with a physical or systemic cause that can be identified through testing or taking x-rays.

Today, there are at least three different sets of diagnostic criteria used to assess whether or not a patient has IBS. There is a constellation of common symptoms (hence we call it a syndrome), but not every person with IBS suffers the same way, and some of the symptoms seem contradictory on the surface.

Exactly what IBS is and how it is caused aren't completely clear. What we do know is that when a person has IBS, the gut doesn't function as it should. The person suffers from altered gut motility and a lowered threshold for pain. The exact way motility is altered varies from person to person, but any irregularity in peristalsis can lead to a variety of problems.

Why peristalsis is altered in patients with IBS isn't particularly clear, either. There is some evidence that communication between the brain and the gut is impaired, and this leads to problems. It may be that the enteric nervous system doesn't function correctly, or it may be that the central nervous system (your brain and spinal cord) doesn't properly receive and interpret messages. Perhaps it's some combination of these factors, or it may be that there are others at play. We just don't know.

Whatever the cause, the symptoms of IBS can include:

- Bloating
- Chronic diarrhea or constipation (often alternating between the two)
- Frequent and recurring abdominal pain (this is the hallmark sign of the condition)
- Loose stools immediately following the onset of abdominal pain
- Mucus in stools
- Stomach cramps

The condition is extremely common. Most studies say that 10 to 15 percent of people in the United States and Europe have IBS, with twice as many women affected as men. However, the numbers may be higher than that. Research suggests that only 10 to 20 percent of people with IBS actually report the condition to their doctor. This is most likely due to embarrassment about the condition, which is tragic because many cases are relatively mild and amenable to self-help treatments.

While the exact biological causes of IBS remain unknown, it is clear that a handful of lifestyle choices trigger the condition. These include:

- Foods in your diet that trigger symptoms (there is a broad range, but we will address some of the more common dietary triggers in Part III)
- Infections from foodborne illnesses and other pathogens
- Stress

An estimated 25 percent of IBS cases begin with a gastrointestinal infection. These are caused either by eating in restaurants where the food has been contaminated or by travel to a country with poor sanitation. This subtype of IBS is thought to involve the chronic release of inflammatory mediators in the gut.

Becoming aware of the triggers can help reduce the frequency of the IBS flareups. So here we have a "disease" that can't be "cured," but one that can be overcome by changing a few aspects of your diet and lifestyle.

Gallstone Disease: Could Excess Saturated Fat Ruin Your Gallbladder?

Gallstones are exactly what they sound like: small stones that form in your gallbladder (or the common bile duct). As you know, your gallbladder stores bile created in your liver and later releases it into your small intestine to help you digest fats. In some cases, stones made of cholesterol and a few other chemicals build up in the gallbladder or common bile duct and keep the gallbladder from doing its job properly.

This doesn't sound like a major problem, and in minor cases it may not be. Many people have gallstones but don't suffer from any symptoms and thus don't require any treatment. But if you have ever seen an image of a gallbladder absolutely packed with gallstones that range in size from a grain of sand to the size of a golf ball, you know that you don't want to have gallstone disease.

When these more severe cases occur, they generally manifest as pain in the upper right side of the abdomen that can then spread into the upper right side of the back and even the shoulder. In very extreme cases (primarily in situations where the bile duct is blocked by stones), you may experience pain, chills, and fever, and the whites of your eyes and your skin may turn yellow. Cases like these also increase your chances of pancreatitis (the swelling of your pancreas).

Gallstone disease is another digestive disorder that is relatively common (13.2 percent of people in the United States have it), and it is much more prevalent in Western countries than in Africa or the East. Many believe that this is due to the higher intake of sugar and saturated fats found in animal products like fatty red meats common in Western diets.

Diverticular Disease: Got Fiber?

Diverticular disease is a matrix of three interrelated conditions: diverticulosis, diverticular bleeding, and diverticulitis.

Diverticulosis is the development of numerous tiny pockets (called diverticula) in the lining of the bowel. These diverticula are caused by gas, waste, or liquid putting excess strain on weakened parts of your intestinal lining. Diverticulosis occurs most commonly in the lower portion of the large intestine, which is called the sigmoid colon.

For some, the condition is relatively harmless. They experience no symptoms and require no treatment. Others have tenderness in the areas where the pockets in the intestinal lining occur. In more extreme instances, the condition is complicated by a number of factors and leads to either diverticular bleeding or diverticulitis (inflammation of the diverticula).

Diverticular bleeding happens when chronic injury to the blood vessels next to the diverticula causes bleeding in the bowel.

Diverticulitis is a condition in which the diverticula become inflamed. This usually happens when the tiny pockets in your bowel get blocked by waste. This allows bacteria to build up in the area and a host of symptoms may result, including:

- Chills
- Constipation

- Diarrhea
- Fever
- Painful cramping
- Tenderness in the lower abdomen

If the condition is left untreated, the bowel can become perforated. When that happens, waste material in your lower intestine leaks into your body with a number of potentially devastating effects, including:

- Abscesses ("walled off" infections in the abdomen)
- Obstructions (blockages in your intestine)
- Peritonitis (a painful infection of the abdominal cavity)

Once the bowel is perforated, surgery is often necessary to repair it. The severity of the complications from diverticulitis will determine the extent of the surgery.

Prevalence rates for diverticular disease vary widely depending on the method of diagnosis and the age of the population being studied. The overall prevalence of diverticular disease in America is estimated to be 20 percent of the population. However, some studies show prevalence between 5 and 45 percent. In any event, the disease is quite common. Its prevalence seems to only increase with age, going from less than 5 percent of the population at age 40, up to 30 percent by age 60, and up to 65 percent by age 85.

The unfortunate commonality of diverticular disease is made all the more poignant by the fact that making one simple dietary change can generally preclude the problem completely: Just add more fiber to your diet.

Pressure changes in the bowel are the primary reason diverticula develop. The problem is mitigated by increasing your intake of plant foods that are high in fiber (in some cases, supplementation with fiber can also be helpful).

The difference between prevalence rates of diverticular disease in the United States and in countries that eat a more traditional diet filled with fibrous plant foods bears this out. Diverticulosis is rare in Africa and Asia (except Japan, which has rapidly become Westernized) and in cultures that consume a high-fiber diet. In Iran, where a high-fiber diet is consumed by the majority of the population, the frequency of diverticulosis was recently reported to be 1.6 percent above age 20 and 2.4 percent above age 50.

Compare these statistics with ours in the West and it's easy to see what a difference a little bit of fiber in the diet can make.

Celiac Disease: Could a Grain Intolerance Be Driving Your Illness?

Celiac disease is defined as an autoimmune disease of the gut that is driven by the ingestion of gluten—the protein found in wheat, rye, barley, and a number of other grains, including triticale, spelt, and kamut. Gluten is also found in many processed foods, in part because these foods contain grains and in part because gluten is used as an additive in some processed foods.

Gluten intolerance is one of the most common and most underdiagnosed chronic diseases in Western countries. The more conservative estimates state that approximately 1 in 133 (about 3 million) Americans are affected by celiac disease. It is also considered the most common genetic disease in Europe. In Italy, about 1 in 250 people have it, and in Ireland, about 1 in 300 people have it.

Some research suggests that celiac disease is actually much more common than this. Dr. Peter Green, an internationally recognized authority on celiac disease, spoke for many when he stated that this condition is grossly underdiagnosed, and he has dubbed it "a hidden epidemic."[1]

Part of the problem with diagnosing celiac disease can be the silent nature of the condition. An intolerance to gluten doesn't normally show up as an acute allergic reaction (an IgE-mediated response—see page 88), like when you are allergic to peanuts. If you are allergic to peanuts, you usually find out about it pretty quickly because as soon as you eat one, either you break out in hives, your throat closes up, or your breathing is compromised. That only has to happen once for you to make darn sure that you never, ever eat a peanut—or anything that contains peanuts—again.

Intolerances to gluten can be more subtle, but if left untreated they can be especially problematic. They may show up as intermittent diarrhea, abdominal pain, or bloating; they may mimic other conditions, such as Crohn's disease, irritable bowel syndrome; or they may show up as symptoms seemingly unrelated to gut function, such as irritability, depression, joint pain, skin rashes, or restless leg syndrome.[2]

This is complicated by the fact that many physicians aren't aware that celiac disease presents itself as such a wide array of symptoms, so they don't connect the dots.

This is unfortunate, because when left untreated, celiac disease can lead to:

- Anemia
- Bone disease
- Cancer
- Neuropathy
- Other systemic conditions

However, you can reduce your symptoms and minimize your risk of developing the condition by eating a healthy, delicious, gluten-free diet. We will teach you how later in this book.

Inflammatory Bowel Disease: The Gut on Fire

Inflammatory bowel disease (IBD) refers to a group of disorders (including ulcerative colitis and Crohn's disease) that cause your inside tract to become inflamed. As its name suggests, ulcerative colitis is generally limited to your large intestine (colon). Crohn's disease can occur anywhere in your gastrointestinal tract, from your mouth to your anus, but it is usually found in the small intestine and the colon. Both conditions result in severe abdominal pain, chronic diarrhea, and rectal bleeding. You may suffer from a few other symptoms as well, depending on the severity and nature of your condition.

While we don't understand all of the mechanisms that lead to IBD, we do know that inflammation is always at the root.

While not all of the mechanisms that cause IBD are known, these diseases are generally thought to be autoimmune reactions—an inflammatory response in which your immune system mistakenly sees your own cells as foreign invaders and begins to attack them. Suffice it to say that when your homeland security team turns against you instead of the enemy cells it's supposed to protect you from, the results aren't good. One of the possible outcomes is IBD.

Again, depending on the methods used for diagnosis and the populations studied, the number of people considered to have IBD can vary
widely. However, approximately 400,000 to 600,000 people in the
United States are thought to be affected with Crohn's disease, and ulcerative colitis is thought to affect about 0.1 percent of the population, or
approximately 300,000 people. Like each of the other diseases discussed
in this chapter, we see higher rates of both of these diseases in North
America and northern Europe than we do in Asia, Africa, South America,
or Australia.

While most doctors say that IBD cannot be cured, we have seen people
make remarkable recoveries. Excessive consumption of refined carbohydrates and unhealthy polyunsaturated fats (like corn oil and margarine)
has been shown to correlate with the development of IBD. Remove these
substances (and a few other pro-inflammatory foods) from your diet, exercise regularly, reduce stress, eat foods with anti-inflammatory properties,
and take a few smart nutrients that cool the inflammatory response, and
the condition can improve.

Colorectal Cancer: A Lifestyle Disease

Colorectal cancer (also called colon cancer or large bowel cancer) is the
growth of cancerous cells in the colon, rectum, and appendix. It is the
most common cancer of the digestive organs, accounting for 60 percent
of all cancer of the gastrointestinal (GI) tract and 25 percent of cancer
fatalities in the United States.[3]

While it is the second most common cancer in Europe and the United
States, it is considered rare in both Asia and Africa (again, barring Westernized Japan). Why is it more common in Western countries? Once again,
we go back to diet and lifestyle.

There are seven behavioral risk factors that have been consistently cor-
related with an increase in colorectal cancer. These are:

1. Smoking
2. Low physical activity
3. Low fruit and vegetable intake
4. High caloric intake from fat[4]

5. Obesity
6. High alcohol intake
7. Sleep deprivation[5, 6]

However, if you make healthy lifestyle choices and follow your doctor's guidance for undergoing screening colonoscopy examinations, you can reduce your risk of developing colorectal cancer.

Obviously this list of digestive diseases is not comprehensive. But by analyzing just these few disorders, we see a pattern beginning to emerge—one that has much to tell us not only about digestive disease but also about disease in general. Later in this book we will further investigate the threads that connect all of these disorders. But first let's turn our attention to the ways in which digestive disease can present itself outside of the gut.

Digestive Disease Outside the Tract

One of the things that is fascinating about your gut is that everything that happens in it radiates to the rest of your body. Like a rose whose petals reach outward from the ovule at the center, your health radiates outward from your gut. Most of us define the beauty of a rose by the quality and shape of its petals. We don't ever look at the ovule. Similarly, you define your health by how you feel, not by how well your gut functions. What most people don't realize is that many chronic health conditions are connected to the gut in some way. If your gut isn't functioning optimally, you are bound to suffer. In this sense, much of illness is actually digestive disease in one form or another.

For many, the first signs of a digestive disease actually appear as symptoms somewhere else in the body. Classic examples include the fever and joint pain that occur during a flare-up of Crohn's disease and the interstitial cystitis or fibromyalgia that are common harbingers of IBS. The table on page 60 shows the relationships between some of the digestive diseases we have discussed in this chapter and symptoms or systemic illnesses that may show up outside the gut.

You may experience chronic health symptoms that you would never think to relate to gut dysfunction, yet digestive imbalances may be at the

Digestive Diseases and Systemic Symptoms and Illnesses

DISEASE	SYSTEMIC SYMPTOMS AND ILLNESSES
Celiac Disease	• Thyroid disease • Neurological diseases[7] • Osteoporosis • Iron-deficiency anemia • Decreased fertility • Low intrauterine weights • Recurrent urinary tract infections • Cardiomyopathy • Autoimmune disorders* • Skin disorders** • Restless leg syndrome[8]
Gastroesophageal Reflux Disease	• Asthma • Hoarseness • Chronic cough • Postnasal drip • Sleep disturbances
Inflammatory Bowel Disease	• Arthritis/joint pain • Fever greater than 100°F • Skin lesions (pyoderma gangrenosum, erythema nodosum) • Eye disorders (uveitis, iritis) • Mouth ulcers (aphthous stomatitis) • Restless leg syndrome[9]
Irritable Bowel Syndrome	• General pelvic pain and urologic disturbances • Interstitial cystitis • Fibromyalgia • Chronic fatigue syndrome • Sleep disturbances • Rosacea • Migraine headaches • Restless leg syndrome

* Including primary biliary cirrhosis, autoimmune hepatitis, autoimmune cholangitis, type 1 diabetes mellitus, autoimmune thyroid disorders, Addison's disease, alopecia areata, and vitiligo.
** Including dermatitis herpetiformis, alopecia areata, vitiligo, and psoriasis.

root of your problems. Restless leg syndrome, migraines, skin problems, asthma, allergies, and arthritis have all been connected to imbalances in the inside tract. Improve your gut function, and in some cases, symptoms seemingly unrelated to the digestive system improve and

Symptoms and Possible Digestive Causes

SYMPTOM	DEFINITION	POSSIBLE DIGESTIVE CAUSES
Restless Leg Syndrome	The compelling urge to move the legs at night, often with discomfort; an estimated 10% of the general population suffers from it.[10]	Irritable bowel syndrome (IBS), small intestinal bacterial overgrowth (SIBO), celiac disease (CD)
Fibromyalgia	Complex systemic pain disorder with palpable tender points for more than 3 months in all four quadrants of the body.	IBS, SIBO
Chronic Fatigue Immune Deficiency Syndrome	A condition of prolonged and severe tiredness of unknown etiology that limits your ability to carry out life activities to 50% of capacity and is not relieved by rest.[11]	IBS, SIBO
Rosacea	A common idiopathic disease that presents with transient or persistent facial erythema, telangiectasia, edema, papules, and pustules, usually confined to the central portion of the face.[12]	IBS, SIBO, *H. pylori* infection
Pyoderma Gangrenosum	A skin condition that causes skin tissue to break down, with large ulcers developing on the lower legs.[13]	Inflammatory bowel disease (IBD)
Erythema Nodosum	An inflammation of the fat cells under the skin (panniculitis). It causes tender nodules that are usually seen on the legs.[14]	IBD
Alopecia Areata	A condition in which hair is lost from some or all areas of the body, though most often from the scalp.[15]	Celiac disease (CD)
Dermatitis Herpetiformis	An intensely itchy skin eruption. It usually shows up in young adults and is more common in men and people originally from some areas of northern Europe.[16]	CD
Vitiligo	A medical condition that causes the skin to lose color.[17]	CD

even disappear. The table on page 61 shows symptoms you may suffer from and some possible undetected digestive disorders that may be leading to those symptoms.

Given the complex and intimate relationship between digestive health and the rest of the body, it's easy to see why digestive disorders sometimes go undetected for a long time. Early clues that there's a problem can be easily missed by both the patient and the physician—sometimes for years. This is unfortunate because if we look closely at the threads that tie these illnesses and health problems together, it's clear that a few simple interventions could prevent a great deal of suffering.

The Patterns of Illness: A Life Out of Balance

The first connection between every disorder in this chapter is that diet and lifestyle choices can have a direct impact on your gut and your health. There is a growing mountain of scientific evidence that proves changing your diet and lifestyle not only helps prevent the diseases previously outlined (along with many others), but actually reverses the progress of these illnesses as well. In many cases, diet and lifestyle treatments are effective, and they are certainly less intrusive.

Consider the typical treatments for GERD, for a moment. If you walk into your doctor's office today and complain of chronic, recurring heartburn, he or she will almost automatically prescribe you a PPI like Nexium or Prevacid. These drugs have one function—they essentially shut down acid production in your stomach.

We have been so trained to think of PPIs as safe that, on the surface, shutting down acid production in your stomach doesn't seem like such a big deal anymore. After all, you wouldn't even have heartburn if your stomach wasn't producing too much acid in the first place, right?

Actually, that line of thinking isn't right . . . at least not always.

As you learned above, GERD is most often a problem with disordered LES function, hypersensitivity to pain, and/or aberrant peristalsis. It is generally not an outcome of "too much acid in your stomach." Regardless of your stomach acid levels, you won't suffer from GERD as long as the LES is doing its job properly and your gut motility is normal.

However, PPIs have become first-line therapy for GERD. Recent evidence has shown that PPIs are not nearly as safe as most doctors make them sound. PPIs can cause an overgrowth of *Clostridium difficile* and a number of other "bad" bugs in your stomach and small intestine; increase your risk of getting pneumonia; increase the likelihood of cardiovascular events by interfering with the blood thinner clopidogrel (Plavix); predispose you to conditions that lead to hip fractures; and inhibit the absorption of calcium, iron, and vitamin B_{12}. And that's just for starters.

The real irony is that there is a cost-effective treatment, the risks of which are so low as to be nearly nonexistent. What is this miracle treatment? Change your diet, lose weight if needed, take a few nutritional supplements, get some exercise, reduce your stress level, and enhance your social support system. Do this, and you will be on the road to good gut health. You have the power to choose foods and habits that will help you overcome your illness and thrive once more. It's time you learned how to heal your inside tract, and in Part II we will teach you how to do that.

The Inside Tract Prescription to Wellness

CHAPTER 4

THE "INSIDE TRACT" TO GOOD NUTRITION

Let thy food be thy medicine and thy medicine be thy food.
—HIPPOCRATES

Despite the fact that in recent years Americans have become much more conscious about how food affects our health, we still don't understand its true power as medicine. In some ways, we are more confused about food than ever.

Every day in the media we hear new claims about which foods make us healthy and which make us sick. For years we were told that a low-fat diet was essential for long-term health, and while that may be true for some, the story about fat turns out to be far more complex. We now know that omega-3 fats perform many important roles in human biology, and getting too few of these essential fatty acids can be extremely detrimental to our health. For some of us, it's not the amount but the type of fat we eat that makes the difference between optimal and ill health. Low-carb, high-protein diets have also seen much press in recent years, but that portrait of a healthy diet was painted in broad strokes and the full truth was lost there as well. Diets rich in whole and unrefined carbohydrates—namely plant foods—deliver some of the most important nutrients in the human diet. Trading these for diets high in animal protein—often unhealthy animal protein that's been processed in giant feedlots where disease runs rampant and antibiotics are overused—is not the best way to achieve good health.

In spite of such conflicting nutrition headlines and murky media reports, there is an emergent consensus among the top scientists and leading nutritionists. This nutritional accord on what constitutes a healthy diet derives from major advances in our understanding of metabolism, nutrition, systems biology, and genetics, as well as studies of the healthiest populations in the world. Interestingly, these scientific advances have, in many cases, proven what ancient systems of medicine have long known. What we've learned tends to reflect traditional eating practices that date back as far as our Paleolithic ancestors. It turns out that humans once knew how to eat. Many Americans, unfortunately, don't.

Though we have something of a national obsession with dieting, Americans have some of the worst eating patterns on the planet. According to a recent study published in the *Journal of Nutrition,* "Nearly the entire US population consumes a diet that is not on par with recommendations."[1] This rather dismal conclusion is underscored by the following:

- ☐ **Fruits and veggies.** Among American adults, only one-third eat enough fruits and a little more than one-quarter eat enough vegetables per day to meet nutritional recommendations set in the Healthy People 2010 national objectives.
- ☐ **Fiber.** We consume about 15 grams of fiber daily, which is below the *minimum* recommended daily intake. The current recommendation for fiber is approximately 20 to 35 grams. Even this is drastically different from our ancestral fiber intake of around 100 grams a day.
- ☐ **Whole grains.** The average American consumes less than one serving of whole grains per day, though My Plate recommends that you make half of your grain consumption "whole."[2] A whole grain is a cereal grain that contains the bran, germ, and endosperm and that provides the nutrient-rich substances that refined grains have been stripped of.
- ☐ **Sugar.** We're drowning in a tsunami of added sugars in a variety of sugar-laden foods and beverages. Sugar contributes more than one-quarter of our total daily calories. We each bank about 22 teaspoons per day!
- ☐ **Calories.** Six foods make up the major sources of calories for kids 2 to 18 years old: soda, fruit drinks, dairy desserts, grain desserts, pizza, and whole milk. It's little wonder that we are seeing such an increase in obesity, allergies, asthma, attention deficit disorder (ADD), and gut problems in this age group.
- ☐ **Eating away from home.** Today, nearly 50 percent of our food dollars are spent on foods prepared outside the home, and much of this is spent in fast-food restaurants. The calorie and fat content

of these foods is far higher, and they tend to be lower in fiber, calcium, iron, folate, and other nutrients critical for digestive health.

We all know there is an epidemic of chronic illness, but it would appear that few of us connect this national health emergency to our diets and environments. We all know there is an obesity epidemic (which in turn contributes to our chronic illness epidemic), but somehow we don't link this to the big burgers, super-sized french fries, and gallons of soda we consume while behind the wheel. Nor do we make the connection with the millions of pounds of pesticides that we spray on our fruits and vegetables or the endless aisles of man-made processed "foods" that line the shelves of our grocery stores.

If you want to know why Americans are so sick, if you want to know why the digestive diseases we have been discussing in this book are often referred to as "Western" diseases, you have only to look at the end of the national fork. That fork can truly be an instrument of mass destruction or an instrument of health instruction!

Our cultural failure to recognize that food is medicine is a detriment not only to our waistlines but also to our entire way of being. Nowhere is this more evident than in the health of our inside tracts. After all, we are all born with an organ whose primary responsibility is to take the foods we eat and break them down into the components necessary to fuel our bodies. Could we really believe that the *kind* of food we choose to put into it would have no effect on how it functions?

The reality is that food contains all of the essential elements you need to sustain cell growth, optimize the speed and efficacy of your metabolism, and even regulate gene expression. Every biochemical reaction in your body is influenced by the foods you consume. The foods we choose to put in our bodies have the power to promote or prevent disease. Choose well, and food can be used to help you heal. Choose poorly, and your chances of getting well plummet.

Given this cultural conditioning, the addictive foods so many of us overconsume, and the fact that altering behavior is rarely easy, changing your diet is no small feat. As author and cultural anthropologist Margaret Mead said, "It is easier to change a man's religion than to change his diet."[3] Confusion over what constitutes good nutrition is one of the chief reasons so many people stay stuck in poor health for so long. In this chapter we will clear up the confusion. The principles of what constitutes a healthy diet are outlined here to provide you with an overview of the growing consensus among medical scientists, doctors, and dietitians. These guidelines form the basis for the food plan in Part III of this book and are the nutritional foundation needed for improving gut function and optimizing health.

Guiding Principles of the Inside Tract Diet

There are 10 simple principles that serve as the foundation for our entire nutrition plan.

Let's review each of these guidelines in detail so you understand exactly what you need to do to begin healing your digestive system.

Eat Whole, Fresh, Unprocessed Foods— Seasonal, Organic, and Local, Whenever Possible

One of the most important things you need to do if you wish to restore and maintain excellent health and well-being is to eat a diet that is rich in whole foods. Whole foods are unprocessed and unrefined, or processed as little as possible before being consumed. Examples include:

THE 10 PRINCIPLES OF NUTRITIONAL INTEGRITY

1. Eat whole, fresh, unprocessed foods—seasonal, organic, and local, whenever possible.
2. Eat a diet that is founded on proven nutritional science.
3. Eat foods that promote good digestion and support your gut flora.
4. Avoid common food allergens and intolerances.
5. Eat foods that taste good, and allow your taste buds time to get used to new foods.
6. Eat in rhythm with meals scheduled at regular intervals throughout the day.
7. Eat until you are no more than two-thirds full.
8. Eat in a relaxed state.
9. Stay happily hydrated.
10. Eat foods *you* cook!

- Fruits and vegetables
- Legumes (beans, peas, and lentils)
- Nuts and seeds
- Organic eggs and poultry, grass-fed lean meat, and wild cold-water fish
- Whole grains

Whole foods are the foods our ancestors ate. They are the foods we consumed as we evolved, and they contain a wide array of healthy components, from the phytonutrients found in fruits and vegetables to the fiber in unrefined grains to the vitamin B_{12} found in lean animal proteins. Each of these natural constituents (and many, many others) found in whole foods supports optimal digestive health.

There's an endless variety of whole foods available, and not all of them can be consumed safely by everyone. In some cases, this can be due to food sensitivities. For example, gluten is found in a number of whole grains, such as wheat, barley, and rye, and even oats can be cross-contaminated with gluten. For many, these grains are safe and even healthy to eat. However, studies suggest that millions of Americans are intolerant of gluten, and research shows that gluten sensitivity in its many manifestations, from mild gluten intolerance to celiac disease, is widespread.[4] Gluten intolerance has been associated with a broad array of digestive complaints such as bloating and diarrhea. It has also been connected with many other systemic symptoms like headaches,[5] joint aches,[6] and even poor mood.[7]

Another factor to consider is the nature of your particular illness. When your digestive tract is unhealthy, this illness may show up as a wide spectrum of symptoms both in the digestive system and in the rest of your body. When determining how to use food as medicine, you need to consider the many ways food impacts gut health in its various stages of illness. For example, an individual with peptic ulcers can become more symptomatic after eating whole foods that can irritate the damaged lining of the gut. These include strong spices like paprika, cayenne pepper, chile pepper, black pepper, and nutmeg. Some individuals with irritable bowel syndrome (IBS) may have more symptoms after eating certain grains, such as whole wheat, and even some fruits and vegetables, such as apples, pears, and onions. In contrast, other whole foods or spices can actually help heal the intestinal lining; these include ginger,[8] the fresh peel of citrus fruits,[9] and aloe vera juice.[10, 11]

So even though some foods are perfectly healthy for many to eat, in the context of a particular illness, you'll need to know what foods you should avoid, at least until the ulcer has been resolved.

The key is to develop an individualized eating regimen that is tailored to *your* symptoms and the stages of *your* illness.

Another important consideration when moving toward a whole-foods diet is how your food is grown and processed. Does a focus on whole foods mean that every food that has been processed is off-limits, that you can't eat a single product that comes out of a box, jar, or can? No. Clearly that would be too extreme. Food processing in the strictest sense has been around for nearly as long as human beings have been eating. Traditional processing methods, like fermentation, can even have digestive health benefits. The important distinction lies in the amount and type of processing done to the food, as well as in the kinds of ingredients used in the creation of the food and the types of chemicals used to preserve it.

What food chemists do to preserve the "foods" we eat today is shocking. You don't even want to know what kinds of chemicals you will find in the dozens upon dozens of varieties of crackers, cakes, colas, chips, and cookies that line modern grocery store aisles. These "foods" are filled with substances that are toxic to your biology and are most certainly *not* good for your gut. You need to limit these highly processed foods if you want to maintain optimal health.

Unfortunately, in today's world it's not only the chemists employed by multinational food corporations who work to add man-made chemicals to our food supply. Some growers are also responsible, to some degree. Conventional farming is now considered one of the most hazardous professions one can practice. The chemicals used as pesticides, herbicides, and fertilizers are poisonous in parts per billion, in many cases, yet they are used liberally on virtually every fruit, vegetable, and herb found in our supermarkets. These chemicals leach into our soil, our water supply, and our air. When we ingest them, they get stored in our bodies and poison our entire biochemistry.

President Franklin D. Roosevelt said, "The nation that destroys its soil destroys itself."[12] Your body and its biological terrain are intimately connected to the earth's terrain, and thus your health is a reflection of the health of your food system. How well the plants are nourished by the soil they are grown in and how the animals are raised influence our health and our inside tracts. Another way to think about this relationship is that we are how *they* ate!

In the past few years, there has been renewed excitement about protecting our planet and greater consideration given to the reformation of our food systems. Documentaries such as *Food, Inc.* and *Fresh,* among others, have stimulated some eaters to reexamine how they are feeding their bodies. People are now thinking more critically about where the food on their plates comes from. Nutrition-minded advocates such as Andrew Weil, Joan Gussow, Marion Nestle, Michael Pollan, Maria Rodale, and Jane Goodall, as well as groups such as the American Dietetic Association's Hunger and Environmental Nutrition Dietetic Practice Group are championing the overhaul of our food supply.

In addition to the impact that modern agricultural practices have had on human health, there is mounting evidence that these same practices have polluted our soil, air, and water; eroded our soil; increased our dependence on imported oil; and diminished biodiversity. A recent article in the *American Journal of Clinical Nutrition* titled "Diet and the environment:

THE NATIONAL ORGANIC STANDARDS BOARD (NOSB) DEFINITION OF *ORGANIC*

The following definition of *organic* was passed by the NOSB at its April 1995 meeting in Orlando, Florida:

Organic agriculture is an ecological production management system that promotes and enhances biodiversity, biological cycles, and soil biological activity. It is based on minimal use of off-farm inputs and on management practices that restore, maintain, and enhance ecological harmony.

Organic is a labeling term that denotes products produced under the authority of the Organic Foods Production Act. The principal guidelines for organic production are to use materials and practices that enhance the ecological balance of natural systems and that integrate the parts of the farming system into an ecological whole.

Organic agriculture practices cannot ensure that products are completely free of residues; however, methods are used to minimize pollution from air, soil, and water.

Organic food handlers, processors, and retailers adhere to standards that maintain the integrity of organic agricultural products. The primary goal of organic agriculture is to optimize the health and productivity of interdependent communities of soil life, plants, animals, and people.

Does what you eat matter?" identified and reviewed six major effects that our dietary choices have on the environment. These choices affect water resources, energy consumption, chemical fertilizer application, pesticide application, waste generation, and land degradation. The authors' conclusion is that because of the ecological pressures that human civilization exerts on our planet, we need to reconsider how much animal food we are consuming and develop more sustainable methods of food production.[13]

This is not only essential for the health of the planet, but for the health of our bodies as well. The ecosystem of human biology is part of the larger ecosystem on this planet. Healing our planet and healing ourselves are the same thing. In Chapter 5, we will discuss the full impact of toxins on the health of your digestive system, as well as how important it is to optimize your detoxification system, given the toxic load of our modern world. For now, suffice it to say that it's best to buy and eat organic, sustainable, seasonal produce (locally grown, whenever possible) and free-range, grass-fed and finished, hormone- and antibiotic-free animal products whenever you can. Though these products are slightly more expensive than their conventionally raised counterparts, the benefit to your health is worth it. Consider it an investment in your inside tract.

Try to become more aware of the ingredients in the foods you eat and the processes used to preserve them. Learn where your food comes from and how it was grown. If you look in your kitchen cabinet and find a bunch of boxes of "food" that have long lists of ingredients with names you can't pronounce or understand unless you are a chemist, you probably aren't eating enough whole foods. If you purchase giant packages of meat from wholesale retailers, you are probably getting a load of toxins, hormones, and antibiotics that your body doesn't need, and your health is being compromised. You can refer to the Environmental Working Group's Web site (www.ewg.org) for updates on important nutrition topics, including organic priorities for vegetables and fruits. You will also find a "Clean, Green and Sustainable Kitchen Checklist" in Chapter 8, page 177. Use it as a reference as you begin the gradual transformation to a greener kitchen and a healthier inside tract.

Eat a Diet That Is Founded on Proven Nutritional Science

A holistic approach to nutrition honors the wisdom of the ages as well as the sophisticated science that has evolved in this era of nutritional genomics (the science studying the relationship between the human genome, nutrition, and health). A thorough review of the origins of the human diet from our Paleolithic ancestors, coupled with extensive analyses of recent proven dietary patterns such as those from the Mediterranean region, clearly reveal critical nutrition factors that promote health and prevent digestive disease. Focusing on these factors will help heal your gut and keep you healthy for life.

Keep Your Plate Plant-Centered

The US Department of Health and Human Services 2010 dietary guidelines recommend a "total diet" approach that is energy balanced, nutrient dense, and very low in solid fats and added sugars. A shift to a plant-based diet that emphasizes vegetables, cooked beans and peas, fruits, whole grains, nuts, and seeds increases the likelihood of achieving the objectives of these guidelines.[14] In spite of this, Americans consume less than 60 percent of the recommended intake of vegetables and less than 50 percent of the recommended intake of fruits, according to What We Eat in America, National Health and Nutrition Examination Survey, 2005–2006.[15]

KEY POINT. Your inside tract depends on a hefty volume of plant material to keep things in working order, so it's important to reach your produce quota of 8 to 10 servings of fruits and vegetables every day.

What's a Serving?

Fruits

- ✓ 1 small whole fruit
- ✓ ½ large fruit (banana, grapefruit, mango)
- ✓ 1 cup fresh berries or melon cubes
- ✓ 4 ounces (½ cup) unsweetened, 100 percent fruit juice
- ✓ 2 tablespoons dried fruit

Vegetables

- ✓ 1 cup raw vegetables
- ✓ 2 cups leafy greens
- ✓ ½ cup cooked or fermented vegetables
- ✓ 4 ounces (½ cup) 100 percent vegetable juice

A higher plant-to-animal ratio on our plates is a smart strategy for keeping inflammatory bowel disease and other digestive disorders at bay.

A semivegetarian diet was found to be highly preventive against relapse in a small study of Japanese patients with Crohn's disease. The meals provided in this trial included traditional Japanese foods, rather than Western foods. The diet included miso soup, vegetables, fruits, legumes, potatoes, pickled vegetables, plain yogurt, and fish. Meat was served about half as often as fish. Subjects were also encouraged to drink green tea and avoid sweets, breads, cheese, margarines, fast foods, carbonated beverages, juices, and alcohol. In addition, other healthy habits were promoted, including eating regular meals, engaging in regular physical activity, and not smoking. The people in the study showed a 100 percent remission rate at 1 year and a 92 percent remission rate at 2 years.[16] Even though this study was limited by the small number of participants, it shows the power of food as medicine for treating inflammatory bowel disease!

This is just an example among dozens that point to the importance of eating a diet consisting primarily of plant foods. Plant foods provide the necessary fiber and anti-inflammatory phytonutrients to keep our GI tracts properly nourished and the genes that influence gut function dancing with joy.

KEY POINT. Meet your vegetable and fruit target each day and you are on your way to achieving your fiber quota. Sprinkle a "seed meal" such as flax, hemp, or chia in a smoothie or on a salad or veggie for a mega-boost of fiber.

EAT NUTRIENT-DENSE FOODS

A nutrient-dense (or nutrient-rich) food contains generous amounts of vitamins and minerals as compared to its total calorie count. Potato chips are nutrient poor. Carrots are nutrient dense. Nutrient-dense foods provide a diverse portfolio of vitamins and minerals and other yet-to-be-discovered bioactive substances. Including them in your diet is a natural, commonsense approach to improving your overall health. The food plan in this book is predicated on nutrient-rich foods. But don't get the wrong idea: As long as you stick to eating whole foods, keep your plate plant-centered, and eat mindfully, you don't need to count calories or calculate nutrient scores to improve your digestive

Fiber at a Glance

The fiber content of whole foods varies tremendously, but here's a quick glance at the approximate fiber content per serving.

FOOD GROUP/SERVING	FIBER (GRAMS)
Fruits, 1 piece, ½ cup	2–4
Vegetables, ½ cup cooked or raw	3–5
Beans, peas, lentils, ½ cup cooked	3–10
Nuts and seeds, 3 tablespoons	2–3
Whole grains, ½ cup cooked	3–8

health. Simply follow the nutrition plan in Part III and you will automatically be eating nutrient-dense foods designed to soothe your inside tract and optimize your overall health.

FOCUS ON FIBER

Dietary fiber, which also goes by the names roughage and residue, consists of the indigestible portion of plant foods. It is not an independent member of the major league of nutrients, which includes carbohydrates, protein, fat, vitamins, minerals, and water. Rather, it is an affiliate of the carbohydrate class of nutrients—that is to say, fiber comes from plant foods. Though it's not counted among the macronutrients, it is undoubtedly the chief operating substance of your inside tract. It helps maintain good peristalsis, feeds your gut flora, and promotes healthy bowel movements. Without enough fiber, your inside tract is at risk for disease, and the fact is that most Americans don't get enough.

Fiber is really a matrix of chemicals including lignin, polysaccharides, resistant starches, inulin, and oligosaccharides. All of these functional fiber components work together to maintain digestive health. Traditionally, fiber has been simply classified as soluble or insoluble, based on its ability to perform vital functions. Soluble fiber is "prebiotic." It is readily fermented and feeds our friendly flora, so physiologically bioactive compounds are created as a result. Insoluble fiber is metabolically inert. It does not ferment, but that doesn't mean it's unimportant. It absorbs water as it passes through your digestive tract, cleanses your gut, and eases defecation.

Plant foods contain both types of fiber, but one is usually bulkier and more plentiful. For example, apples, pears, oats, barley, and beans are all loaded with soluble fiber, while whole wheat, nuts, seeds, and the skins of fruits are packed with insoluble fiber. Both types are instrumental to the health of your inside tract, and fortunately, Mother Nature endowed all plants with these fibrous twins.

The Inside Tract nutrition plan is designed to meet your daily quota of fiber and is rich in prebiotic soluble fiber, which is readily fermented in your colon to produce those gut guardians, the short-chain fatty acids (SCFAs). Our plan is also rich in insoluble fiber, which absorbs water throughout your GI tract, resulting in first-class elimination.

MAINTAIN ACID-ALKALINE BALANCE

Anthropologists and nutrition scientists have been enthusiastically studying our early ancestors' dietary patterns to find evolutionary clues that might lead to a cure for our epidemic of chronic diseases. Numerous studies of our hunter-gatherer, preagricultural forbears have contributed to our understanding of another crucial nutrition factor that influences health and the prevention of digestive diseases: the net acid-base yield of our diet, or what is sometimes referred to as acid-alkaline balance.

Though the studies in this area are relatively complex, the basic principle is that your blood pH must be maintained within a relatively narrow range. If it isn't, you begin to suffer from "metabolic stress" as your body works harder to rebalance its own pH. Generally, your body likes to be in a slightly alkaline environment. How do you maintain this? Consume a primarily plant-based diet. Data points to a strong link between a diet with a high plant to animal (P:A) ratio and a more alkaline state.[17] The highly valued practice of eating more vegetables and fruits prevents an acid-prone, highly disruptive state and protects your bones in the process.

☞ **KEY POINT:** Acid-base balance is a critical factor in preventing osteoporosis and preserving kidney function.

Maintaining a healthy body weight and performing a physical activity that incorporates good breathing dynamics to prevent the buildup of lactic acid promotes a healthy physiological state. Shoma Berkemeyer, a noted researcher in acid-base physiology, summarized it impressively by noting that "what we eat and how we breathe are two important cornerstones in acid-base maintenance."[18]

BE ATTENTIVE TO THE SODIUM-TO-POTASSIUM RATIO

Minerals are essential nutrients that perform many functions in the body. A nutrient-dense, plant-based diet provides an array of superstar minerals like calcium, magnesium, chromium, zinc, selenium, and others that participate in a whole host of activities to keep us alive and well. But what you may not be aware of is the dramatic change in what is referred to as the sodium-to-potassium ratio that has occurred in recent years.[19] This is another critical nutrition factor that plays a major role in the health of your cells, including your GI tract, since these two minerals work in concert to help maintain fluid and electrolyte balance. Electrolytes are important because they carry information across cell membranes and affect the functioning of your muscles, nerves, and organs.

The sodium-stuffed processed foods that dominate supermarket shelves and fill our grocery carts have resulted in a menacing move in our cellular milieu to an unfavorable balance of sodium and potassium. What this means is that our cells can become overwhelmed by this flood of sodium and scant supply of potassium, resulting in all kinds of problems ranging from fluid retention to high blood pressure. Our lopsided sodium-to-potassium ratio is alarming, but it's easily remedied by a big boost in consumption of vegetables and fruits. Produce packs a high-potassium punch while contributing sparse amounts of sodium. Our nutrition plan has been carefully crafted with respect to the sodium-to-potassium ratio. Through its rich supply of plant foods and absence of processed foods, potassium predominates to restore the cellular relationship that safeguards your health.

BALANCE YOUR MACRONUTRIENTS

The macronutrients are carbohydrates (carbs), protein, and fats, and there are macro debates in the scientific community as to what percentage of each we should eat for better health. Popular diet books often proclaim their own unique magical trifecta of carb-protein-fat percentages based on your particular metabolic type or the need to get you in the right "zone." But the science is far more complex than these "express lane" diets reveal.

Some of us may need to be more in tune with the carbs in our diets, while others may have to be more mindful of total fats. At least, this is what the new science of nutritional genomics is uncovering.[20] Doesn't this make sense to you? You almost certainly know individuals who are blessed with an inherent macronutrient calibrator—people who don't need to be as careful about what they eat. You probably know others who seem to possess more carb- or fat-sensitive genes and who have to pay attention to their intake of each.

When it comes to gut health, some carbs, such as the lactose found in dairy products or the fructose found in high-fructose corn syrup–soaked foods, or even those found in whole foods with a high fructose load (such as grapes), might contribute to annoying symptoms such as gas, bloating, abdominal pain, and loose stools if you can't tolerate those carbs. In Part III, we'll talk more about this and how you can modulate how much of these sugars you consume.

The macronutrient combo on your plate is another crucial factor that supports good health. A fuss-free approach both for energy balance and gut health is to include foods from all three categories at each meal. The Inside Tract menus have been planned with smart macronutrient economics in mind. So rest assured, you do not need to keep a calculator by your plate!

CONSUME A LOW-GLYCEMIC-LOAD DIET

Eating too many high-glycemic, highly processed carbohydrates and sugars affects not only the size of your gut (giving you that extra belly fat around the middle), it also has a very serious impact on gut function. These foods cause your pancreas to misfire and create surges of insulin. When there is a gush of insulin, the blood sugar dynamic is disturbed and chaos results. Eventually this constant chaos will affect your appetite regulation, energy metabolism, and cardiovascular health, and can also result in type 2 diabetes. Incidence of this disease has doubled over the last three decades.[21] At least 24 million Americans now suffer from diabetes, and an additional 57 million people over the age of 20 struggle with prediabetes.[22] This is obviously a serious health concern, and all of the evidence points to this epidemic being the result of dietary and lifestyle changes, especially the massive amounts of sugar and refined carbs that have found their way into the fiber-deficient American diet.

Blood sugar imbalances also have an impact on your inside tract. Long-term imbalances can damage the nerve cells that work with your digestive system's motility center. When this happens, peristalsis may slow and the foods you eat may take longer to move through your digestive tract. This can lead to small intestinal bacterial overgrowth (SIBO) and various other gut disorders, as we discussed in Chapter 2. Blood sugar imbalances that are left unchecked can also have an impact on your liver. The metabolic havoc that comes from squalls of insulin may result in the all too common condition called nonalcoholic steatohepatitis (NASH), which now afflicts both children and adults. NASH is characterized by inflammation and fat accumulation in the liver. When this happens, your liver has a much harder time detoxifying your blood, and various problematic health outcomes can result. In some untreated cases, it can even lead to cirrhosis.

Maintaining steady blood sugar levels is essential, not only for the health of your gut but also for the health of every organ and system in your body. To maintain these levels, you need to consume a diet that has a *low glycemic load*.

KEY POINT: To better manage your blood sugar, you simply have to balance the overall glycemic load of your meals. Doing this is quite easy. Maximize your plate with whole plant foods—vegetables, fruits, whole grains, and legumes—all of which come naturally packaged with fiber. These foods convert to sugar slowly and steadily, which is what your body prefers.

The nutrition plan in this book has been deliberately created with glycemic balance in mind. Each meal in Part III provides a blend of fiber-rich carbohydrates paired with smart proteins and healthy fats for the ultimate in glycemic balance and satisfying portions.

GET PLENTY OF ANTI-INFLAMMATORY FOODS

Inflammation conjures up images of heat, fire, swelling, redness, and pain. When you get cut, are bitten by an insect, or sprain an ankle, your body naturally initiates a set of biochemical processes to protect and heal the injured area. But sometimes this compensatory process gets out of hand, like a wildfire. Recent discoveries have shown us that systemic inflammation of this nature is one of the chief causes of everything from heart attacks to cancer to Alzheimer's to other diseases. Some of the most challenging digestive diseases are essentially the outcome of runaway inflammation. This includes inflammatory bowel disorders (like ulcerative colitis and Crohn's), nonalcoholic steatohepatitis (NASH), and others.

There has been a deluge of diet books targeting inflammation. Geneti-cists have identified genes that make some people especially prone to "itis" or inflammatory conditions. In addition, pharmaceutical companies have developed battalions of anti-inflammatory drugs to combat the condition. However, the best way to keep inflammation at bay is to eat foods that are high in anti-inflammatory compounds. Getting the right balance of healthy fats is particularly important, in this regard.

We used to think that fat was simply a way to store energy, that it didn't have a biochemical impact on biology. We now know that this isn't true. Some fats are "essential," meaning they must be supplied through the foods we eat because our bodies cannot manufacture them. These essential fatty acids, called omega-3s and omega-6s, are important because they are involved in eicosanoid production. Eicosanoids are powerful signaling molecules that send messages throughout the body; these messenger molecules impact our health on a number of levels, mainly through their influence on inflammation and immunity. The fats we eat can become biological dictators of inflammation—some fats ignite fires in the body, others act as coolants to the physical inferno and protect against inflammatory processes. Interestingly, these dynamic, multifunc-tional nutrients are also responsible for cell membrane integrity, which allows for vigorous communication into and out of the cell. This ulti-mately influences your mood, your energy, your aches and pains, your brain power, and your resilience.

Eat healthy fats in moderation; they are vital components of re-establishing good gut function. Some examples are:

- Avocado
- Coconut
- Nut and seed butters
- Nuts and seeds
- Oils, cold-pressed (extra-virgin olive oil and grape seed oil)
- Organic soy foods
- Olives
- Wild cold-water fish (salmon, black cod/sablefish, and sardines)

These immune defensive and anti-inflammatory fats are built into the nutrition plan in Part III.

We suggest that you keep your plate plant-centered by loading it with fruits and vegetables. Beyond that, you should make intelligent protein choices, like beans or wild cold-water fish; obtain an optimal amount of healthy fats; and season your foods liberally with herbs and spices (including ginger, rosemary, turmeric, and others that provide natural anti-inflammatory relief).

Eat Your Antioxidants

Another delicate dance that takes place in our bodies is the tango between molecules involved in metabolism. This chemical concept is referred to as reduction-oxidation or, more affectionately, as "redox." As calories are burned in your mitochondria (the tiny energy factories in your cells) to produce energy, free radicals or reactive oxygen species (ROS) are produced. These free radicals are kind of like exhaust from the engine of a car—they're pollution, and they need to be cleaned up. Left unattended, these free radicals build up to unhealthy levels in the body, damaging your cells and eventually leading to *oxidative stress*—a condition that is a common feature in many digestive diseases, including pancreatitis, inflammatory bowel disease, and gastric and colorectal cancer.[23]

The key to reducing and overcoming oxidative stress is to keep the redox process in balance. You do this by maintaining enough antioxidant reserves to capture the harmful ROS before they can destroy your tissues. Your body produces its own supply of antioxidants, but when it's burdened by too much oxidative stress, supply cannot keep up with demand.

Luckily, there is a food-based solution. Plants must defend themselves against environmental stressors, temperature extremes, pests, and insects, and because of that they've developed an intricate antioxidant defense system. When we consume plant-based foods that have *not* been sprayed with pesticides or other harmful chemicals, we ingest these valuable antioxidants and can make use of them ourselves against the onslaught of free radicals that threatens our health. Pack your plate with a plethora of colorful plant foods (red-blue-purple, dark green, yellow-orange, and white-green), and you'll be supplying your body with these natural antioxidants to help it fight its battle against the free radicals.

Invest in Phytochemical Diversity

Phytochemicals (sometimes called phytos) are a vast group of plant-derived compounds that have been under intensive investigation because of their probable role in health. They are grouped together based on their chemical structure. One diverse family of phytos that appears to confer some particularly healthful properties is the flavonoids. Foods that are high in flavonoids include berries, grapefruit, apples, onions, soy, tea, and even dark chocolate and coffee!

Recent research has revealed the multiple roles these diverse chemicals play in protecting our health. In addition, numerous public health nutrition organizations, including the American Cancer Society and the American Heart Association, have started encouraging people to consume a variety of plant foods in order to obtain enough of these important chemicals.

Foods particularly high in phytochemical diversity include dark berries (cherries, blueberries, and blackberries), brassica or cruciferous vegetables (broccoli, kale, cabbage, cauliflower, and Brussels sprouts), alliums (garlic, onions, leeks, and scallions), tomatoes, soy foods, extra-virgin olive oil, and herbs and spices. All of these have been built into the meal plan in Part III. Even our few sweet treats, like the Chocolate Cherry Chews on page 273, have been carefully concocted to provide phytochemicals with an antioxidant boost!

EAT FUNCTIONAL FOODS

"Functional foods" are foods or dietary components that may provide a health benefit beyond basic nutrition. That is to say, they confer one or more specific physiological benefits that reduce your risk of disease. Grapes (and yes, red wine, too) are a popular example of a functional food because the skin of these delicious little fruits contains resveratrol, a powerful antioxidant that promotes cardiac cellular functions and prevents cardiovascular disease.

Food from almost any food group can be considered a functional food, as long as the food in question contains elements that benefit human function beyond that of being a calorie source. Given this, most foods and spices in their natural or "whole" states fall under this rubric. Whole foods like fruits, vegetables, whole grains, nuts, seeds, and high-quality sources of protein like wild cold-water fish are all functional foods.

However, there are now plenty of processed and manufactured foods that fall under the definition of "functional foods" as well. Some of these are healthy, some aren't. In our "age of nutritionism," as Michael Pollan, author of *In Defense of Food*, calls it, the food chemists are hard at work creating new foods that are considered "functional foods," even though in some cases, their effect on human function may be questionable at best.

Examples of processed functional foods targeted at digestive wellness include cereals, bars, yogurts, and beverages. These products are promoted for gut health since they contain beneficial bacteria or probiotics and may contain other gut-friendly prebiotic ingredients. However, when you read the ingredient fine print and the nutrition facts, you'll find that many of these functional foods contain way too much sugar.

We promote the use of functional foods to optimize digestive function because you can take greater control of your health by choosing foods that you know provide specific health benefits. The vitamins, minerals, enzymes, antioxidants, and other cellular nutrients in these foods can help you optimize digestive function.

But you must choose wisely. Use a discriminating eye when choosing functional foods to add to your diet. Stay away from highly processed foods that tout questionable health claims. Instead, choose whole foods that you know have specific gut-healing effects. Here are a few examples of healthy functional foods that have powerful, positive effects on the function of your inside tract.

- Colorful foods such as blackberries, blueberries, curry powder, ginger, green tea, and olive oil contain polyphenols that attenuate gut inflammation and may help prevent cancer. Polyphenols have beneficial effects on the digestive system and throughout the body. More and more research indicates that they also have regulatory effects on cell signaling pathways and help to regulate energy metabolism and overall gastrointestinal health.
- Flavonoids are a class of polyphenols that also have powerful antioxidant properties and that prevent free radical damage to cellular constituents such as DNA, cell membranes, lipids, and proteins. Apples, citrus fruits, dark chocolate, and onions are dietary sources of flavonoids.
- Foods that have natural enzymes to facilitate digestion include pineapple (contains bromelain) and papaya (contains papain).
- Green, leafy vegetables (such as kale, spinach, and Swiss chard) are high in folate, which can help prevent digestive tract cancers.
- Healthy sources of fiber (soluble and insoluble) benefit the growth of friendly gut bacteria, help prevent digestive tract cancer, and provide bulk to stools, which facilitates elimination. Apples, beans, brans (rice, oat, and wheat), citrus fruits, lentils,

peas, psyllium seed husk, and seeds (hemp, flax, and chia) are all good options.

- Wild cold-water fish, flax, extra-virgin olive oil, and coconut oil are all rich in fatty acids that can help treat inflammatory gut disorders. Coconut oil is particularly interesting because it contains medium-chain triglycerides (MCTs), a type of fatty acid that is more easily digested and absorbed in the GI tract.

Do you see a pattern here? The functional foods we recommend are by and large plant foods, wild cold-water fish, and healthy fats and oils—the very foods we have been discussing throughout this section. We strongly advocate using these foods to heal your gut, not only because mounds of scientific evidence indicate that they have a positive impact on gastrointestinal function, but also because human beings have used these foods as the core of a healthy diet and a way to heal the body, mind, and spirit for thousands of years.

Eat Foods That Promote
Good Digestion and Support Your Gut Flora

As you learned in Chapter 2, your gastrointestinal system does an extraordinary amount of work and takes care of a plethora of functions we don't normally attribute to it. But its main job is still to digest the foods you eat, pure and simple. Here are some foods that help foster good gut health by facilitating digestion.

- Cardamom
- Celery seeds
- Cinnamon
- Coriander seeds
- Cumin
- Fennel
- Fenugreek
- Gingerroot
- Lemon
- Orange peel
- Papaya
- Peppermint
- Pineapple

PROBIOTIC-RICH FOODS

✓ Cultured dairy products (buttermilk, yogurt, cottage cheese, kefir) and cultured nondairy products (soy or coconut yogurt and kefirs)
✓ Fermented beverages
✓ Fermented grains
✓ Fermented vegetables (sauerkraut, beets, green beans, etc.)
✓ Kimchi
✓ Miso
✓ Natto
✓ Tempeh

In order to help maintain a healthy inside tract, you should consider eating plenty of foods that contain probiotics. These beneficial bacteria, found in fermented foods that are often a component of traditional diets, help to replenish the good bacteria in your gut and fend off unfriendly invaders that lead to conditions like SIBO. Try incorporating some fermented foods into your diet. (See "Probiotic-Rich Foods" for suggestions.)

Other foods help sustain the growth of your gut flora and have "prebiotic" potential, meaning that these foods pass undigested through your stomach and small intestine and are then fermented in your colon. As they are fermented, short-chain fatty acids (acetic acid, butyric acid, and propionic acid) are created. These are critical for maintaining good caloric health, and are anti-infammatory and help prevent cancer.

Prebiotics

Certain prebiotics, when used in adequate amounts, have been shown to improve digestive function and intestinal environment, immunity-enhancing benefits, and improved absorption of dietary minerals. They complement probiotic functions in addition to supporting the growth of probiotics. (See "Prebiotic Power," on page 88, for suggestions.)

By eating foods that support your digestion and sustain your gut flora, you will provide your inside tract with the materials it needs to renew and repair itself.

Avoid Common Food Allergens and Intolerances

The impact of adverse food reactions (including both food allergies and intolerances) on health is a much-debated subject in medicine today. Classic food allergies like the anaphylactic reactions seen in IgE-mediated responses, where even a tiny drop of honey (or another allergen) causes your throat to swell shut and endangers your life, are not in question.

However, a growing body of literature is now proving what practitioners of integrative, complementary, and alternative therapies have long known to be true: Adverse reactions to foods come in many different shapes and sizes and are not limited to the IgE-mediated response. Some are nonimmune mediated. Some are pharmacologic, toxic, or metabolic. Some are due to enzyme deficiencies, like a lack of lactase, which is needed to digest lactose. For some, they cause gastrointestinal symptoms. For others, gastrointestinal symptoms are not present, but other systemic symptoms like headaches, alterations in mood, neurological changes, and even bone loss can occur.

Not everyone reacts adversely to the same foods, and not everyone who reacts to a particular substance will respond in the same way. Adverse food reactions are not a single disease but a complex of factors that, when

---

PREBIOTIC POWER

These foods help feed the good bacteria in the gut.

- ✓ Almonds
- ✓ Asparagus
- ✓ Banana
- ✓ Burdock
- ✓ Chicory root
- ✓ Endive
- ✓ Garlic
- ✓ Greens (beet, chicory, dandelion, endive, mustard, or turnip)
- ✓ Jerusalem artichoke
- ✓ Jicama
- ✓ Kiwifruit
- ✓ Leeks
- ✓ Oats
- ✓ Onions
- ✓ Salsify
- ✓ Whole wheat

put together, can cause suffering and disease for many. However, there is one force that ties all of them together—the gut.

As you learned in Chapter 2, the gut harbors the largest collection of immune tissue in your body. For more than two decades, science has shown that the immune system of the gut is primed to read and react to foreign invaders in the digestive tract while being nonreactive to the constituent flora and other nonpathogenic materials that dwell in it. This notion of gastrointestinal sensing and sampling is called "GI intelligence," and the process by which the gut reads and reacts to foreign substances while not reacting to food and friendly flora is called "oral tolerance."[24]

Food allergies occur when the gut's immune system reacts to what it perceives to be foreign antigens (proteins) that can harm you. Even though these proteins may come from substances that are harmless to most people—wheat, dairy, shellfish, and other common food allergens (see the complete list on page 91)—*your* gut may get "confused." It may read and react to these substances as though they are harmful, even though they aren't under normal circumstances.

How does this happen? Why do some people react to certain substances while others don't? How can your gut-immune system make mistakes like this?

While the mechanisms are complex and more research needs to be done, one hypothesis has been the "leaky gut" theory. Simply put, a breakdown in the intestinal barrier occurs and substances such as food allergens that are normally unable to cross the epithelial barrier gain access to the circulation, resulting in a host of disturbances.[25] Dr. Allesio Fasano, world-renowned expert on celiac disease, is one of many doctors who have proposed that the breakdown of the gut barrier may play a role in the initiation of gastrointestinal autoimmune disease.[26] A very recent paper published by Dr. Fasano suggests that the intestinal barrier operates as the "biological door" to inflammation, autoimmunity, and cancer.[27] Together this doorway along with the gut immune system and neuroendocrine network controls the delicate equilibrium between our ability to tolerate substances that we take in from our outside environment. Simply put, adverse food reactions can result from a breakdown in barrier integrity when the doorway in our inside tract is left wide open.

Swift Tip About Gluten Sensitivity

In my practice, I (Kathie) see many clients who have problems with gluten intolerance. If you are sensitive to gluten and you consume gluten-containing foods, you may experience abdominal distention and pain, increased frequency of bowel movements, and chronic constipation.

Celiac disease is now considered a multisystem disorder instead of primarily a gastrointestinal one. It has been shown that the existence of gluten sensitivity is associated with a number of disorders both within and outside of the gastrointestinal tract. Everything from irritable bowel syndrome (IBS) to type 1 diabetes to autoimmune thyroid disorders may be connected to celiac disease. While more research is needed to fully understand the relationships between celiac disease and other disorders, the incidence of correspondence makes it clear that there may be a connection. Five to 10 percent of people with celiac disease also have type 1 diabetes and/or thyroid disorders.[28]

Understand that when we use the terms *gluten sensitivity* and *celiac disease,* what we are really talking about is a spectrum of immune responses ranging from minor gluten sensitivity to full-blown celiac disease. While you may not meet the specific criteria needed for a diagnosis of celiac disease, you may still have a sensitivity to gluten. There are differences in response to dietary antigens among different people. Not everyone reacts the same way to every food, and some may be more sensitive than others.

These same basic concepts apply not only to gluten, but to many other foods (for example, dairy) as well. The exact biochemical pathways that lead to the adverse reactions as well as the reactions themselves may differ from food to food, antigen to antigen, and person to person. But the basic principle remains the same: People can be sensitive to foods, and consuming those foods can set off a complex sequence of events that leads to a wide array of symptoms and diseases.

Many people aren't aware that what they are eating every day may be making them ill. We have become so disconnected from our bodies that we may not realize how much the foods we eat can have an impact on the way we feel. Understanding the relationships between what we eat and how we feel is made even more complicated by the fact that symptoms can be subtle or even silent (as with gluten), they can occur anywhere from a few hours to a few days after you eat the food you are sensitive to, and the testing available for food sensitivities is often inconclusive.

So how do you know if food allergies or intolerances are leading you off track?

It's actually surprising to learn that you can track down adverse food reactions if you know how. You simply eliminate foods you suspect you may be sensitive to and then systematically reintegrate them into your diet and watch for symptoms. This is called an elimination diet, and it is an extremely powerful tool that will help you determine whether or not the foods you eat are contributing to your health problems.

Although you could react adversely to any food, including fruits, vegetables, and meats, there are eight foods that account for 90 percent of all food-allergic reactions.[29]

- Eggs
- Fish
- Milk
- Peanuts
- Shellfish
- Soy
- Tree nuts (like walnuts or cashews)
- Wheat

There are also some "usual suspects" that are responsible for many adverse food reactions, including:

- Additives and preservatives, including colorings, monosodium glutamate (MSG), and sulfites
- Gluten
- Sugars: fructose, lactose, and sucrose
- Yeast

We will give you the exact steps you need to take to eliminate some of the foods that we have found to be most problematic in adults, and we'll show you how to successfully reintegrate them (see Part III of this book). For now, simply be aware that adverse food reactions could be contributing to your health concerns, they could be the very source of your digestive disease, and tracking down your trigger foods is an essential part of healing your inside tract.

Eat Foods That Taste Good,
and Allow Your Taste Buds Time to Get Used to New Foods

One of the most profound nutrition statements was coined by chef and gourmand Julia Child, who said: "In matters of taste, consider nutrition and in matters of nutrition, consider taste." Taste and nutrition are intimately linked, and taste plays an important role in health and disease, as research at the Monell Chemical Senses Center in Philadelphia is now showing. As noted by Dr. Beverly Cowart, clinical director of the Monell-Jefferson Chemosensory Clinical Research Center, taste is the body's vigilant gustatory gatekeeper. It evolved to reject harmful substances and promote useful ones. Interestingly, taste's communication system with the brain is unique. There are multiple information pathways that connect this sense to your brain. This deliberate, redundant design lessens the chances that an injury or infection will shut down the entire system.[30]

There are five basic tastes—sweet, salty, sour, bitter, and umami or savoriness. (Some scientists think "fatty" merits a place on the table of tastes as well.) All other flavors are actually smells. Each of these primary flavors contains specific information about the foods they are related to. For example, bitter and sour tastes signal the presence of potentially dangerous dietary toxins, especially in the plant world. Sweet, salty, umami, and even fatty flavors provide us with very different information. Humans have developed preferences for these tastes because they confer evolutionary advantages for our survival.

Consider what "sweet" meant for Paleolithic humans. When trucking across the savannah, where little food was available, an encounter with a sweet, natural food source like a delicious apple could mean the difference between life and death. Due to this, we have a primal desire for foods that deliver these taste attributes. We are especially fond of sweet and salty. Babies like sweet tastes at birth, and within a few months also develop a taste for salty.

Part of the problem with the modern food supply is that our taste buds have been deluged with highly processed foods polluted with mega amounts of sweet and salty, unlike the natural sweet and salty tastes derived from a whole foods diet. The advent of artificial sweeteners is a prime example. These supersweeteners were created in the 19th century during a freak accident when a chemist at Johns Hopkins fell asleep at his desk and accidentally dropped his cigar into a petri dish, setting in motion the birth of saccharin.[31] Since then, the proliferation of these high-intensity sweeteners in our diets has contaminated our palates and incited the modern pursuit of sweeter and sweeter foods. The result is that we have developed a taste for foods so sweet that the apple our Paleolithic ancestor encountered on the savannah is no longer sweet enough. We want more.

Artificial or nonnutritive high-intensity sweeteners trick the gustatory system into listening to their siren song of sweetness. Some individuals—by nature of their genetics—are more prone than others and thus more susceptible to the song. This wouldn't be so bad if artificial sweeteners were safe, but recent evidence suggests that they aren't. Research on inflammatory bowel diseases has pointed to a connection between high consumption of sugar and sweet-laden foods in the diet and the later development of Crohn's and ulcerative colitis.[32]

In addition to artificial sweeteners corrupting our palates with their overly sweet taste, some researchers believe that they are hormetic agents, meaning that even when they are ingested in small amounts they can have major effects by introducing "new to nature" molecules into our cells. Our bodies don't quite understand what to make of these novel molecules and may react defensively by hoarding calories or engaging in other negative responses.

One class of sweeteners—the polyols, or sugar alcohols (xylitol, maltitol, sorbitol, isomalt, etc.)—is particularly worrisome in the context of digestive disease. Sugar alcohols, present in many "sugar-free" foods, chewing gums, oral-care products (such as toothpaste and mouthwash), and medications seem to wreak havoc on individuals with irritable bowel syndrome, contributing to gas, bloating, abdominal pain, and diarrhea.

The science of taste and the evolving research on our gustatory systems warrants a reorientation of our taste buds toward nutrient-rich foods that we may have tried once, rejected, and never tried again. It's important to eat foods that taste good, but you may need to "reboot your palate" to undo the conditioning our standard American diet has imposed on so many. Food preferences are shaped by repeated experiences with food over time. For example, there are people who have a strong aversion to the bitter compounds found in brassica vegetables such as broccoli or Brussels sprouts (or as some say, Brussels pouts!). With time, these folks can overcome this by including these foods in their diets in small amounts—for example, by adding some broccoli to a healthy stir-fry.

The alchemy of taste reveals that this sense is highly influential to our well-being and that preferences for sweet and salty can be diminished with time and effort. This can be a huge challenge in our current food environment, where sugar and salt are heralded as national treasures by food manufacturers and well-trained chefs. Not to mention the explosion of beverages and foods that are infected with artificial ingredients.

However, it's essential that you prepare your taste buds to be open-hearted, open-minded, and open to the recipes that we've created with your digestive wellness in mind. Prime your taste buds to enjoy the Inside Tract Smoothies, which are unadulterated with sweeteners (see page 287). Prepare them for a flavorful wake-up call and a sweet-and-salty sabbatical. You'll get used to it, and you'll even enjoy it, in time. Don't believe us? Dark chocolate might change your mind. This food of the gods is naturally bitter, but many of us have learned to relish it.

It's time to realign yourself with your nutritional lineage and the tastes of that ancestry. In time, you will taste the difference and savor the satisfaction of better digestion.

Eat in Rhythm

The human body is designed to eat and digest in a rhythmic pattern. This helps maintain metabolism, because when you eat this way your body is processing a manageable amount of food. When you eat just one or two megameals per day, it leaves you feeling sluggish afterward; your body must allocate precious and oftentimes limited resources to digesting those excessive quantities of food.

Most people in our society eat one or two medium-to-large meals per day. For some, this diet is nearly unavoidable in today's culture. It is certainly more efficient from a time and convenience standpoint to eat just a couple of times per day. The "start-up cost" of transportation to and from a restaurant or time spent shopping for and cooking food makes it hard enough to have three meals per day, let alone five or six.

To the angst of our bodies, our society is engineered to feed us in nearly the exact opposite manner as is necessary for us to achieve optimal health. Fast-food restaurants meet the demand for a quick, filling, but usually unhealthy meal. Most people just don't care to spend a portion of their day dealing with the task of staying well nourished.

More often than not, a large meal triggers an exaggerated insulin response, which makes your appetite surge and your blood-glucose levels drop. This makes you feel tired and contributes to the blood sugar imbalances discussed above. The supersized meal also diverts a substantial amount of blood to the gut in order to digest the sudden presentation of large amounts of food. This means less blood and vitality for your brain, which results in sleepiness, fatigue, and even brain fog.

In order to maintain a steady level of blood glucose and optimize your energy levels and metabolism, you need to eat at regular intervals. This is the best way to avoid the peaks and dips in blood sugar that can adversely affect gut function and your overall health and well-being. Dr. Wayne Callaway, noted endocrinologist and former director of nutrition at the Mayo Clinic, said it best: You want to avoid "starving, skipping, and stuffing," not only for permanent weight control but also for the health of your gut. So let's talk about how you can avoid stuffing.

Eat Until You Are No More Than Two-Thirds Full

Another essential component of good gut health and well-being is the ability to assimilate and digest foods properly. As we have already seen, when foods are poorly digested, bacterial fermentation and the maldistribution of bacteria in the digestive system can result. One of the most common reasons for poor digestion is overeating. Too much food entering your body at once overwhelms your upper digestive system and results in digestive upset, gas, malodorous stools, diarrhea, and plenty of other unpleasant symptoms.

🗝 **KEY POINT:** Eating too much is akin to smothering a flickering flame. Drowning your digestive flame in excessive quantities of food can only lead to poor digestion. The key is to eat until you are about two-thirds full. You don't want to be stuffed after a meal, but you don't want to leave the table feeling hungry, either.

Here's an easy way to avoid overeating: As you eat, rate your satisfaction level on a scale from 1 to 5, where 1 is extremely hungry, 2 is a little hungry, 3 is gently satisfied, 4 is full, and 5 is completely stuffed. As often as possible, you want to stop eating when you hit 3. You want to be gently satisfied, but not too full.

This obviously goes hand in hand with eating rhythmically, with meals spaced at regular intervals. Adjusting your dietary patterns to a more nourishing rhythm of eating will help heal your inside tract and optimize your energy.

Eat in a Relaxed State

Your digestive system pays very close attention to your brain, and there are sound reasons for it to do so. In times of stress, our bodies are designed to focus on the things that can help us stay alive. When our ancestors had to fight off wolves or run away from cave bears, they didn't want to waste any energy on less important things, such as proper digestion. We were not designed to digest our food during periods of stress!

But most of us in today's society are stressed-out basically all of the time, and Americans are culturally conditioned to eat under stressful conditions—while we are on the run, at our desk, in front of a television, or staring at a computer screen working on a report. Our minds are not concentrating on eating with awareness, and as a result, we do not digest our food properly.

You learned about the importance of the cephalic phase of digestion in Chapter 2. When your eyes feast on food and your sense of smell stimulates your taste buds to start the flow of saliva, the process of digestion is ignited. Eating with relaxed awareness and staying conscious while you eat is a digestive health practice that you need to embrace. The problem is that most of us don't know how to relax, much less how to eat in a relaxed yet fully conscious state. Luckily, there is a solution that will allow you to relax, optimize your digestion, and enjoy your food more fully, all at the same time. It is called "mindful eating."[33]

MINDFUL EATING: LEARNING TO BE AWARE WHILE YOU EAT

Mindfulness is the simple, moment-by-moment awareness of life. Eating with awareness is great practice for living with awareness. Mindfulness is a return to paying attention to life. When we are fully present while enjoying a meal, we efficiently extract the available nutrition and naturally avoid consuming foods that are toxic. When we pay attention to our food—really pay attention—we begin to notice all sorts of wonderful aspects of the food, and we become aware of how much we're putting into our bodies.

The basic techniques for mindful eating are very simple. Try the mindful eating technique below and see how it changes your experience with food and eating.

Inside Tract Mindful Eating Practice: Be, Breathe, and Break

1. **Be. Just be.** Before you eat, enjoy a meditative moment. Look at your food and smell your food. You may also want to whisper a quiet grace. A lovely Native American Arapaho proverb reminds us, "Before eating, always take time to thank the food."
2. **Breathe.** Take three relaxing, slow breaths before you start eating. To breathe means *to inspire,* and by breathing in this manner, you are setting the stage for a leisurely digestive tempo.
3. **Break.** Once you ingest your food, focus on the tastes, textures, and mouthfeel of your food. Allow it to become more liquid before you swallow. After your first few bites, take a break, rest your hands in your lap and repeat Steps 1 and 2: Be and breathe again. Savor the pause at your plate. Like yoga, this practice requires discipline and training, but it will be well worth the effort as your digestive health improves.

When you eat mindfully, you set the stage for excellent digestion. Eating this way is an integral part of our nutrition plan. Work to be more mindful of your food and you will watch your entire experience with eating and digestion transform.

Stay Happily Hydrated

The next principle for good gut health isn't about eating but about drinking. Drinking enough water is absolutely necessary for good digestive health. Our muscles are approximately 70 percent water—and slightly more than that, in women—so hydration is key if you want to heal your gut and achieve optimal health and well-being. It is essential for cellular health and detoxification, and it is especially important where digestion is concerned. One of the major functions of water in your body is to bulk up your stool and keep it moving along. That means that if you want to poop properly (which is extremely important for good gut health), you've got to drink an adequate amount.

There's a simple rule of thumb where water is concerned: Let thirst be your guide. There is also a general guideline: Drink ½ ounce of water every day per pound of body weight. So if you weigh 180 pounds, you need to drink 90 ounces of water each day. You should also drink extra water when eating fiber-rich foods like legumes, nuts, seeds, and whole grains. And be aware, if you work out or you live in a warm climate, you need more fluids.

We recommend drinking purified water because you can avoid unnecessary exposure to toxins and other pathogens by doing so. You can either purchase a water filter or buy bottled water. Water filters are cheaper in the long run and are an excellent investment in your health. If you choose bottled water, try to avoid plastic bottles. Many plastics contain phthalates—toxins that can leach into the water and contribute to hormone disruption. Buy water in glass bottles. Mineral waters and sparkling waters can be included in your total daily consumption.

While drinking water is the preferred choice for hydration, other beverages and foods contribute to your fluid account as well. Generally, about 80 percent of our total water comes from drinking water and beverages, while the other 20 percent is derived from the plant foods that we eat.

You may be wondering about other beverages—fruit juices, coffee, tea, herbal teas, and so on. The consumption of these beverages does contribute to your total fluid needs, but we're selective about choosing those that work for, not against, your health goals. Our nutrition plan favors purified water, with additional fluid coming from herbal teas and decaffeinated teas and coffee.

When it comes to alcohol, you're in the driver's seat of responsible decision making. Some kinds of alcohol, like red and even white wine, do have health benefits. However, everyone reacts differently to alcohol. Some individuals should abstain from alcohol entirely, while others can drink in moderation and not suffer ill effects. Since alcohol can affect gut permeability, we recommend that you limit alcohol in Track 2 and avoid it completely in Track 3, to optimize healing.

In the end, water is truly the liquid of choice. It is absolutely vital to your health, so raise a glass and hydrate your inside tract!

Eat Foods *You* Cook!

Many gut-related diseases are directly linked to our time-compressed lifestyles, express-lane eating, fast-food feasts, and desktop dining. We hope that by now you are eager to better plan and organize your eating by following the nutrition plan in Part III. What this means is eating food *you* cook.

Jean's Story

Jean came to see me, Gerry, for a history of fatigue, loose stools, and abdominal pain. She had been diagnosed with IBS but could not find relief through prescription or over-the-counter medications. Jean was in pain and spending a lot of time in the bathroom, and her condition was having a serious impact on her quality of life.

During my initial meeting with her, I was struck by a few red flags in her history. Jean ate the typical SAD diet full of highly processed foods; she skipped meals or ate on the run; and she snacked on junk food and caffeinated beverages (coffee and sodas) while at work. When she did eat at home, she ate large meals late at night, right before going to bed. Jean was also under a great deal of stress at work and at home, and she gave herself far too little downtime to relax and revitalize her mind, body, and spirit. Clearly, her diet and lifestyle were in need of attention.

Since Jean had already been through extensive testing and medication trials by other digestive disease specialists, my immediate goal was to focus on Jean's diet. I first placed Jean on a Track 2 elimination diet, which provided her with a method of eating that cut out many allergens and sugary foods and beverages. After only a few weeks on this diet, Jean started to feel the difference. She had less abdominal pain and her energy was slowly returning.

Gradually, we moved Jean from a Track 2 diet to a Track 1 whole-foods diet that consisted of lots of vegetables, whole grains, fruit, wild cold-water fish, grass-fed lean meats, organic poultry, and eggs, along with plenty of water. I also provided additional beverage choices such as peppermint tea, organic decaffeinated green tea, and ginger tea. I encouraged Jean to eat more mindfully and to permit at least 30 minutes for her meals in a relaxed environment. We also worked on her stressful lifestyle. Jean budgeted more downtime to relax, sleep, and pursue hobbies that she enjoyed. She went for weekly massages and took hot baths in mineral salts and lavender oil twice a week. After 8 weeks on this program, she came for a visit to see me at the clinic without a single complaint. She came just to share the good news of her newfound health.

In order to heal your inside tract, it is essential that you take back your kitchen—it is your healing center. In the kitchen, we hope that you will rediscover the joy of cooking. You will begin to understand the delights of food and learn how to nourish yourself once again.

Nourish—just the sound of the word is soothing. According to Webster's, to nourish means to:

1. Sustain with food or nutriment; supply with what is necessary for life, health, and growth
2. Cherish, foster, keep alive
3. Strengthen, build up, or to promote

The cross-pollination between the science of nutrition and the art of nourishment is the ultimate soothing soup for your body, mind, and spirit, and it is in the kitchen that this soup can be made. Unfortunately, at the accelerated pace of our everyday lives, the way we eat and our eating patterns do not foster healthy digestion or promote good health. We are too often hurried and harried and may skip meals or eat at a breakneck pace. We hunger for some daily downtime, but we continue to push instead of pause.

Take some downtime in your kitchen and immerse yourself in it's delights. Scope out your pots and pans, check out your pantry, clean out your fridge, line up your equipment, and sharpen your knives. Enjoy each and every experiment and experience along the way. Be patient with yourself as you experiment, learn, discern, and decide what nourishes you most. And most importantly, take some time to plan and organize, for it is a key to success. Your inside tract deserves this nourishing attention.

One patient, Jean, took the steps outlined in this chapter and the results were dramatic. Her story appears on page 99.

In Part III, we will offer a more in-depth explanation of exactly how to do all of this, as well as provide you with menus, recipes, food charts, recommendations on the tools you'll need, and more. We hope it delights your senses as much as it heals your inside tract.

But before we get to that, there are a few more items we need to cover. Diet is not the only thing that has an impact on your inside tract. Stress, the amount of exercise you get, your relationships, and other lifestyle factors also play crucial roles in gut health. Can a spiritual connection actually reduce digestive symptoms? Does the quality of your relationships have an impact on your gut? Are those butterflies you feel under stressful circumstances really in your stomach, or are they in your head? Turn to the next chapter to find out. That's where we'll provide you with concrete steps you can take to optimize your GI health by improving your life.

CHAPTER 5

The "Inside Tract" to a Better Life

The essence of health is inner balance.
—Andrew Weil, MD

As a society, we're stuck on the notion that healing begins with a trip to the doctor's office and a concoction scribbled on a prescription pad. We've been trained to believe that when our bodies break down and we become ill, it's because we've caught a bug or have finally succumbed to genetic weaknesses we were programmed with from birth. We think illness is something that happens to us, out of the blue, that we have no defense against. Rarely are we taught that the solution to illness is to make healthy dietary and lifestyle choices.

The truth is that we are dynamic creatures whose interactions with our environments affect every level of our health. For the vast majority of people with a chronic digestive disease, it is not genetic predisposition or infection alone that has led them to illness. There is a highway to health as well as a pathway toward pathology. Illness is a journey—an unfortunate one, perhaps, but a journey nonetheless. In order to recover, one needs to take a step back and look at their journey toward that illness from a lifestyle perspective.

For thousands of years, traditional forms of medicine like Traditional Chinese Medicine (TCM) and Ayurveda have taught us that health is our body's natural state and that it results from the maintenance, organization, and balance of the energies and life forces that govern our vitality. It is when this balance is lost that illness sets in.

We all have a healing force within us that holds the key to our recovery. Understand that this isn't a mystical or metaphysical statement. It's not something we simply believe—it is a biological reality. Your body was built to be healthy and to heal itself when illness occurs. But to take advantage of your body's inherent healing energies, you need to find balance again. In seeing countless patients over the years, we have seen the best results when the anatomy of illness is seen not only as a physical ailment but also as a matrix of imbalances in the mind, body, and spirit. Recognizing this, realigning your lifestyle, and rebalancing your whole self will give you your best chance at healing.

The first and most important step is to address your diet. In Chapter 4 we outlined the principles of good nutrition and the practices we recommend for optimizing your diet. In Part III you will find an eating plan tailored to the severity of your illness. Embarking on a healthy eating plan is a powerful strategy for healing.

The second step is nearly as important as the first: assessing your lifestyle and making the necessary changes so you can achieve balance once again. What life events or lifestyle perturbations preceded your illness and led you off track? How have the events in your life altered the life force that lies within you, and how has that manifested itself in your physical body?

In this chapter, we will provide you with tips, techniques, and tools that will help you rebalance your mind, reduce stress, rebuild relationships, and revitalize your body, mind, and spirit. We will focus on seven of the most common lifestyle areas that people need to work on.

1. Reducing stress
2. Reprogramming your mind
3. Getting regular exercise
4. Getting restorative sleep
5. Returning to spirit
6. Repairing relationships
7. Removing toxins

By assessing your level of imbalance in each of these areas and using the steps we recommend for making changes in them, you will rebalance your lifestyle and set the stage for your digestive problems to be resolved.

The Inside Tract Lifestyle Survey

The first step in healing is to find out where you are out of balance. This survey will help you determine that. In the chart that follows, circle the number that best describes your state of being with respect to each of the categories below. The lowest number, 1, represents the best-case scenario in that category; 10 represents the worst-case scenario. Here are some guidelines that will help you decide how to score yourself. You might give yourself a 1 if you:

- **Mental/emotional:** Have a very positive outlook and a balanced state of mind.
- **Stress:** Rarely get stressed-out and practice active relaxation regularly.
- **Exercise:** Exercise for 45 to 60 minutes per day regularly.
- **Sleep:** Regularly get 7½ to 9 hours of sleep per night and wake up feeling refreshed.
- **Spirituality:** Feel a sense of fulfillment and peace and a connection to a nurturing guiding energy source.
- **Relationships:** Have meaningful and supportive relationships.

Once you've completed the survey, you can use the following as a guideline for how much change you need to make and in what areas of your life you need to make it.

The Inside Tract Lifestyle Survey										
	☺				☺				☹	
MENTAL/EMOTIONAL	1	2	3	4	5	6	7	8	9	10
STRESS	1	2	3	4	5	6	7	8	9	10
EXERCISE	1	2	3	4	5	6	7	8	9	10
SLEEP	1	2	3	4	5	6	7	8	9	10
SPIRITUALITY	1	2	3	4	5	6	7	8	9	10
RELATIONSHIPS	1	2	3	4	5	6	7	8	9	10

Total Score: _____

- **Total score:** If your total is less than 15, little, if any, lifestyle adjustment is required; if it's greater than 15 but less than 30, some changes are required; if your score is greater than 30, significant changes are required; and if it's greater than 50, a complete lifestyle overhaul is required.
- **Individual categories:** Any category in which you score greater than 5 requires considerable attention.

Now that you have some sense of where your imbalances lie, let's look more carefully at each of the seven key areas of change listed above.

Reduce Stress

> *Tension is who you think you should be. Relaxation is who you are.*
>
> —CHINESE PROVERB

Your mind influences the way your body functions. In fact, your mind and your body are one dynamic unit. If one is out of balance, the other likely will be, too. Your thoughts, feelings, and perceptions *do* have an impact on your health. In this sense, there is really no such thing as "psychosomatic illness." There is now a wide body of research that supports this statement, and we are beginning to understand more about the biological mechanisms by which the mind influences the body and the body influences the mind all the time. Rebalancing your mind and body is a sophisticated dance, and it isn't until both have found stability and peace that you will fully heal.

An important part of doing this is reducing your stress levels. We have been emphasizing the impact of chronic stress on your digestive system throughout this book because the epidemic of gastrointestinal (GI) illness and the unremitting stress so many suffer from today are intimately related. This stress isn't good for you or your gut. But then you don't need us to tell you that stress is hard on your stomach or that social isolation makes you feel ill. Those feelings happen in your gut, and that's where they hit you the hardest.

You may remember from Chapter 1 that at least 60 to 70 million people in the United States suffer from a digestive disease. It's interesting to note that more than 40 million Americans between the ages of 18 and 64 have an anxiety disorder. These are overlapping problems, and the relationship between stress and digestive dysfunction is not arbitrary or incidental. Stress is a contributing factor to some of the most prevalent digestive disorders, such as irritable bowel syndrome (IBS) and gastroesophageal reflux disease (GERD).

The medications doctors and psychiatrists typically prescribe for these problems have come under growing scrutiny in recent years.[1] However, antidepressants continue to be the second-highest-selling class of medications on the market and can even cause digestive symptoms. The Inside Tract antidote to stress is balance and relaxation. The other six lifestyle areas we discuss in this chapter will give you tips on how to achieve that, but before we dive into the details, let's start with one very simple relaxation exercise. Just do this every day, and you will soon be on the road to reducing your stress and healing your gut.

Deep Breathing

> *Practicing slow, deep breathing or "soft belly" allowing your belly to rise with the in breath and fall with the out breath, while you focus on the image of a soft, relaxed belly is a powerful relaxation technique.*
>
> —James Gordon, MD

Proper breathing is a key to good health and breathing exercises should be, a part of a wellness regimen. On page 106 is a Relaxing Breath practice for you to try in addition to Soft Belly.

Reprogram Your Mind

> *What you believe yourself to be, you are.*
>
> —Claude M. Bristol

In order to get well or heal, we need to have a positive outlook. This is because our perceptions and outlook on life can impact health outcomes. The first physicians in the West were integrative healers who used

DR. ANDREW WEIL'S 4-7-8 (OR RELAXING BREATH) EXERCISE [2,3]

Sit with your back straight while performing this exercise. Place the tip of your tongue against the ridge of tissue just behind your upper front teeth, and keep it there throughout the entire exercise. You will be exhaling through your mouth around your tongue; try pursing your lips slightly if this feels awkward.

- ✓ Exhale completely through your mouth, making a whoosh sound.
- ✓ Close your mouth and inhale quietly through your nose as you mentally count to four.
- ✓ Hold your breath while you count to seven.
- ✓ Exhale completely through your mouth, making a whoosh sound as you count to eight.
- ✓ This is one breath. Now inhale again and repeat the cycle three more times for a total of four breaths.

This exercise is a natural tranquilizer for the nervous system. Do it at least twice a day. If you feel a little lightheaded when you first breathe this way, do not be concerned; it will pass.

all of the behavioral, biological, and pharmaceutical knowledge available to them to promote wellness and to cure illness. Hippocrates, for example, recognized very clearly that emotional health and physical health are connected. He understood the impact that a person's social environment had on his or her health and promoted a biological *and* psychological understanding of the diagnosis and treatment of illness and disease.

A large clinical study completed in 2006 looked at 840 general medical clinic male patients in Rochester, Minnesota, to determine whether or not their thinking style had an impact on their health and longevity. Researchers identified whether the patients were optimists or pessimists, and then followed up 30 years later to determine how their views on life had impacted their health. They found that optimists, on average, lived 19 percent longer than pessimists. This translates to roughly 15 additional years of life.[4]

We are clearly governed by our thoughts. They can lead us to acts of kindness or brilliance in our careers, or they can mire us in depression and despair. Your gut is exquisitely sensitive to your thoughts and moods.

You learned about the "second brain" in Chapter 2, so you know your gut is in constant communication with your brain. There is an ongoing, bidirectional highway of information that flows between these two systems and connects them. In some sense, they aren't two separate systems at all, they are simply separate branches of one organism: you!

Have you ever noticed how a great meal can put you in a good mood or that being upset or depressed radically alters your appetite? This isn't an illusion. These experiences are mediated by biochemical signals between your brain and your gut. When your gut feels good, your brain feels good, and vice versa. Perhaps that's why mental and emotional imbalances are strong contributors to digestive illness today.[5, 6]

If you scored high in this area of the survey, it's likely that your negative thinking is contributing to your gut problems. Here are some tips and techniques to help you overcome negative thought patterns.

Five Tips to Reprogram Your Brain

These five tips come from the very heart of cognitive-behavioral therapy—a school of psychotherapy backed by a great deal of research and clinical studies. Try them and see if they make a change in your thinking.

1. **Self-monitoring.** Keep a daily record or journal for a week or two. Include significant events, thoughts, and feelings that have an impact on you. This will help give you a better sense of what troubles you and what is leading to your negative thoughts; it will also highlight some things that bring you joy and stimulate healthy behaviors.
2. **Self-regulation.** Regulate your behavior, thoughts, and feelings after you've used self-monitoring to identify the origin of the problem. When negative thoughts come up, you can try using the breathing exercise mentioned on page 106 or using laughter as medicine, described on page 108.
3. **Self-calming and self-soothing.** People who are emotionally well-balanced are typically good at soothing and calming themselves. Try using deep breathing, progressive muscle relaxation, visualization, meditation, and other techniques to achieve a feeling of calm. Investigate these methods to calm your mind and soothe your gut.

4. **Cognitive modification.** You *can* modify the thoughts that have been causing so much distortion and grief in your life. Try challenging your thoughts using the three previous techniques, or look into other forms of cognitive modification.
5. **Installing positive mental software.** Get rid of your old, malfunctioning mental software and replace it with positive thinking, values, beliefs, and attitudes. Positive self-affirmation is a great place to start. Rather than focus on the negative, look at your good attributes. (Yes, you have some—everyone does!)

Laughter Is the Best Medicine

Laughter has a number of important health benefits. A good, hearty laugh relieves physical tension and stress, leaving your muscles relaxed for up to 45 minutes afterward. Laughter boosts the immune system, decreases stress hormones, and increases immune cells and infection-fighting antibodies, thus improving your resistance to disease. It also triggers the release of endorphins—the body's natural feel-good chemicals that combat pain and promote an overall sense of well-being.[7] There are good clinical studies that show laughter protects the heart by improving the function of blood vessels and increasing blood flow.[8] Laughter truly is powerful medicine. It not only gives you perspective, it also helps rebalance your body, mind, and spirit. If you get stuck in stress or trapped in negative thinking, try to take some time to laugh. Watch a funny movie or show (such as a sitcom) that you know will make you laugh, look at photos of friends you have fun with, or perhaps go to a comedy club for the evening.

If these tips for reprogramming your mind don't help, or you don't feel like you are making progress, consult with a psychotherapist who can help put you on the track to good health. You deserve it, and it will not only help your mind, it will help your inside tract as well.

Get Regular Exercise

Patients frequently ask, "How will exercise affect my digestive condition?" This is an excellent question, and the answer is actually slightly more complex than the general advice to "get more exercise" we so often hear. The truth is that your exercise program needs to be individually tailored to your needs, goals, and overall health.

Most Americans do not get enough exercise. In 2007, 78 percent of Americans were not meeting basic activity level recommendations and 25 percent were completely sedentary. The medical costs of this inactivity now tower at $76 billion annually. Lack of exercise contributes to weight gain, which in turn can lead to digestive diseases and many other chronic illnesses. Many people today do, indeed, need to get more exercise.

There can be no question that exercising appropriately has many health benefits. In fact, regular moderate exercise is one of only a handful of lifestyle choices that have been shown to improve health over and over in the scientific literature. Regular exercise:

- Improves heart and lung function
- Reduces cardiovascular risk
- Increases metabolic rate
- Enhances strength and conditioning
- Strengthens bones
- Improves lean body mass
- Enhances and balances immunity
- Promotes a positive outlook
- Reduces stress, anxiety, and depression
- Lessens fatigue
- Facilitates better sleep
- Improves quality of life
- Accelerates stomach emptying
- Reduces constipation
- Reduces the risk of colon cancer and prevents recurrence after treatment
- Improves nonalcoholic fatty liver disease
- Improves pain and altered bowel function related to IBS[9, 10]

However, it's important to remember that not everyone needs to exercise more. On the flip side, excessive exercise can have dramatically negative effects on health—especially on gut function. For example, 25 to

(continued on page 124)

GARY'S STORY

Gary was a 26-year-old athlete who had begun experiencing heartburn every time he exercised; this began a couple of years before he came to see me, Gerry. Gary owned a gym, was a full-time trainer, and competed in triathlons as a hobby. He ran 10 miles a day and, needless to say, was in extraordinary physical shape, except for one problem: His gut problems were becoming debilitating.

After 2 years of experiencing heartburn nearly every time he exercised, Gary eventually began having bouts of diarrhea in the morning. He learned to live with this condition and went on for an additional 2 years without seeking treatment. It was only when Gary was admitted to the hospital because his diarrhea became bloody and he developed severe anemia, which limited his ability to exercise, that he finally realized how serious his condition was.

After performing a series of tests including a flexible sigmoidoscopy to view Gary's colon, I discovered that he had a severe case of ulcerative colitis and required intravenous corticosteroids to control his symptoms. On the evening following his colonoscopy, I visited Gary to have a serious discussion about how his stressful life and his overexercising needed to be curtailed if he wanted to have a healthy gut.

Gary admitted that he often became "stressed-out" in the days prior to an event and that he would push himself to train even harder in very hot weather in the hopes of outperforming the competition. Training this way not only over-activated his adrenal system but also led to dehydration that only served to further complicate his health problems. All the while Gary was convincing himself that if he lived "clean" and worked out hard, he could overcome his gut problems. What he didn't see was that it was this very ethic that was leading to his digestive ill health in the first place. Gary had a very difficult time accepting that his passion may have been poison to his inside tract.

What Gary did not understand is that marathon-level exercise short-circuits the gut's blood supply and diverts it to the muscles to meet their intense energy demands. This produced a fight-or-flight response, shunting blood away from his gut and causing an injury to his inside tract.[11]

Surprisingly, people who push their bodies too hard are at risk of developing health problems just like those who don't exercise enough. In addition to the strain overexercising puts on the body, many athletes today take nonsteroidal anti-inflammatory drugs like ibuprofen—after a minor bone lesion or joint sprain, for example—in an attempt to maintain their highest level of performance. Overusing these kinds of medications significantly raises the risk for several digestive disorders.

We recommend 30–45 minutes of light to moderate exercise daily to improve one's well-being, mood, and gut health. This appears to be the most effective amount for improving all three of these areas.

So make sure you exercise enough, but not too much. Here are some recommendations on how to effectively integrate exercise into your life.

1. **Create a joy list of exercises.** Do what you love. These activities can range from sports to jumping rope to brisk walking to swimming to cycling on level terrain. After a short recovery period (5 to 10 minutes), you should drink at least one 8-ounce glass of purified water for every 20 minutes of exercise until you have to urinate.

2. **Consider yoga.** Yoga increases blood flow to your digestive tract and stimulates peristalsis, so digestion is more efficient. Yoga also calms you, which in turn relaxes your digestive system and leads to more effective elimination.

3. **Tone your abdomen.** Today, you hear a lot about "building your inner core" through exercises that focus on your abdomen.[12] This is a good practice for general and digestive health. We recommend training your abs every other day. All you have to do is choose two or three different exercises that focus on the abs and perform 4 or 5 sets of 10 to 12 reps for each exercise. Exercises aimed at toning the abs include situps, crunches, cable side crunches, and twists. Many yoga poses tone the abs as well.

4. **Keep moving.** No matter how hectic or mundane our lives become, the key to promoting health and vitality is to simply keep moving! In many disciplines of energy medicine (any discipline of medicine that manipulates the movement of energy with a therapeutic intention, such as Traditional Chinese Medicine, qigong,[13] and tai chi), it is believed that the life force, or chi, becomes stagnant when we adopt sedentary lives.[14] Regular exercise facilitates the flow of these energies.

5. **Be consistent, but don't overdo it.** Reshaping your habits needs to happen slowly over time. If you are like Gary and exercise all of the time, start by limiting your training time to one 45-minute or two 20- to 25-minute periods of training per day. If you don't exercise at all, begin with one 20-minute period and gradually increase to 45 minutes of exercise. Start with moderate-intensity exercise unless you are already in outstanding physical condition.

40 percent of long-distance runners experience abdominal cramps or diarrhea in association with competitive endurance running.[15] In extreme cases, excessive exercise can even lead to an increased leakiness of the gut lining (permeability) and gastrointestinal bleeding from lack of circulation. It has been shown that marathon runners are at a higher risk for GI bleeding—as many as 23 percent of marathon runners suffer from microscopic bleeding of the digestive tract.[16] This is a startling figure, and it calls into question how much more exercise some people really need.

When you engage in intense exercise, your enteric nervous system is impacted by the surge of adrenaline and other neuroendocrine hormones. The result is that gut motility slows down and your stomach empties more slowly. The lower esophageal sphincter also relaxes; this, along with the slowed emptying of the stomach, can contribute to heartburn and even GERD—a common complaint in runners.[17]

We have seen many individuals over the years who are in outstanding physical shape but who develop a digestive illness or have it worsen as a result of overexercising.

If you have doubts about your current exercise regimen or are confused about the program outlined above, seek the assistance of an exercise physiologist or certified personal trainer to help you design and monitor a quality exercise program. If you have a health condition that may be adversely affected by moderate exercise (like a cardiovascular condition), consult with your physician prior to starting an exercise program.

Get Restorative Sleep

Sleep. We all love it, especially when we wake up from a great night's sleep feeling refreshed and ready to take on the world. It's strange, then, that so many of us are sleep deprived and so few of us truly respect how important sleep is to our long-term health and well-being.

Approximately one-half of the adult American population has been reported to suffer from some degree of sleep disturbance, and over 40 million Americans are reported to be chronically sleep deprived.[18] Lack of sleep increases stress, worsens mood disorders, and has a severe impact on gastrointestinal symptoms.[19] The relationship between sleep and digestive function is actually quite intriguing. There is a dynamic interplay between the digestive system and sleep.

Recent research has shown that neuropeptides called orexins are one of the biochemical links between sleep and gut function. Orexins are produced in both the brain and the gut, and they help regulate the sleep/wake cycle and appetite, as well as stimulate gastric acid secretion and gastrointestinal motility.[20] This may be one of the reasons so many digestive disorders are linked with sleep disturbances.

There is actually a bidirectional relationship between digestive illness and sleep disruption—the more your sleep is disrupted, the worse your gut function becomes, and the worse your gut function becomes, the more your sleep is disrupted. This relationship has been best studied in GERD.[21] The prevalence of sleep disturbances in GERD patients has been reported to be as high as 55 percent. Poorly controlled nighttime GERD has been causally linked to sleep apnea. Interestingly, sleep apnea has been reported to reverse upon proper treatment of GERD. Furthermore, nighttime GERD is a major risk factor for the development of adenocarcinoma of the esophagus, a form of cancer that's rapidly on the rise in the United States. Unfortunately, this association between sleep disturbance and digestive dysfunction is not emphasized by many clinicians.

Yet there can be no doubt: Sleep has a profound impact upon digestive health, and vice versa. Sleep is more than simply a period of rest; it is an essential time for your body to perform routine maintenance and repair damage done to itself during the day. That's why restoring proper sleep habits—often referred to as "sleep hygiene"—is an important part of any digestive health program. The following are some guidelines to help you do that.

Improving Your Sleep Hygiene

Your goal should be to get 7½ to 9 hours of quality, uninterrupted sleep each and every night. Every adult needs this much sleep to function optimally, regardless of age or gender—and missing an hour or two here and there *does* have an effect on your health and your life.

For most people, disturbances in sleep are primarily the result of lifestyle habits that interfere with sleep. Improving your sleep hygiene in the following ways will most likely improve your sleep.

1. **Establish a fixed time for sleeping and waking.** Consistently getting the same amount of sleep at the same time each night—including on weekends—will vastly improve your quality of sleep.

2. **Slow down your mind and body before bedtime.** Engage in activities that relax you and slow down your mind and body. It's essential to avoid stimulating activities before bed. Watching the news or other television shows as you fall asleep or right before bed is likely to have a negative impact on the quality of your sleep. Drop the media fix before bed and pick up a book or magazine, instead.

3. **Be careful about napping.** Despite popular belief, naps are not a waste of time, and for some they can be wonderfully rejuvenating. In many cases, a 20-minute afternoon nap does more than that 3:00 p.m. cup of coffee will, and napping at the right time can actually improve your sleep rhythms overall. There is a reason something akin to siesta (a rest period after lunch) exists in so many cultures.

   However, if you have trouble sleeping at night, watch your naps. Make it a point not to nap for more than an hour, and never take naps after 3:00 in the afternoon. If you do, it will likely affect your ability to fall asleep at night.

4. **Avoid stimulants and alcohol just before bed.** Caffeine, sugar, and alcohol before bedtime can disrupt your sleep and leave you waking up unrefreshed. Avoid them for 2 to 3 hours before bed. Also avoid strenuous exercise for at least 3 hours before bed. While regular exercise facilitates sleep, working out right before bed is probably going to disrupt it.

5. **Try supplementation.** Consider temporarily taking a natural supplement that may help restore sleep while you are working on improving your sleep hygiene. You may want to consider one of the following: 3 milligrams of melatonin, 300 milligrams of hops with 500 milligrams of valerian root, or 400 milligrams of gamma-aminobutyric acid (GABA).

Remember that improving your sleep hygiene significantly will benefit your overall health, quality of life, mood, and digestive health.

Return to Spirit

> *The greatest mistake in the treatment of disease is that there are physicians for the body and physicians for the soul, although the two cannot be separated.*
>
> —Plato

> *It is better to believe than to disbelieve; in so doing you bring everything to the realm of possibility.*
>
> —Albert Einstein

Balance and harmony are among the keys to a healthy and fulfilling life. Without having a higher purpose, it is easy to get "caught up in the rat race" and become discouraged by life. When this happens, recovering from an illness is that much more difficult. For many, discovering a spiritual path has proven to be a way out of this trap, and doing so can be an essential step in recovering from illness.

According to integrative medicine expert Deepak Chopra, spirituality is a natural self-expression that goes beyond a focus solely on ourselves.[22] It is a state of being whereby the individual is filled with peace and happiness while experiencing spontaneous love and compassion for others. It is an intuitive awareness that gives us a sense of connection to a life force of supernatural source. And we now know that spirituality can have a profound impact on health. One of the primary mechanisms by which this occurs appears to be through stress management.

Many studies have demonstrated a connection between spirituality and lower rates of stress and even depression. Maintaining a spiritual practice can help people cope better with stressful situations, thus reducing their anxiety levels and lessening the impact of chronic stress. Numerous researchers have documented a link between spirituality and depression: Spiritually healthy practices like finding meaning and purpose in life, having an intrinsic value system, and belonging to a supportive community with shared values may reduce depressive symptoms. Since stress and mood disorders such as anxiety and depression have such a profound impact on gut health, it stands to reason that engaging in a spiritual practice could have a positive impact on stress-related digestive disorders, too.

We have all heard stories of people who prioritized their faith while recovering from catastrophic illnesses and experienced profound results. Prayer, for example, is now considered a powerful tool you can use to improve health outcomes, though its impact has been "studied" with mixed results. One of the most stunning of these studies was a report in which patients who regularly prayed and were admitted to a coronary care unit were observed to have improved survival rates and less adverse cardiac events compared to those who did not pray.[23]

Harvard cardiologist Dr. Herbert Benson was one of the first to study the relationship between spirituality and health. He revolutionized the field by showing that meditating in a trancelike state reduces stress and improves health while simultaneously raising consciousness and spiritual awareness. Though this finding is still considered groundbreaking by many in the West, ancient cultures have integrated spirituality into healing for millennia. Shamanic priests were regarded as "healers" long before the development of pharmaceuticals, and meditation and prayer have been at the very center of healing practices since the dawn of time.

It is important to take time to quietly reflect on your life and connect with the higher energies and spirits that refresh your soul and renew your sense of peace and calmness. Doing this is a profound part of healing for many. If you are interested in including spirituality in your path toward overcoming illness, here are some suggestions to get you started.

1. **Consider prayer.** If you are rooted in an organized religion, prayer can help you feel more calm and grounded, and this acts as a buffer against stress.
2. **Express gratitude.** Gratitude has been linked to improved health outcomes and can reduce the experience of stress as well.
3. **Become a member of a spiritual community.** Sharing one's sense of spirituality with a community serves as a form of social support that can impart a sense of belonging and reduce stress and social isolation.
4. **Be the optimist.** Believing that the glass is "half full" invokes a sense of positivity and energy that reduces stress and attracts positive people into your life. Consider using mantras of positive affirmation, tailoring yours to suit your life ("I love my wife," "Life is great," etc.). This is a way to program your brain with a rosy outlook.
5. **Find the "silver lining" during difficult times.** As noted above,

people who practice spirituality tend to adapt better in times of stress. One reason may be that they tend to see stressful situations as tests of strength or even as valuable lessons. This belief can be empowering, and it helps moderate stress levels if you can see stressful situations as less threatening. Remember, illness *can* be a great teacher. It's your choice to use it that way.

6. **Consider meditation.** Meditation is the process of intentionally shifting your attention and consciousness toward a specific objective. This typically means removing yourself from thoughts about everyday life in favor of some other focus that produces a relaxing effect. Being able to intentionally relax your body, mind, and spirit in this way is highly effective for stress control and acccelerates recovery from illness. Today, the efficacy of meditation is so widely accepted that even conventional digestive disease specialists are advocating its use to treat stress-related digestive conditions such as IBS. Meditation is a technique you can use anywhere, and it's easily learned.[24] Do some research to find a form of meditation that suits you.

7. **Go on a spiritual retreat.** You might want to try a spiritual retreat to help you return to spirit. You can go to a spiritual retreat center or you can simply try relaxing on the beach with a book that raises your consciousness and distracts you from your everyday life for a weekend.

Whatever approach you take, returning to spirit can lead you to better health and a more meaningful and fulfilling life. Michael's story, on page 118, is a good example of this.

Repair Relationships

> *The power of love to change bodies is legendary, built into folklore, common sense, and everyday experience. Love moves the flesh, it pushes matter around . . . Throughout history, "tender loving care" has uniformly been recognized as a valuable element in healing.*
>
> —LARRY DOSSEY, HEALING WORDS

MICHAEL'S STORY

Michael came to see me, Gerry, complaining of knifelike abdominal pain shortly after his engagement to his beloved fiancée ended. He found that while he was busy at work, his pain was unnoticeable, but at home it was unbearable. Michael had experienced many sleepless nights, and he began to lose weight. He was having panic attacks, and this eventually began affecting his work. Michael began taking lorazepam to control his anxiety and especially to help him sleep.

He was looking for relief from his pain and help getting his life back on track. He made it clear that his life felt empty without his ex-fiancée. During one of our visits, we began exploring some alternative ways for him to find a way out of the darkness he was experiencing. Bikram Yoga, silent meditation, and fly-fishing were helpful, but they were not enough. He continued to feel alone and empty, but the feeling of loss continued to drive his sadness. Michael then met another doctor who incorporated spirituality into his practice through a technique called *Natural Force Healing*. Michael and I had many discussions about how faith and spirituality could bring the sense of inner peace he was looking for.

Through his friend Kenny and other people in his life, Michael explored spirituality through a branch of Judaism known as kabbalah. He attended an introductory class and felt a path open for him when the instructor said, "Don't ask for an easier life, ask for a greater capacity to deal with the things that come to you in your life." Within a few weeks, there was a dramatic shift in Michael's self-esteem, perspective, and health. He began sleeping without medication and was no longer so anxious. His abdominal pain quickly became a bad memory, thanks to the connection he formed outside of himself and with others who shared his beliefs and values. Kabbalah teaches that in darkness there is light. We need to see the lessons that are brought to us through this process for transformation to take place. Michael continues to practice kabbalah and helps his patients navigate toward good health by using an integrative approach to wellness. The last time we spoke, he told me that doctors work on seeking the minutia of illness, but in reality, we are spiritual beings living in physical bodies with emotions and a biochemistry, and it is the integration of these systems that is really necessary to create wellness.

> *Unconditional love is the most powerful stimulant of the*
> *immune system. The truth is: love heals. Miracles happen to*
> *exceptional patients every day—patients who have the cour-*
> *age to love, those who have the courage to work with their*
> *doctors to participate in and influence their own recovery.*
> —BERNIE SIEGEL, LOVE, MEDICINE & MIRACLES

Let's face it, relationships make us or break us. The research in this area is tremendous. Social isolation and stressful relationships can depress our immune systems. A study in the *Journal of the American Medical Association* showed that, even after controlling for risk factors like smoking, alcohol consumption, poor diet, and lack of exercise among poverty-stricken communities, the one thing that had more influence over health than all other factors was a lack of social relationships or support groups.[25] Numerous other studies have shown that social isolation is associated with adverse health outcomes and that self-expression, education, and a sense of community can lower levels of stress hormones, improve quality of life, and enhance immune function.[26] People who are socially isolated often have an overactive stress response.[27] In fact, social isolation alone has been identified as an independent, major risk factor for all causes of mortality.[28]

Social connection, on the other hand, has been shown to positively influence disease outcomes including: all-cause mortality, depression,[29] heart disease,[30] disease susceptibility,[31] diabetes mellitus,[32] and survival from breast cancer[33] (even metastatic breast cancer[34]). The study done on the last of these is absolutely fascinating. Researchers surveyed 6,900 participants about their contact with friends and relatives, church membership, membership in clubs or groups, and marriage, and then followed them for 17 years. Those without close ties or frequent social contact had an overall death rate that was 3.1 times higher than those who did have those contacts.

Of course, not just any relationship will do the trick. Stressful relationships have been linked to a number of adverse outcomes, ranging from cardiovascular disease to cancer. They also have an impact on digestive disease.

Despite the importance of relationships, establishing them and repairing those that are broken are two of life's most challenging tasks. But doing so is fundamental to recovering from an illness, as Bernie Siegel pointed out in *Love, Medicine & Miracles.*

Dysfunctional relationships put us in a state of chronic stress in part

ADAM'S STORY

Adam was a 35-year-old entrepreneur who was in the process of plan-ning his wedding. He fell ill and came to see me, Gerry, because of recur-rent stabbing abdominal pains at night; the pains worsened with meals.

Adam ate what I would call a "hole foods" diet: spicy foods, alcohol, pizza, hot dogs, and sandwiches from the deli almost every day. And indeed, there was a hole in his stomach. After looking at his stomach during an upper endoscopy, I found marked erosion and inflammation in his stomach—signs of a peptic ulcer that was not healing. Interestingly, Adam did not have an infection with the *H. pylori* bacterium. (Presence of *H. pylori* is one of the major risk factors for peptic ulcers.)

As I was discussing his illness with him, it suddenly came to me that Adam had come in with a woman earlier in the day, just before the endos-copy, and that their relationship had seemed strained. I was struck by the woman's abrasiveness and rudeness both to Adam and to my staff. When I asked Adam about her, the floodgates opened.

He admitted that the girl was his fiancée and that they constantly fought. Adam then went on to tell me that he was having second thoughts about their upcoming wedding and was losing sleep over whether or not to call it off.

Just as Adam and I finished talking there was a call for me in the recov-ery room, and I had to excuse myself. It was Adam's fiancée. Though Adam was in no condition to talk with her, she threatened to come to the hospital and throw us both through a wall if I didn't put him on the phone immediately. I politely refused, and after hanging up reached into my pocket for my prescription pad as I headed back to Adam's room.

As I jotted down notes, Adam asked, "Doc, what are you doing?" I said, "I'm writing your prescription." I handed him a paper that said:

1. Get rid of fiancée: ASAP.
2. Find someone nice.
3. Rent some funny movies and laugh!
4. See a therapist for stress management counseling if Steps 1 through 3 fail.
5. Eat a whole foods diet instead of "hole" foods.

Adam laughed for several minutes. He took my advice and never had an ulcer again! To this day, he laughs while recalling how I saved his life with my unique prescription. (By the way, Adam found a nice girl a few months later and has been happily married with children for more than 10 years.)

because we tend to "internalize" emotions that arise from these unhealthy relationships. Anger is one of the most common emotions that comes up in situations like these, and it is one of the most harmful to human health. When you are angry, a profound stress response is set off that is measurable biochemically, and it impacts your health on a number of levels.

Chronic anger causes hypertension, high blood pressure, and depression.[35] Myocardial infarctions have been linked to fits of rage and arguments.[36] And even angry words have been shown to adversely affect intestinal reactivity as well as gut transit in IBS sufferers.[37, 38]

It's fascinating to note that in some cultures, anger and irritability are seen as signs of digestive illness. For centuries, anger was considered a reflection of stagnation and distortions in liver chi in Traditional Chinese Medicine. Dispersion of these negative emotions through acupuncture (to redirect the flow of the related stagnant chi) and nutritional support are the cornerstones of therapy for many digestive ailments in the ancient Eastern healing arts.

Relationships thrive on a healthy exchange of ideas, gestures, deeds, and words. Words can range from healing to hurtful. Wounding or hurtful words from a loved one can cause emotional trauma that manifests itself internally as digestive symptoms.

In order to heal, you need to shift your consciousness toward nurturing relationships. It may be difficult to build good relationships or repair those that have been broken, but it can be done. Good relationships thrive on a dynamic exchange of energy between beings. When we become stressed, irritable, angry, or introverted, we give off "vibes" that may attract similar responses from others. This leads to friction and throws us into isolation. On the other hand, when we are in a state of balanced emotional health, we project positive energy that appeals to others, attracts similar energies, and fosters a sense of connection with those around us. Feeling compassion toward ourselves and others is an important step in a healing journey.

When all is said and done, the best guarantee of a long and healthy life may be the connections you have with other people. In isolation, there is little hope; without hope, life can be bleak. Healthy relationships sustain us and help us thrive. Here are some tips to help you develop and maintain good relationships and find your way out of social isolation.

Choose Love

Your gut will love you for it. If you feel unloved and struggle to show love, this is a prime area to work on. Many authors have noted the studies showing that people who engage in loving relationships have less heart disease, survive cancer better, and generally live longer than those who feel isolated. For example, in his book *Love & Survival,* Dr. Dean Ornish demonstrates that personal intimacy and other aspects of emotional well-being—all the elements that make up what we call "love"—are as important to your physical condition as to your mental health.[39] Dr. Ornish emphasizes that we must deal with our own negative emotions, such as anger, in order to nurture loving relationships and heal heart disease.

Love is the most powerful of the positive emotions, and positive emotions can motivate us to make better lifestyle choices; strengthen our immune systems; calm our nervous systems; and reduce gut illness. The benefits of opening your heart to others go beyond curing your body; it's actually the first step toward healing your entire life.

Work on Family Unity

Family can provide you with social support and reinforce your sense of meaning and purpose in life. Lisa Oz,[40] in her book *Us,* provides some suggestions for improving connection with your family by scheduling set times for family meals and expressing gratitude together and toward one another. Affirming the family unit this way will help your relationships become stronger, and your life will become more meaningful as a result. She also suggests having a family date night that involves something like bowling, rather than watching movies, to foster communication and promote togetherness.

Avoid Isolation and Loneliness

Loneliness and isolation foster stress and anxiety, and they set the stage for depression. Take the time to connect with others. There are many ways you can do this. You might try:

1. Joining a cultural group focused on a background similar to yours or connecting with other cultures by investigating groups you are interested in.

2. Getting involved in a spiritual community.
3. Seeking out a support group for people with the same illness you have.
4. Locating community groups or clubs that are involved with activities or topics you are interested in.
5. Asking someone out for coffee. You never know, it might lead to something even more interesting!

Whatever you do, seek out ways to make friends and create community. It's essential not only for the health of your gut but also for the health of your life.

Seek Zen at Work

For some, the workplace can be the most challenging environment in which to form stable relationships, given the tendency for egos, different temperaments, and politics to polarize even the best of us. In truth, it's best not to get sucked into other people's negativity. It will drain you mentally, emotionally, and—eventually—physically. Try to keep a Zen-like calmness about yourself, and keep your composure. Friction at work will only worsen your gut problems. Calmness is a vital asset to maintaining emotional stability in the workplace.

Engage in Calming Exercises
Before Going to Work and Before Coming Home

If you want to maintain healthy relationships, one of the best ways is to maintain your own sense of emotional stability. A variety of calming and empowering mind-body exercises have been proven to help people decrease anxiety and pain, enhance sleep, strengthen their immune systems, increase their sense of control and well-being, and enhance their ability to heal. These include deep breathing exercises, progressive muscle relaxation, and guided imagery, among others. (Belleruth Naparstek, a mind-body therapist and the founder of Health Journeys, has a number of excellent resources, including an especially helpful guided imagery CD for irritable bowel syndrome and inflammatory bowel disease.) Try engaging in these activities before leaving for work in the morning and before coming home in the evening. If you do, your life will change for the better, and so will your relationships.

Remove Toxins

The last topic we want to address in this chapter is one that concerns most of us: toxins. Toxins are chemicals that have the potential to interfere with your body's physiological processes. These toxins may come from the environment (exogenous toxins) or from within your own body (endogenous toxins). Removing toxins essentially means reducing your exposure to toxins and enhancing your body's natural ability to remove harmful substances from your body with the help of your intestines, lungs, lymph, liver, kidneys, and skin. This process is called detoxification, and when this system is compromised, impurities aren't properly filtered out of your body. This can adversely affect every cell in your body. The link between toxins and disease is highlighted by the President's report on cancer, which stated that the "public should be well aware of the link between toxins and cancer."

If you're like most people, you probably don't realize the number of toxins you're exposed to every day. We are inundated with toxins in our environment. Some, like cyanide, poison our cells immediately, so it's easy to track the relationships between these toxins and negative health outcomes. However, there are many thousands of other chemicals that we are exposed to on an ongoing basis (like pesticides, herbicides, and organochemicals) that have known carcinogenic, neurotoxic, hormonal mimetic, and immunomodulatory properties that affect us more slowly over long periods of time. Science is uncovering the relationships between these chemicals and their impact on our health. Environmental toxins have been associated with dozens of diseases ranging from cancer to autoimmune diseases and more.[41]

For example, pesticides, insecticides, plasticizers (such as bisphenol A, or BPA), and polychlorinated biphenyls (PCBs) all cause hormonal disruptions in the body by directly stimulating receptors on the cells of the immune and endocrine systems. This wreaks havoc on the body in the long term. Disruptive chemicals can be found in conventionally grown fruits and vegetables, on our lawns, in our water supply, in dental sealants, and in food packaging. BPA is used to line metal cans, beverage cups, the plastic packaging used for foods, and more. Studies have shown that BPA is released from the plastic into food products over time and is catalyzed by heat. That's why it's found in such significant amounts in hot beverages, such as teas and coffees kept in plastic containers.[42, 43]

Despite their prevalence, a growing body of research shows that only tiny amounts of environmental toxins like these are required to cause hormone disruption or have an adverse effect on the immune system. They wind up stored in fat cells, where they slowly release tiny but dangerous doses and cause untoward effects systemically over the course of years.

Our problems with toxins are only compounded by the fact that, as a nation, we consume more factory-made and processed foods containing these chemicals than we ever have before. We add toxic chemicals to our foods simply for the sake of taste and presentation. Food colorings such as red and yellow dyes have been linked to a variety of illnesses, and the consumption of high-fructose corn syrup (HFCS) has been linked to the rise in diabetes and obesity—conditions that directly cause digestive disease.[44] HFCS is also a leading cause of nonalcoholic fatty liver disease in America.[45]

Today, even things we would normally consider "real food" cannot escape the reach of toxicity. Nonorganic poultry, red meat, and dairy products have detectable levels of hormones that adversely affect immune function, as well as antibiotics. Nonorganic fruits and vegetables contain pesticides, fungicides, and heavy metals that disrupt immune and endocrine balance. If you think you are eating "healthy" by eating salmon several times a week, think again. Farm-raised salmon has been shown to be significantly contaminated with many of the aforementioned toxic chemicals, including PCBs.[46]

As educated and intelligent consumers, it is hard for us to ignore the plethora of evidence that links illness to toxic exposure, and the good news is that we don't have to. We can make better choices about the foods we eat and the chemicals we expose ourselves to. No, we probably can't eliminate all environmental toxic exposure in our modern world, but we can reduce the load dramatically.

However, the story becomes a little more nuanced when we consider endogenous toxins—toxins that are produced in the body as part of our cell metabolism. These are somewhat harder to avoid, though we can swing the balance in our favor here as well. Every moment of the day, our cells are breathing, working, and generating waste by-products. When our cells are unhealthy or there is biochemical interference, these waste products can accumulate to harmful levels and place us at risk for injury or illness.

Let's consider how this process works by looking at the intestinal flora once more. As they digest your food, the bacteria in your gut produce toxins that may lead to systemic illnesses if they are released into your bloodstream. However, when you have the right balance of beneficial bugs in your gut, those bugs transform these toxins into harmless chemicals. Conversely, when your gut flora is out of balance and there are microbes in your gastrointestinal tract that shouldn't be there, those bad bugs can release poisonous chemicals such as amines, ammonia, hydrogen sulfide, indoles, phenols, and secondary bile acids. To make matters worse, some of these microbes damage the microvilli in the intestine and their toxins can be absorbed into the bloodstream, leading to a whole range of problems.

The key here is to rebalance the microbiota and rebuild good gut flora. Although we "inherit" these bugs at birth, there are many diet and lifestyle decisions we make that impact their health. Excessive alcohol intake, stress, and antibiotic use kill off the good bacteria and set the stage for evil invaders to get a foothold in the inside tract's microbial rainforest. Get rid of these invaders using a comprehensive dietary and lifestyle change program like the one outlined in this book, and you will be limiting your exposure to endogenous toxins as well.

It's true that eliminating toxins from your everyday life can be challenging, but it's essential that you do so to achieve optimal health. Here are some tips to help you do that.

Limit Toxins from Your Diet and Environment

You change your automobile's engine oil, coolant, fluids, and filters, knowing that pollutants lead to wear and tear and suboptimal performance. The body is no different, in that respect. For millennia, ancient medicine emphasized "purification" as an important part of the healing process. The first step in any purification process is to limit your exposure to "pollutants." Think of your body as a Rolls-Royce—you want to maintain its integrity and provide it with the very best fuel. Get rid of the junk. Consider eliminating or limiting your exposure to these common environmental toxins.

> **Diet:** Artificial sweeteners; colorings and unsafe additives; excess caffeine; excess alcohol; foods cooked at very high temperatures (fried foods, char-grilled/

blackened foods); foods that are known allergens or that you have intolerances toward; highly processed foods; high fructose corn syrup; partially hydrogenated oils; and sugar laden foods

Environmental: Moldy environments, tobacco, toxic personal care products, cleaners and pesticides, herbicides and other organochemicals, excess ionizing and electromagnetic radiation (EMR)

Medications: Unnecessary use of acetaminophen, ibuprofen, and other over the counter medications

Swift Tips for Optimizing Your Body's Elimination and Detoxification Pathways

Bolstering your body's detoxification pathways is actually much easier than it sounds. Here are a few ways to amplify your body's natural detox pathways.

1. **Promote daily bowel movements**. Get plenty of fiber and stay well hydrated. We also encourage the use of psyllium seed husks (*Plantago ovata*) diluted in a mixture of water and pineapple juice to add some bulk to the stool and ease passage. Interestingly, psyllium husks have been shown to improve constipation-predominant IBS.
2. **Take saunas for detox (unless advised not to by a physician).** Toxins are stored in fat. Recent evidence has shown that regular saunas help release these stored toxins and improve health.
3. **Practice deep breathing.** Doing so fosters the elimination of toxins and promotes a sense of calmness that has positive effects throughout the body.

Exercise and Drink Plenty of Purified Water to Enhance the Elimination of Toxins

Among the many benefits of exercise is the potential to enhance the body's detoxification through a "good sweat."[47] Use the strategies outlined earlier in this chapter to start a regular exercise routine and amplify your detoxification.

Both while you are exercising and after your routine, drink plenty of purified water. Adding a fresh citrus splash such as lemon, lime, or orange to your water will add flavor and promote alkalinity. We recommend that you drink at least 2 liters of purified water with the freshly squeezed juice of two lemons each day.

Detoxifying the Body with Healthy Foods and Juices

Ultimately, cleaning up your diet is *the* key to detoxifying your body. Following the plan in Part III and eating the delicious recipes for detoxifying broths, soups, salads, smoothies, and entrees helps aid your detoxification system. In addition, you may want to focus on a few foods and techniques that are renowned for enhancing detox pathways.

THE DETOX POWER HITTERS

There are a few foods that are thought to be particularly good for detoxification. They are:

- Alliums (garlic, leeks, onions, and shallots)
- Brassicas (broccoli, broccoli sprouts, Brussels sprouts, cabbage, cauliflower, kale, kohlrabi, mustard, rutabaga, turnip, and watercress). In a recent study, people who had *H. pylori* infection showed fewer bugs and reduced stomach inflammation when eating broccoli sprouts every day for 8 weeks.[48]
- Decaffeinated green tea
- Herbs and spices (cilantro, curry, dill, ginger, oregano, parsley, mint, rosemary, and turmeric)
- Red and green fruits (avocado, berries, pink grapefruit, pomegranates, purple grapes, and watermelon)
- Red and green vegetables (arugula, artichokes, beets, collards, dandelion greens, mustard greens, radicchio, red cabbage, and Swiss chard)

JUICE YOUR WAY TO A CLEAN BODY

We commonly recommend juicing with fresh and organic fruits and vegetables such as apples, beets, beet greens, carrots, celery, cilantro, dandelion greens (including the root), ginger, lemon, mint, parsley, red chard, spinach, Swiss chard, and watercress.

If you have a blender or juicer, making delicious, detoxifying juices from these fruits and veggies is simple. Here's what to do:

1. Wash all fruits and vegetables well.
2. Chop up the fruits and veggies according to the directions for the equipment you are using.
3. Juice using interesting combinations until you land on one you love.
4. Enjoy immediately to gain the most benefits from juicing!

The strategies outlined in this chapter have been at the heart of healing practices since ancient times. Reducing stress; seeking out mental and emotional well-being; eating a well-balanced, wholesome diet; creating healthy relationships; developing a sense of connection to the divine; exercising in moderation; and eliminating impurities are not only the cornerstones of recovery from illness but also the key features of a happy, healthy life. If you want to get on the inside track to health and well-being, we hope that you embrace and integrate some of these practices.

In the next chapter, we will explain what supplements you can add to your plan to support your digestive health, and we'll explain why these special nutraceuticals may be essential to helping you rebalance your gut function.

CHAPTER 6

Supplements
to Heal Your Inside Tract

The cornerstones of digestive health are your lifestyle and eating habits. There are no magic bullets when it comes to maintaining good gut health and preventing digestive disease. Nothing can ever prevent digestive discord more effectively than a good diet and a healthy lifestyle.

However, there are some nutritional supplements that may further assist you on your journey to health. The use of supplements is one of the hottest and most debated topics in modern medicine: Are they useful? Can they help you overcome your digestive disease? What does the research say? What should you take? Who should you believe about supplements? And are they really worth spending your hard-earned dollars on?

In this chapter, we will give you a basic overview of how supplements work. We'll explain how they can be extremely effective adjuncts in healing gut disorders, and we'll provide you with the details you need to take the right supplements for your specific digestive disease.

Supplements 101

Dietary supplements are products that contain substances like vitamins, minerals, foods, botanicals, amino acids, and fatty acids; they are available in pill, tablet, capsule, powder, or liquid form. They are called supplements because they are designed to "supplement"—not replace—a healthy diet and lifestyle.

Dietary supplements used therapeutically are sometimes referred to as nutraceuticals. This word, which combines the terms *nutrition* and *pharmaceutical,* refers to a food or food-derived product that is useful in the prevention or treatment of disease. As we stated in the last chapter, food is medicine. When considered from this perspective, you could call your salmon a nutraceutical. From a medical perspective, the fish oil in the salmon is a nutraceutical. The salmon itself is a functional food—a food that has a health-promoting or disease-preventing property beyond the basic function of supplying nutrients.

There are a variety of nutraceutical supplements available today, and many of them have been shown to affect digestive health in profound ways. We support the use of dietary supplements as part of a holistic plan for healing the gut, and we encourage you to consider using supplements in *your* digestive healing plan. When used strategically, they can help with healing your inside tract.

On page 133 we begin to outline our recommendations for specific supplements that you can use to heal your gut, but first there are some guidelines you need to keep in mind when starting a supplement protocol of any kind. Refer to these tips as you integrate the supplements on the next few pages into your plan.

Your Smart Supplementation Guidelines for Good Gut Health

1. **Consult with your health-care provider or nutritionist** before starting a supplement program, and check in with them along the way.
2. **Keep records.** Record the dosages, dates started, and effects (positive or negative) of any supplement you use.
2. **Be aware of any potential supplement interactions with medications** (e.g., drug-herb, drug-nutrient).
3. **Know what benefits to expect.** Supplements used therapeutically to treat a condition are intended for short-term use, thus it is important to periodically reevaluate what supplements you're taking and whether they're working. We suggest that you do so at least every 3 months.
4. **When you're beginning a supplement program, start with one supplement and wait 1 to 2 weeks before you add another supplement.** This will let you monitor for any potential adverse effects. If you do experience an adverse effect, be sure to let your health-care provider know so he or she can make modifications to your regimen.
5. **Carefully follow the dosage guidelines in this chapter (unless**

instructed otherwise by your health-care provider or nutritionist).
Individuals with digestive dysfunction may want to start with a
half dose, working up to a full dose as tolerated. If you use more
than one supplement or a combination formula, check the labels
to ensure that you do not exceed total dosage guidelines for individual substances.

6. **Check with your doctor before surgery, anesthesia, and other
   medical procedures.** Some supplements (including vitamin E,
   ginger, ginkgo biloba, and fish oils) can decrease the body's ability to form blood clots, while others can alter the effects of
   anesthesia.

7. **Store capsules and tablets in a cool, dark, safe place at home.**
   Fresh herbs can be frozen in airtight containers.

Supplements for Your Inside Tract

In the remainder of this chapter, we will outline the supplements that
have been shown to help resolve digestive symptoms in research studies and in clinical practice. For each common digestive condition, we
will provide a brief overview of the supplement, along with dosing
information.

Starting on page 152, you will find a chart where we have compiled the
essential information you need in order to make informed decisions about
what supplements may be best for you. In Chapter 7, we will explain how
to integrate these supplements into your plan. Understand that supplements, like food, affect different people differently. What works for someone else may not always work for you. We encourage you to find what
works best for your body and your illness in partnership with your physician and health-care team.

DYSPEPSIA AND GASTROESOPHAGEAL REFLUX DISEASE

Dyspepsia is one of the most common gut disorders in America. It affects an
estimated 20 percent of the population. Symptoms such as bloating, nausea,

belching, and abdominal distention—what is often referred to as "indigestion"—are all manifestations of dyspepsia. It is a functional digestive disorder that is usually the outcome of disordered gut movement (gastroparesis), and it is often compounded by stress.

We discussed gastroesophageal reflux disease (GERD) in Chapter 3. In GERD, the stomach contents reflux into the esophagus, causing pain and discomfort. This condition is shockingly common in America. Interestingly, many people suffer from both dyspepsia and GERD at the same time. Luckily, there are a group of supplements that can be used to treat both conditions.

Artichoke Leaf

A number of studies have demonstrated that artichoke leaf extract can reduce upper gastrointestinal symptoms and improve quality of life in those suffering from dyspepsia symptoms, such as fullness, flatulence, nausea, early satiety, and pain in the stomach region.[1, 2]

DOSE: 320 to 640 milligrams three times daily for dyspepsia only.

Bitters

Bitter compounds are known to promote *many* beneficial physiological responses. In fact, bitter tastes are specifically sought in traditional medicine because of their perceived therapeutic value.[3] As a result, bitter-tasting herbs have been used for millennia as digestive aids. Bitter tastes actually stimulate sensory responses in the tongue, which in turn increase the production of gastric acid, and stimulate bile flow. Some of the most commonly used bitter herbs include artichoke, bitter orange peel, dandelion root, gentian, and hops. Swedish bitters are a well-known formulation that combines many of the bitter herbs; its use is very popular among alternative practitioners. Of the most common bitters, artichoke leaf (discussed above) has been studied the most in clinical trials.

DOSE: Seek out a quality combination of the bitters noted above. Follow the dosage instructions on the bottle and take them 20 to 30 minutes before your main meal.

 CAUTION: Bitters should be used cautiously by people who suffer from reflux esophagitis, which may be aggravated by bitters.

Caraway Seed Oil

Caraway is an essential oil that is well-known for its medicinal properties. It's a natural antihistamine and antioxidant that can also be used to reduce spasms and facilitate the expulsion of gas. It's an excellent diuretic. It helps fight parasites in your gut and protects your liver. Interestingly, it can also be used to reduce anxiety, tension, and irritability.[4, 5] Caraway is a very powerful medicinal agent in a convenient, plant-based package.

When administered at a dose of 50 milligrams daily, it enhances gastric motility as well as the medication cisapride does.[6] This is stunning, considering the fact that few digestive health specialists are aware of it. Caraway seed oil is one of the best-kept secrets for improving gut motility, and that means it is an excellent addition to a comprehensive program for dyspepsia and GERD.

DOSE: 1 to 4 drops daily of the essential oil taken according to the package directions in water.

Curcumin

Curcumin is derived from the spice turmeric, and it conveys a number of beneficial health effects that range from cancer prevention to inflammation and pain reduction. It also induces a "calming effect" in the gut and stimulates proper bile flow for fat digestion. In Ayurvedic medicine, it was traditionally used to treat "stomach upset."[7]

The effectiveness of curcumin in the treatment of dyspepsia has been demonstrated by two well-designed clinical trials,[8] and the World Health Organization (WHO) now recommends turmeric for the treatment of acid, flatulence, and dyspepsia.[9] We also highly recommend it for dyspepsia.

DOSE: 500 to 1,000 milligrams of powdered turmeric root three times per day.

D-Limonene

D-limonene is a major constituent in several citrus oils, including orange, lemon, mandarin, lime, and grapefruit. It has antimicrobial, anti-inflammatory, and anticancer effects. (D-limonene has been shown to reduce the incidences of stomach and colon cancer.) Because of its pleasant citrus fragrance, it is widely used as a flavoring and fragrance additive in perfumes, soaps, foods, chewing gum, and beverages. However, its real power lies in its ability to help the inside tract.

D-limonene is also a cholesterol solvent and has been used to dissolve cho-lesterol-containing gallstones when taken as a supplement.[10, 11] It also coats and protects the gut and promotes normal movement of the upper digestive tract. Limited clinical studies have shown that it is useful for relieving heartburn and GERD.[12] While these studies are promising, D-limonene alone isn't enough to treat GERD.

⚊ KEY POINT: We prescribe D-limonene for dyspepsia and gastroparesis as well.

DOSE: 1,000 milligrams once daily.

Deglycyrrhizinated Licorice

For centuries, licorice root has been used for the treatment of peptic ulcer, and GERD. Research and clinical effectiveness bear out the wisdom of these practices.[13, 14, 15] The only downside is that prolonged use of licorice root can lead to fluid retention and hypertension. However, a special preparation called deglycyrrhizinated licorice (DGL) has had the glycyrrhizin removed, and therefore it may be taken without worrying about these side effects. Though there are no clinical trials evaluating the use of DGL for GERD, widespread effective use across the globe shows it to be a successful method of treatment.

DOSE: Take 350 to 1,000 milligrams three times daily with meals.

Demulcent Herbs

Marshmallow and slippery elm bark are classic demulcents. These herbs soothe and protect irritated tissues and are used to alleviate irritation of the mouth, throat, esophagus, stomach, and bowels. Although there are no clinical studies that support their use, there is a longstanding tradition of using them in the treatment of irritable bowel syndrome (IBS), GERD, and IBD.

The **British Herbal Compendium** recognizes the use of marshmallow root or leaf for treating duodenal ulceration, ulcerative colitis, and enteritis. It also suggests slippery elm for inflammation and ulceration of the gastrointestinal tract that occurs with conditions such as esophagitis, gastritis, colitis, gastric or duodenal ulcers, and diarrhea.[16] The Food and Drug Administration (FDA) recently approved slippery elm as a safe, nonprescription product for soothing the gastointestinal (GI) tract.

DOSE: The usual starting dose is two drops of slippery elm tincture, two cap-sules three times daily of marshmallow root, or 1 or 2 teaspoons of 1:5 tincture in 25 percent alcohol three times daily. Demulcents are usually taken at least 1 hour after prescription medications, to prevent interference with absorption.

Digestive Enzymes

An absence or insufficient production of any of the digestive enzymes can lead to indigestion and produce many bothersome symptoms. (Lactose intolerance from a deficiency in the enzyme lactase is a classic example.) Supplementation with the enzyme lactase in milk or capsule form prevents bothersome digestive symptoms. There are also prescription enzyme formulations for individuals with severe pancreatic insufficiency. Digestive enzyme insufficiency may show up in other, less-evident ways. A double-blind study recently showed that individuals with IBS who used pancreatic enzyme replacement in conjunction with a high-fat meal experienced an improvement in digestive symptoms.[17]

References to the medical use of proteolytic (protein-digesting) enzymes actu-ally stretch back well over 100 years. Early explorers in the Caribbean Islands noted that native groups used fresh pineapple juice as a digestive aid. Pineapple contains the proteolytic enzyme bromelain, meaning it breaks down proteins when used as a digestive aid. We know that this has been a useful treatment for many people across the globe for a long time.

Most people fare well using a broad-spectrum plant-based enzyme formula that contains proteases (enzymes that digest protein), carbohydrases (enzymes that digest carbohydrates), and lipases (enzymes that digest fats). Some enzyme formulations also contain dipeptidyl peptidase IV (DPP-IV), which may help break down casein and gluten for those with a known sensitivity or intolerance to these substances.

DOSE: One or two tablets or capsules at the beginning of a meal. Do not take with hot beverages, which may deactivate the enzymes. Individuals with gastritis, an active ulcer, or GERD should discuss the use of proteolytic enzymes with their physician.

Ginger

Ginger is a popular home remedy for dyspepsia and has been clinically studied for hyperemesis gravidarum, motion sickness, and chemotherapy-induced nausea and vomiting.[18, 19] It reduces vomiting, nausea, and flatulence; relaxes the bowel; is an anti-inflammatory; enhances gut motility; and reduces spasms. Ginger also restores proper electrical conductivity to the stomach, which results in more efficient emptying of the stomach.[20] All of these beneficial properties are useful for digestive tract conditions such as gastroparesis, GERD, dyspepsia, IBS, and IBD.[21]

Ginger has even been used in intensive care units to improve gastric emptying and decrease the incidence of pneumonia.

☞ KEY POINT: It takes 14 grams of gingerroot to produce 120 milligrams of powder. For this reason, it's best to take ginger as a supplement instead of in tea form for a therapeutic effect.

DOSE: 1,000 to 2,000 milligrams daily of ginger powder, divided into three or four doses. (Capsules typically contain 500 milligrams of gingerroot.) Since ginger is a known blood thinner at these doses, you should check with your physician if you are already on anticoagulant medications.

Lemon Balm

Lemon balm is a member of the mint family. It has many healthy flavonoids, is a rich source of antioxidants, and is considered a "calming" herb. It was used as far back as the Middle Ages to reduce stress and anxiety, promote sleep, improve appetite, and ease pain and discomfort due to indigestion (including gas, bloating, and colic). Lemon balm has been best studied for its tranquilizing and sedative effects on the nervous system and has been used to treat sleep disorders.[22]

DOSE: In capsule form, take 300 to 500 milligrams three times daily or as needed; as a tea, steep 1.5 to 4.5 grams (¼ to 1 teaspoon) of dried lemon balm in hot water and drink it up to four times daily; as a tincture, take 2 to 3 milliliters (40 to 90 drops) three times daily.

Mastic Gum

Chios mastic gum is a resin produced by the **Pistacia lentiscus** tree, an evergreen shrub from the pistachio tree family. It has been used for a variety of gastric ailments in Mediterranean and Middle Eastern countries for at least 3,000 years. Several studies have been published on mastic gum's effectiveness in treating **H. pylori,** healing peptic ulcers, improving functional dyspepsia, and reducing the intensity of gastric mucosal damage caused by antiulcer drugs and aspirin; they've also examined its antacid and cellular-protective qualities.[23, 24] Mastic gum appears to have important healing properties for the gut and can be considered as adjunctive therapy for patients with functional dyspepsia and *H. pylori*–associated gastropathy.

DOSE: 1,000 to 2,000 milligrams daily.

Melatonin

Three studies have consistently shown that 3 to 6 milligrams of melatonin daily relieves GERD symptoms. In these studies, symptom reduction starts at 4 weeks and optimizes at 8 weeks.[25] Melatonin improves GERD by preventing acid from being regurgitated into the esophagus. It does so by bolstering the lower esophageal sphincter. Interestingly, melatonin also reduces gastric acid production (to a milder degree than proton pump inhibitors [PPIs]). A recent study found melatonin to be *more* effective than PPIs in the treatment of GERD.[26] Melatonin certainly has fewer negative side effects than PPIs. This is a stunning finding that if reproduced should encourage us to rethink our position on nutraceuticals for this condition.

DOSE: 3 to 6 milligrams daily.

IRRITABLE BOWEL SYNDROME

Irritable bowel syndrome (IBS) is a complex disorder characterized by abdominal discomfort and altered bowel habits. Medications for IBS are typically aimed at reducing symptoms. Often, they do not provide significant benefits. Two decades ago, only 16 percent of IBS patients took dietary supplements, but recent data indicates that up to 51 percent of patients currently do so. This is good, because clinical data backs up this practice. Here are some supplements to consider for IBS.

Artichoke Leaf

This multipurpose plant (see page 146) has also been shown to improve IBS symptoms.[27, 28] In one trial, the severity of all symptoms decreased significantly at doses of 320 milligrams taken three times daily. Approximately 84 percent of physicians and patients rated the overall effectiveness of artichoke leaf extract as good or excellent. Another IBS trial experimented with increasing the dose to 640 milligrams three times daily, and the results were even more impressive: The total symptom score decreased by 41 percent and the total quality of life score increased by 20 percent after treatment.[29]

DOSE: 320 to 640 milligrams three times daily.

Fiber Products

Many millions of people suffer from chronic constipation as a result of eating a processed-foods diet that is lacking in fiber, a vital substance for a healthy GI tract. Fiber is a bulk-forming agent that helps foster elimination and prevents GI diseases such as colorectal cancer and diverticulosis. There are many fiber products on the market. Psyllium seeds contain a type of fiber called mucilage. In the digestive tract, mucilage absorbs and expands to provide increased bulk and moisture content to the stool. Bulkier stools trigger contractions of the colonic walls and encourage normal motility, leading to better bowel movements. Psyllium is also a prebiotic and is broken down in the gut as a food source for your friendly bacteria. Because it is a prebiotic, you should be careful when you introduce it into your system.

There are other fiber products on the market that do not ferment, such as methylcellulose (found in Citrucel) and calcium polycarbophil (found in Fibercon). These are used strictly as bulk-forming agents, and because they are nonfermentable, they don't form gas.

In addition to these products, we also recommend increasing fiber through the use of powdered seeds, including chia, flax, and hemp. Not only do they contribute both soluble and insoluble fiber, they also contain essential fatty acids and valuable vitamins and minerals.

DOSE: Start with ½ teaspoon of powder with 8 ounces of water or juice once daily, gradually increasing to 1 rounded teaspoon once or twice daily. Gently mix the powder and water together, and drink the mixture right away to make sure you get the entire dose. Some brands also offer fiber capsules. You need to take several capsules with water to achieve the same results you'll get from the powder.

 CAUTION: Be sure to drink plenty of water every day, or else fiber supplements can actually make your constipation worse. Avoid taking prescription medications within 2 hours of ingesting fiber supplements to avoid any interference with the absorption of your medicines. If you have a history of intestinal blockages or have had a surgical ostomy (colostomy or ileostomy), consult your physician before using fiber products.

German Chamomile

These aromatic and mildly bitter flowers have been used to support digestive health since ancient times. Chamomile is an anti-inflammatory that reduces spasms, encourages the expulsion of gas, and may help prevent ulcers. The efficacy of chamomile for the relief of diarrhea has been verified through two double-blind, placebo-controlled trials.[30, 31] Likewise, chamomile has been shown to be effective for colic in a number of randomized control trials.[32, 33]

DOSE: The typical dose is 1 heaping tablespoon (approximately 3 grams) in 8 ounces of hot water as a tea three or four times daily. The tea should be taken between meals.

Iberogast

This proprietary blend of nine herbs was developed in Germany in 1961 and is available without a prescription in many countries, including the United States. Several randomized, controlled clinical trials have shown that Iberogast improves symptoms and pain in IBS sufferers and functional dyspepsia.[34, 35] Several studies suggest that the efficacy of Iberogast could be due to its complex composition of nine standardized herbal extracts that target different areas to improve IBS symptoms. This principle of multitarget therapy is quite popular in clinical medicine for treating functional bowel disorders. Iberogast can be helpful for IBS and functional dyspepsia. We highly recommend it.

DOSE: 20 drops in a beverage three times daily.

Magnesium

This mineral has been used for centuries as a laxative for those who suffer from constipation.

DOSE: 500 to 1,000 milligrams of magnesium citrate daily.

Melatonin

Melatonin decreases pain and hypersensitivity in people with IBS. Two clinical studies have shown that 3 milligrams of melatonin daily improves these symptoms in women with IBS.[36, 37]

DOSE: 3 to 6 milligrams daily at bedtime.

Peppermint Oil

Peppermint oil is one of the most extensively studied and widely used alternative treatments for IBS patients. It works like a calcium channel blocker and helps relax GI smooth muscle. This effect helps relieve the cramping and pain associated with IBS. Enteric-coated peppermint oil is usually recommended over other forms because it dissolves lower down the GI tract; this reduces the risk of esophageal reflux. Studies have also shown that peppermint oil is an effective treatment for pain and spasms in IBS patients.[38, 39] In one study published in the *Journal of Gastroenterology*, enteric coated peppermint oil was matched against an inactive placebo in over 100 patients with symptoms of IBS. After 1 month, 79 percent of those taking the herbal remedy had relief from pain and well over half were pain free. In the placebo group, only 43 felt better and less than 10 percent were pain free.[40] Many additional studies have shown the benefits of using peppermint oil to treat IBS. If you have IBS, you should consider this safe, effective, and cost-effective treatment for global symptoms and pain related to this condition.

DOSE: 0.2 to 0.4 milliliter of enteric-coated peppermint oil three times daily.

 CAUTION: Peppermint oil that is not enteric-coated should be avoided if you have diagnosed GERD or are experiencing heartburn.

Probiotics

In addition to their uses in other conditions outlined above (see pages 99 and 164), these little bacterial helpers have been shown to regulate gastrointestinal motility, prevent and treat GI infections (including traveler's diarrhea), and improve idiopathic constipation. They are also useful for preventing and treating antibiotic-associated diarrhea, including *C. difficile* and rotavirus infection.[41, 42] These are all reasons probiotics have been shown in numerous trials to help improve IBS.[43]

DOSE: No strains appear to be any more effective than others. We recommend 10 to 25 billion colony-forming units(CFU) of multistrain probiotics daily.

CHRONIC LIVER DISEASE

Viral hepatitis, nonalcoholic steatohepatitis (NASH), alcoholic liver disease (ALD), and cirrhosis of various causes have been the most studied liver disorders in clinical trials. Here are the supplements may be helpful with diseases of the liver.

Dandelion

This fascinating plant is known by cultures around the world as an edible delicacy and an important medicine. Dandelion's Latin name is derived from the Greek and means "disease remedy." This is exactly how it was used in Europe for centuries. Traditionally, dandelion roots were used for improving liver function and dandelion leaves and flowers were used as bitter digestive stimulants and diuretics. Unfortunately, that practice has been lost and most people in the United States consider dandelion little more than a pesky weed that should be purged from the lawn with herbicide. Perhaps our inside tracts would be happier if we learned to eat this weed!

When eaten as a vegetable, dandelion is rich in inulin, the prebiotic we discuss on page 147. When taken as an extract, dandelion has been shown to protect the liver against alcohol and chemical-induced liver injury,[44] and we know that it has many anti-inflammatory and anticancer effects.[45]

DOSE: 1 dropperful of liquid tincture 1:5 three times daily.

 CAUTION: Because it is a bitter, dandelion should be used cautiously in people who suffer from reflux esophagitis, which may be aggravated by bitters.

Magnesium

Magnesium is an essential mineral involved in multiple enzyme systems, muscle function, and insulin/glucose metabolism. It is found in dark green leafy vegetables, beans, and nuts and seeds; however, most people do not get adequate dietary magnesium. Because of this, there are many patients with digestive disorders (inflammatory bowel disease, pancreatitis) and liver disorders (cirrhosis) whose magnesium status is compromised. Furthermore, having too little magnesium has been implicated in the development of a number of liver diseases, including nonalcoholic fatty liver disease and nonalcoholic steatohepatitis. There is a significant relationship between low magnesium concentrations and liver inflammation and fibrosis in nonalcoholic fatty liver disease.[46] Alcoholics, including those without liver disease, and patients with cirrhosis frequently have low total body magnesium levels, even though they sometimes have normal magnesium levels in their blood.[47]

Magnesium glycinate is used for the treatment of muscle cramps in patients with liver disease. Magnesium citrate can be helpful for stimulating bowel motility and aiding constipation.

DOSE: 200 to 400 milligrams once daily.

 CAUTION: Magnesium is eliminated by the kidneys. Therefore, if you have kidney impairment, you should cut back on your dose of magnesium.

Probiotics

Probiotics are live strains of gut flora that can be obtained from supplements. These are the "good" bacteria that you need in your gut. When taken in adequate amounts, they can confer a wide range of health benefits.

While there are no human studies on probiotics and liver disease, there are animal studies that support the use of probiotics to treat liver conditions. Probiotics appear to reduce inflammation, oxidative stress, and insulin resistance, and to improve metabolism. *Bifidobacteria* in particular seems promising in the treatment of nonalcoholic fatty liver disease.[48, 49]

Using probiotics in this capacity is likely effective due to the bowel and liver interactions in liver disease. For example, heavy alcohol use leads to increased gut permeability, which in turn allows bacterial toxins to leak into the circulatory system.[50] The gut bacteria create byproducts called lipopolysaccharides, which stimulate inflammation in the liver.[51] The probiotics not only restore normal bowel flora balance but also help the gut lining heal so that it is less "leaky."

DOSE: We recommend 10 to 25 billion CFUs once daily in capsule or powder form.

S-adenosylmethionine

S-adenosylmethionine (SAMe) is a nutrient that is involved in many biochemical reactions throughout the body. People with liver disease often cannot synthesize SAMe in their bodies, and some preliminary studies suggest that taking SAMe may help treat chronic liver disease caused by medications or alcoholism by helping normalize levels of hepatic enzymes. Studies in mice support this and show that SAMe protects against and can also reverse liver damage.

Being deficient in either vitamin B$_{12}$ or folate may reduce levels of SAMe in your body.

DOSE: Start with a low dose— approximately 200 milligrams daily—and increase slowly to 200 to 400 milligrams three times daily. This helps avoid stomach upset.

Silymarin (Milk Thistle)

Silymarin is the active ingredient extracted from *Silybum marianum* (also known as milk thistle). Historical references to using this herb for treating liver and gallbladder diseases date back more than 2,000 years. Pliny the Elder, the 1st-century Roman writer, recommended a formulation of milk thistle, which involved an extract of the juice in combination with honey, for improving digestion by stimulating the flow of bile. Milk thistle is a powerful antioxidant and anti-inflammatory, and it also reduces the development of excess fibrous tissue in the liver, fights cancer, and works as an antiviral agent.[52]

Many Europeans still routinely use milk thistle extract for protection against environmental pollutants, over-the-counter medications (such as acetaminophen), and other common chemicals that adversely affect the liver (including alcohol). In Germany, it is a popular treatment for numerous liver conditions, including viral hepatitis, alcohol-induced cirrhosis, and toxin-related liver injury (such as from acetaminophen or

> *The herb most commonly used to treat hepatitis C is milk thistle.*

alcohol). And the mortality of those with alcoholic liver disease is lower with silymarin than with a placebo.[53]

Studies are currently being developed to evaluate the use of milk thistle as a liver-protective agent in patients undergoing chemotherapy.

DOSE: 100 to 200 milligrams twice daily.

Vitamin E

This all-star antioxidant is also a powerful anti-inflammatory. Some theories suggest that oxidative stress may play a role in the development of many forms of liver disease, including nonalcoholic fatty liver disease. Vitamin E has been shown to diminish oxidative injury in experimental liver injury (performed in a lab setting). When compared with a placebo, vitamin E has been associated with a significantly higher rate of improvement in liver function for nonalcoholic steatohepatitis.[54]

DOSE: 400 to 800 IU of vitamin E complex with mixed tocopherols once daily.

Zinc

Zinc has been shown to decrease abnormalities in gut barrier function caused by alcohol; decrease the release of gut bacterial toxins; reduce inflammation and oxidative stress; and preserve the function of critical liver proteins.

A deficiency of this essential mineral has been documented in multiple types of human liver diseases.[55] Too little zinc appears to increase your susceptibility to several forms of liver toxicity, and extensive recent research has shown that zinc supplementation protects against alcohol-induced liver injury.[56]

DOSE: 15 milligrams of zinc glycinate capsules or tablets once daily.

INFLAMMATORY BOWEL DISEASE (CROHN'S DISEASE AND ULCERATIVE COLITIS)

As you learned in Chapter 3, inflammatory bowel disease (IBD) is characterized by unremitting chronic intestinal inflammation. This inflammation injures the intestinal lining and causes numerous complications including malabsorption of minerals and nutrients, diarrhea, and abdominal pain. Our approach to supplementation for inflammatory bowel disease is to cool off the intestinal inflammation, facilitate healing of the gut lining, and rebalance the enteric flora. The following supplements will help you do that.

Aloe Vera

Most people are familiar with aloe vera. It has been used medicinally for over 5,000 years in Egyptian, Indian, Chinese, and European cultures. Aloe is an anti-inflammatory and antioxidant,[57] which makes it an appealing treatment option for gut inflammation. It contains an enzyme that inactivates bradykinin—a potent mediator of inflammation—and produces pain-reducing, anti-inflammatory, analgesic effects much like aspirin does.[58] Aloe vera also contains the antioxidant vitamins A, C, and E, which facilitate the reduction of oxidative stress throughout the body. Interestingly, this succulent also facilitates short-chain fatty acid production by the "friendly flora,"[59] and this has immune-regulating effects and gut healing benefits.

The use of aloe vera as a medicinal agent for the treatment of digestive illnesses has been formally studied in animals and humans. It has been shown to help prevent and treat chemical-induced colitis in animals[60] and to help induce remission in inflammatory bowel disease,[61] mucositis in chemotherapy patients, and peptic ulcers.[62, 63, 64, 65]

DOSE: Take 100 milliliters(3.4 fluid ounces) of aloe gel twice daily for colitis.

Boswellia

Boswellia, also called frankincense, is a traditional Ayurvedic remedy. It has been used in Asia and Africa for at least 3,500 years to treat a wide variety of digestive ailments including diarrhea, constipation, flatulence, and liver disease.[66] This species of plant has anti-inflammatory and antioxidant properties, and it fights tumors as well as microbes. It has been shown to behave in similar ways as corticosteroids do in chemical-induced colitis in animals. It is an excellent treatment for inducing remission in inflammatory bowel disease and collagenous colitis.[67, 68, 69, 70]

DOSE: 350 milligrams three times daily for IBD or other inflammatory conditions of the inside tract.

Curcumin

As mentioned above, curcumin is derived from the rhizome of turmeric and has a number of beneficial health effects. Interestingly, the average daily intake of turmeric in India, where IBD is rare, is approximately 2 to 2.5 grams per day. The power of curcumin as an anti-inflammatory has been demonstrated in several studies, and it has also been shown to be extremely effective at maintaining remission of inflammatory bowel disease.[71, 72]

DOSE: The typical dosage is 500 to 1,000 milligrams of powdered turmeric root three times daily.

Glutamine

Glutamine is an amino acid that is vital for maintaining a healthy lining in your small intestine because cells turn over daily in that part of the gut. The need for glutamine dramatically increases when there is injury or chronic inflammation in the small intestine. Glutamine appears to have a special role in restoring the integrity of the small bowel lining and improving immune function.[73] Patients with intestinal mucosal injury due to chemotherapy or radiation benefit from glutamine supplementation and have less injury to the gut lining, increased mucosal healing, and decreased passage of bacterial endotoxins through the gut wall.[74]

Glutamine has also been studied as a therapeutic agent in Crohn's disease. The results of these studies are generally disappointing to date; however, recent evidence suggests that new formulations and targeting could enhance glutamine efficacy at the site of mucosal lesions.[75, 76] Medical foods that contain glutamine in combination with other healing nutrients may work better than glutamine does when used by itself.

DOSE: Begin with 500 to 1,000 milligrams three times daily. Monitor the effects, as some individuals require higher dosages.

Omega-3 Fatty Acids

Essential fatty acids (EFAs) are healthy fats that are anti-inflammatory by nature. They build the walls of your cell membranes, and they cause a wide variety of positive health effects throughout your body. There are two EFAs: alpha-linolenic acid (ALA), an omega-3 fatty acid, and linoleic acid, an omega-6 fatty acid.

Alpha-linolenic acid is found in plant foods such as dark greens, purslane (an edible garden weed!), walnuts, flaxseed, hempseed, and soybeans. ALA is biochemically transformed into two other omega-3 fatty acids, EPA (eicosapentaenoic acid) and DHA (docosahexaenoic acid). However, it has been shown that this conversion is limited in many individuals. Thus, it is best to obtain EPA and DHA

INULIN

Inulin is a naturally occurring polysaccharide found in plants. Plants that possess high levels of inulin include chicory, dandelion root, leeks, onions, garlic, and asparagus. Inulin is also an ingredient in many processed foods. The label may list inulin, chicory root extract, oligosaccharide, or oligofructose. Most healthy people can tolerate up to 10 grams of native inulin and 5 grams of the "sweet" inulin a day. Too much inulin can cause bloating and digestive symptoms for some.

directly from fish (deep-water fatty fish, such as sardines, anchovies, and wild-caught salmon) or fish oil supplements. There are a number of "functional foods" now on the market that have been fortified with EPA and DHA, including omega-3 eggs (which come from hens fed a diet rich in flaxseed), cereals, bars, spreads, beverages, and other items. Omega-3s help to cool inflammation whether they're eaten in foods or taken in supplement form.

Though the overall results are mixed, laboratory studies and a number of clinical trials support the use of fish oils for the maintenance of remission for inflammatory bowel disease.[77, 78, 79, 80, 81, 82, 83] While it is unclear whether fish oil supplements by themselves maintain remission in Crohn's disease and ulcerative colitis, the evidence to date is promising.

O→ KEY POINT: We recommend using fish oils as part of a comprehensive therapeutic program with other anti-inflammatory agents.

DOSE: 4,000 to 6,000 milligrams of combined EPA and DHA daily.

Prebiotics

We introduced you to prebiotics (also called soluble fiber) in Chapter 4. These indigestible food ingredients stimulate the growth of or modify the metabolic activity of your intestinal flora. Your flora produce increased amounts of short-chain fatty acids as a result, and these have a variety of healthy benefits. Your goal is to include prebiotic foods in your diet to feed your flora; however, supplements may also be helpful.

To date, the research on prebiotics is limited but promising. They have been shown to improve outcomes of ulcerative colitis in particular, and given their general health benefits, it's highly likely that they have other positive effects on digestive function as well.

Prebiotics that have proven beneficial in the treatment of ulcerative colitis include:

- Oat bran (60 grams daily, which supplies 20 grams of dietary fiber)[84]
- Germinated barley foodstuff (GBF) containing hemicellulose-rich fiber (20 to 30 grams daily)[85, 86, 87]
- Inulin-derived fructooligosaccharides (FOS) (3,000 to 5,000 milligrams daily)
- Larch arabinogalactan (3,000 to 5,000 milligrams daily)

PROBIOTICS AND H. PYLORI

Research is emerging supporting the use of probiotics in the treatment of *Helicobacter pylori* (*H. pylori*) infection as well. As noted, probiotics are used to prevent antibiotic-associated diarrhea and *Clostridium difficile* infection. New preliminary evidence reveals that probiotics appear to work synergistically with antibiotics in resolving *H. pylori* infections.

Prebiotics can help improve a healthy gut environment by restoring the proper friendly flora and producing short-chain fatty acids, which reduce inflammation and repair colonic cells.

DOSE: We recommend trying Larch arabinogalactan at 3,000 to 5,000 milligrams daily. It is recommended that you begin with a half dose and gradually increase to a full dose.

 CAUTION: Many people experience gas and bloating when introducing prebiotics, especially people with existing GI problems, so ease into these by starting off with a very low dose and gradually increasing.

Probiotics

As we have discussed, these beneficial microorganisms influence a number of physiological functions. Consuming a diet that includes prebiotic foods and some cultured food products will help maintain a good gut microflora population. However, for many with digestive illnesses, taking additional probiotics supplementally may have many additional benefits. Probiotic supplements may:[88, 89, 90]

- Promote intestinal healing
- Rebalance your immune system
- Reduce inflammation
- Prevent and treat GI infections
- Maintain remission in ulcerative colitis
- Induce remission in pouchitis (inflammation in the surgically created pouch following a total colectomy for ulcerative colitis)

DOSE: The vast majority of studies related to inflammatory bowel disease have utilized a probiotic preparation referred to as VSL#3. The dose of VSL#3 has varied, but most studies have used 450 billion colony-forming units (CFU) per day. Clinical trials for probiotic use to treat Crohn's disease have successfully utilized *Saccharomyces boulardii*—a special strain of yeast that kills other "bad" strains of yeast in the gut. *S. boulardii* is taken in capsule form, and is known as SBC; the common dose is 250 milligrams once or twice daily. There are many quality preparations on the market to consider as well. When starting on probiotics, start with a smaller dose and gradually increase to a full dose, since you are changing your gut flora.

Short-Chain Fatty Acid Enemas

Enemas have been used for the treatment of inflammatory bowel disease of the distal colon for decades. Topical aminosalicylates, available in the form of mesalamine enemas or suppositories, are the first-line treatment for ulcerative colitis, with few associated side effects.

We are facing an epidemic of vitamin D deficiency, with recent studies showing that as much as 90 percent of the US population is getting less than the recommended daily allowance of this crucial vitamin.

Short-chain fatty acids have a number of beneficial properties that may benefit people who suffer from colitis. They are anti-inflammatory, fight tumors, and promote the integrity, growth, and repair of cells in the colon. Their direct application to the rectum and sigmoid colon has been shown to induce remission of colitis in cases of ulcerative colitis that are resistant to conventional medical therapy.[91, 92, 93, 94, 95] Short-chain fatty acid enemas can be used in hard-to-treat cases of ulcerative colitis that are resistant to conventional medical therapy and that may otherwise require intense immunosuppressive therapy.

DOSE: 60 to 100 milliliters of 80 to 100 millimoles per liter rectally twice daily for 4 weeks for resistant left-sided ulcerative colitis. (Your doctor will need to contact a compounding pharmacy to prepare this for your use as an enema.)

Vitamin D

Vitamin D has widespread effects throughout the body, and intake of adequate amounts has been associated with lower risks of colorectal cancer, autoimmune disease, cardiovascular disease, and all-cause mortality.[96] Unfortunately, due to our modern lifestyle, most of us don't get enough vitamin D. There *are* a few dietary sources of vitamin D, but they are very uncommon in the American diet. Your body synthesizes it when you are exposed to sunlight. However, since most of us live and work indoors, few of us produce enough on our own.

Several studies have reported an association between low bioactive vitamin D in people living in northern latitudes and the development of autoimmune diseases, including multiple sclerosis, diabetes mellitus, and Crohn's disease.[97, 98] As the incidence of autoimmune diseases rises with increasing latitude, a "hot hypothesis" has been proposed, indicating that the development of an autoimmune disease is associated with low vitamin D levels.

Since vitamin D rebalances immunity and most individuals with IBD are deficient in this nutrient, there is intense interest in the use of vitamin D for the prevention and treatment of relapses in inflammatory bowel disease.[99] Studies using vitamin D to treat animals with IBD have shown that vitamin D has potential for use in treating humans with IBD.[100] Recently, investigators from Denmark reported that daily intake of 1,200 IU of vitamin D reduced the annual risk of relapse in individuals with Crohn's disease from 29 to 13 percent.[101] Vitamin D has a profound influence on proper immune function, and sufficient levels appear to protect against autoimmunity. Vitamin D also holds promise as a potential therapeutic agent for inflammatory bowel disease.

DOSE: We recommend taking 1,000 to 2,000 IU of vitamin D_3 daily and that you see your doctor twice each year to have your vitamin D levels checked.

Zinc

Zinc is an important element in antioxidant defenses, and it is important that you have enough. However, in some digestive disorders, like Crohn's disease, zinc absorption is impaired and it is lost from your gut. Low blood levels of zinc are common in patients with Crohn's disease. In one study, supplementation with zinc significantly decreased small intestinal permeability in patients with Crohn's disease for a period of 12 months,[102] and correction of zinc deficiency provided improvement in folks with IBD.[103]

Zinc L-carnosine—a form of zinc that is bound to the amino acid L-carnosine—has a number of properties that guard the lining of your digestive tract. Clinically, zinc L-carnosine has been found to protect the gut's mucosal lining.[104, 105]

DOSE: 30 milligrams of zinc L-carnosine daily.

Smart Supplementation: Final Thoughts

This chapter is an overview of some of the nutraceutical supplements for the management and treatment of digestive disease. Along with diet and lifestyle changes, they can be extremely powerful tools for treating—and in many cases overcoming—the symptoms of a wide array of digestive diseases. You may need to experiment to find what works for you, but once you do find the right supplements, they can have very beneficial effects.

Supplement Chart

For your convenience, we have included all of the important dosing details regarding supplements and what conditions they can be used for in one chart. Use this as a quick reference as you integrate these important nutraceuticals into your plan.

SUPPLEMENT	CONDITION(S)	THERAPEUTIC EFFECTS	DOSE(S)
Aloe Vera	IBD	Mucosal healing Anti-inflammatory	100 ml (3.4 fluid ounces) of aloe gel, 2 times daily
Artichoke Leaf	Dyspepsia, IBS	Promotes bile flow Antinausea Antiemetic	320–640 mg daily
Boswellia	UC, CD	Anti-inflammatory	350 mg, 3 times daily
Caraway Seed Oil	Dyspepsia, GERD	Anti-spasmodic	1–4 drops daily of essential oil
Curcumin	Dyspepsia, IBD (UC, Chron's Disease)	Anti-inflammatory	1,500–3,000 mg daily
D-Limonene	GERD, peptic ulcer disease	Promote gut motility	1,000 mg daily
DGL-Licorice Root	GERD, hepatitis	Gut lining repair	350–1,000 mg 3 times daily
Dandelion Root	Chronic liver disease	Improves bile flow Liver tonic	5 to 10 ml of a 1:5 tincture in 45% alcohol, 3 times daily

(Continued)

Supplement Chart (cont.)

SUPPLEMENT	CONDITION(S)	THERAPEUTIC EFFECTS	DOSE(S)
Demulcents: Slippery Elm tincture or Marshmallow Root capsules	GERD, IBD, IBS	Soothe irritated intestinal lining	2 drops of tincture; 2 capsules, 3 times daily; or 1–2 teaspoons of 1:5 tincture in 25% alcohol, 3 times daily
Digestive Enzymes	IBS	Antimicrobial properties Reverse maldigestion	1 or 2 capsules or tablets with meals
Fiber	IBS-induced constipation	Improves motility	1 tablespoon with water on an empty stomach
Fish Oils (Omega-3 Fatty Acids)	IBD	Anti-inflammatory	4,000–6,000 mg of EPA/DHA daily
German Chamomile	IBS	Relaxes gut smooth muscle Calms the mind Anti-ulcerogenic	1 heaping tablespoon (about 3 g) in hot water as a tea, 3 or 4 times daily, between meals
Ginger	Dyspepsia, gastroparesis	Antiemetic Improves motility Anti-inflammatory Antispasm	1,000–2,000 mg daily
Glutamine	Crohn's disease	Gut lining repair	2,000–3,000 mg daily
Iberogast	Dyspepsia, IBS	regulates motility anti-spasmodic	20 drops 3 times daily
Lemon Balm	Dyspepsia	Gut calming agent	900–1,500 mg daily
Magnesium	IBS-induced constipation	Hydroscopic Promotility	500–1,000 mg daily
	Chronic liver disease	Prevents muscle spasms	200–400 mg daily
Mastic Gum	Dyspepsia, Peptic ulcer	Kills H. pylori, antiacid	1,000–2,000 mg per day

(Continued)

Supplement Chart (cont.)

SUPPLEMENT	CONDITION(S)	THERAPEUTIC EFFECTS	DOSE(S)
Melatonin	IBS, GERD	Stress reduction Sleep aid	3–6 mg daily
Milk Thistle	Hepatitis	Anti-inflammatory	200–400 mg daily
Peppermint Oil	IBS	Antispasmodic Analgesic	0.2–0.4 ml of enteric-coated peppermint oil, 3 times daily
Prebiotics: Larch arabinogalactans	IBD	Promotes growth of friendly flora Fosters motility and healing	3,000–5,000 mg daily
Probiotics	IBS and IBD (Crohn's disease, ulcerative colitis)	Regulates the immune system Restores motility Rebalances flora Gut repair Improves barrier function	10–25 billion CFUs daily; 250 mg daily of *S. boulardii*, 450 billion CFUs of VSL#3 daily; other preparations vary in peak effective concentrations of live bacteria
S-Adenosyl Methionine	Chronic liver disease	supports methylation	200 mg daily start, increase to 600–1,200 mg daily
Short-Chain Fatty Acid Enemas	Ulcerative colitis	Regulates motility Gut lining repair	60–100 mL of 80–100 millimoles per liter twice daily for 4 weeks for resistant left-sided ulcerative colitis
Vitamin E	Non-alcoholic fatty liver disease	anti-oxidant, anti-inflammatory	400–800 IU daily
Vitamin D	General health, IBD	Immune balancing Bone health	1,000–2,000 IU daily (see page 150 for details)
Zinc (Elemental)	Chronic liver disease	Gut lining repair Antioxidant	15 mg daily
Zinc L-carnosine	IBD	Gut lining repair	30 mg daily

An extensive line of professional formulations ofr many of these products by www.mnmwites.com and www.swiftnutrition.com.

PART III

Food As Medicine
for Digestive Health

CHAPTER 7

Getting on the Inside Track to Optimal Digestive Health

Now that you understand the basic scientific underpinnings of the dietary and lifestyle changes we recommend for healing your gut, it's time to get on the Inside Tract plan for optimal digestive health—a 2- to 12-week holistic healing plan designed to help you regain balance and heal your gastrointestinal (GI) tract. The plan is founded on three basic steps.

1. **Complete the GPS and get on track.** We've developed a three-track nutrition plan that provides you with everything you need to make the dietary changes necessary to heal your particular digestive ailment.
2. **Improve your lifestyle.** You'll learn how to optimize your lifestyle and support your detoxification system so you can support your gut and your health for the long term.
3. **Add gut-healing supplements.** You'll add gut-healing supplements to your program to help you heal from your digestive disease.

In this chapter, we will explain how to integrate these three elements into a comprehensive program that will help you heal your gut and rebalance your life. Along the way, we will teach you how to adjust the program to your needs so that you can get the most out of your time on the plan. Let's get started.

Step 1: Complete the GPS and Get on Track

> *Knowledge of any kind . . . brings about a change in awareness from where it is possible to create new realities.*
> —Deepak Chopra

Before you start a journey, you need to have a plan. You need to know where you are going and how you will get there. You don't hike a mountain, take a vacation, or even run to the grocery store without a plan. The journey to digestive health is the same. You know where you want to go. You want to heal your gut. The question is, how will you get there?

Our Gastrointestinal Patient Symptom tool (or the GPS, as we like to call it) takes into account a number of validated tools to assess digestive symptoms. In the clinical setting, integrating them into one tool as we've done here has proven extremely effective in accurately assessing the severity of a patient's condition as well as determining the dietary and lifestyle interventions needed to heal it. The GPS will help give you the direction you need to go from poor digestive health to optimal gut function. However, it does not replace diagnosis by a medical professional.

To use the GPS, simply rate the severity and frequency of the digestive symptoms listed below on a scale from 0 to 10. Depending on how severe your symptoms are, the GPS will put you on one of three dietary tracks.[1,2,3,4]

- **Track 1: The Foundational Food Plan.** This is an eating program rooted in proven, whole-foods dietary patterns that are typical of the healthiest regions in the world. It is designed for people with periodic minor digestive symptoms or for those who simply want to maintain optimal health. It provides a model for how you can eat healthy for life. We recommend you spend a minimum of 2 weeks on this program to experience its benefits.
- **Track 2: The Exclusion Food Plan.** This entails a comprehensive elimination diet, which you should be on for at least 2 weeks, followed by reassessment and gradual food reintroduction. The purpose of Track 2 is to reduce the burden on your immune system by avoiding foods that are sending possible "alarm and harm" messages with each bite that you take. It is for people who have established low- to mid-level digestive symptoms.
- **Track 3: The Specific Food Plan.** This is for people with a digestive disease who have moderate to severe symptoms. We've designed a lower-residue elimination diet to help mitigate the

symptoms of irritable bowel syndrome (IBS), Crohn's disease, ulcerative colitis, and other GI conditions. The diet should be followed for a minimum of 2 weeks, but many of the people who end up on this plan may need to stay on it longer and then progress to Track 2 as they heal.

These dietary changes form the core of the program. Once you have completed the GPS, you will know which track you should be on. All you have to do is follow the instructions for your plan in the corresponding chapter. As you work through the program and your digestive symptoms improve, you can move from plan to plan accordingly. We'll give you plenty of instruction along the way about how to do this, so don't worry!

To get you started on your journey, rate your symptoms as instructed below.

How Severe Are Your Symptoms? A GPS for Digestive Health

In the table on page 161, rate your digestive symptoms on a scale from 0 to 10, where:

- 0 = Symptom is infrequent and/or not noticeable
- 10 = Symptom is very frequent and/or unbearable

You should rank your overall experience with these symptoms over the last 2 to 4 weeks. Digestive problems tend to come and go in cycles for most people, so the severity and frequency of your symptoms may change over time. Considering a 2- to 4-week period usually provides a broad enough time frame to get a good assessment of your condition.

Note that you should rate your symptoms as outlined below even if you have already been diagnosed with a digestive illness. As long as you rate your symptoms accurately, the GPS will place you on the correct track no matter what digestive illness you are suffering from.

To get a better sense of how the GPS will help you, here is a story from one of the many clients who have used this program to overcome their digestive illness.

(continued on page 162)

MARIA'S STORY

Maria had been suffering from recurring, cyclic bouts of diarrhea and abdominal pain for more than 6 months. She went to see her physician, who quickly diagnosed her with irritable bowel syndrome and sent her away with a prescription for Lotronex.

While the medication did reduce her diarrhea, after a couple of months of taking it, she began to get constipated, instead. In addition, her abdominal pain was replaced with a persistent feeling of nausea, and she broke out in hives. Though these are side effects of the medication (and warning signs that should be taken seriously), her doctor noted that at least she wasn't "spending all of [her] time in the bathroom anymore."

Luckily, Maria followed her instincts, quit taking the medication, and sought out a second opinion. That's when she came to see me, Gerry. In addition to performing a complete clinical workup, I had her fill out the GPS tool you will use.

Maria hadn't been suffering from her usual symptoms for about a week when she came to my office. But the week before had been one of the worst she'd ever faced in her life. She'd had severe diarrhea that she rated an 8. The recurrent nature and the overall severity of her symptoms made her feel terribly depressed, and needless to say, it was having a severe impact on her quality of life. Standing for long hours in a courtroom was out of the question.

Her total score after completing the GPS was 75—which is extremely high—and I assigned her to Track 3 of the program. She went on a strict, lower-residue, specific-food elimination diet that included healing soups, smoothies, and broths. In addition, I placed her on a high-quality probiotic and a few other nutritional supplements, and I asked her to regularly engage in relaxation exercises, including deep breathing, and mindful eating.

This program was exactly what Maria needed. In 8 weeks, her GPS scored dropped from 75 to 12. Her diarrhea and abdominal pain were completely resolved, as were her nausea and depression. Aside from a bit of gas and some residual concerns that her symptoms might return, Maria's IBS symptoms were dramatically improved.

When I saw her at our 1-month follow-up appointment, Maria reported that she had never felt better. Her GPS score was down to a 2, she was back in the courtroom and not running to the bathroom all day, and she said she had more energy than she'd had since she was a teenager. Where medication had failed, diet and lifestyle changes had succeeded. I was pleased, but unsurprised. This is the kind of change I see when people take an integrative approach to healing.

Gastrotestinal Patient Symptom Assessment Tool

SYMPTOM	DESCRIPTION	SEVERITY 0–10
Abdominal Cramps or Pain	Discomfort in the abdominal region	
Constipation	Hard, pelletlike, or infrequent stools	
Diarrhea	Loose, watery, or mushy stools—often more than twice a day	
Gas	Flatulence or burping	
Heartburn	Gastroesophageal reflux disease	
Mood	Any negative alteration in mood, including irritability, anger, anxiety, depression, and others	
Impact on Quality of Life	Any effect your digestive symptoms have on your lifestyle	
Dyspepsia	Early sense of fullness/bloating (particularly after meals)	
Queasiness	Nausea/vomiting/suppressed appetite	
Systemic Symptoms: • Asthma • Fatigue • Hoarseness • Joint aches • Migraines • Myalgias • Poor Sleep • Restless leg syndrome • Skin lesions/rashes • Tongue/mouth sores • Weight loss	These are common symptoms associated with digestive imbalance that show up outside the gut. Review these, see if they are a problem for you, then take an average of your overall experiences with any or all of them as a group	

Take some time now to rate your symptoms, as Maria did. It is the first step on your journey to digestive wellness.

Once you have rated your symptoms, add up your score and use the scoring key below to determine your track.

Scoring Key

YOUR SCORE	SEVERITY OF DIGESTIVE SYMPTOMS	YOUR TRACK
0–25	Mild	Track 1: The Foundational Food Plan
26–50	Moderate	Track 2: The Exclusion Food Plan
51 and up	Severe	Track 3: The Specific Food Plan (We recommend you seek the help of a qualified physician if you are on Track 3.)

After 2 weeks on your plan, you will come back here and take the GPS again. Reassessing your symptoms after 2 weeks will give you a concrete sense of how your symptoms are changing—or aren't. Knowing this will give you critical information that you need in order to take the next steps. If your symptoms improve (which will likely be the case), you can scale back the dietary restrictions. For example, move from Track 3 to Track 2, and so on. If you don't see the improvement you'd like after 2 weeks, you may need to move to a more aggressive dietary program. For example, if you don't see a significant change in your GPS score after 2 weeks on Track 1, it may be time to try Track 2. You will receive complete instructions on how to make these decisions in the chapter that outlines the track you are on. But before you get started on the diet, we want to briefly explain how to integrate lifestyle changes and gut-healing supplements over the next 2 weeks.

Step 2: Improve Your Lifestyle

After altering your diet, the next important step you need to take is improving your lifestyle. It's important that you begin to integrate the lifestyle changes we outlined in Chapter 5. Excess toxic exposure, stress, being too sedentary (or exercising too much), social isolation, and other lifestyle factors can wreak havoc on your gut. In Chapter 5, we reviewed some of the research that connects lifestyle to poor digestive health and outlined detoxification strategies, relaxation techniques, and other lifestyle changes to optimize your gut function, heal your body, and refresh your spirit.

Obviously, it won't be possible for you to integrate all of these changes over the next 2 weeks. However, you can take the time to start analyzing the ways in which your lifestyle has contributed to your illness and begin to make changes that lead you toward a healthier way of being in the world. For example, in Maria's case (see page 160), she began using mindful eating to slow herself down during mealtimes and then used deep breathing exercises to destress. We recommend you begin taking the same kinds of steps she did.

In Chapter 5, you completed The Inside Tract Lifestyle Survey (see page 103). This survey should guide you toward the changes you need to focus on over the next 2 weeks. We recommend that you start by addressing the lifestyle areas you scored highest on in that survey. If you scored high in all of them, just work on one change during the next 2 weeks and gradually integrate more lifestyle changes over time, just as Maria did.

Step 3: Add Gut-Healing Supplements

If you have a diagnosed digestive disease, it's a good idea to add supplements to your whole-foods eating plan to provide your body with some additional healing nutritional support. There is an excellent body of research that supports the use of nutraceutical supplementation as a means to heal a wide variety of digestive diseases. Nutraceuticals are effective and typically do not present the health risks that medications do.

You should begin taking your supplements at the same time that you start on the dietary plan you were assigned in Step 1. If you were assigned to Track 1, you probably don't need to take any other supplements except perhaps a good multivitamin/multimineral supplement (look for one with natural instead of synthetic folic acid) and vitamin D_3 (1,000 to 2,000 IUs each day). Otherwise, the vitamins and minerals you need should come from a wholesome diet. If you do have a diagnosed digestive illness, there are some additional supplements you can integrate that may help heal your GI tract. Those who are on Track 2 may require one or two supplements to improve. And those on Track 3 often require two or more supplements taken in combination.

Start by taking one of the supplements associated with your digestive illness as specified in the condition-specific supplement chart in Chapter 6. For example, in the case above, Maria first chose to take 3 milligrams of melatonin each day to help with her IBS symptoms, sleep, and mood. Although she experienced tremendous benefits from the melatonin, she was still having intermittent intestinal cramping. After 2 weeks had passed without abatement of her intestinal spasms, she then elected to begin supplementation with enteric-coated peppermint oil. This gave her an excellent result: relief!

Responses to supplement therapy are highly individualized, and not all supplements work the same for all people. That means you will need to experiment and test these supplements for yourself one at a time to find out what works best for you. With a bit of time and patience, you will find that some of the supplements in Chapter 6 provide powerful support on your path toward healing.

We have provided the Web sites for professional formulations that are designed to support digestive wellness and vitality in the supplements appendix at the back of the book. These products are from trusted sources who adhere to good manufacturing practices (GMPs) and maintain the highest quality standards.

Now turn to the chapter that corresponds to your dietary plan and start down your path toward a healthy gut and better life. We wish you well on the journey.

CHAPTER 8

TRACK 1:
THE FOUNDATIONAL FOOD PLAN

The Foundational Food Plan is built on nourishing foods that support your health and help heal mild digestive disorders. You arrived here because you scored between 0 and 25 on the GPS (see page 161). This indicates that Track 1 is your initial pathway to optimizing your gut health.

We recommend that you stay on this track for a minimum of 2 weeks. During that time, we highly encourage you to keep a journal, and we've included a sample for you to use to record your food and beverage intake along with physical, emotional, and lifestyle factors such as your elimination patterns, mood, and the quality of your sleep (refer to the Inside Tract Journal at www.theinsidetract.org). Tracking these factors will help you make connections between the foods you eat and how you feel.

At the end of 2 weeks, we recommend that you reassess your score. If your symptoms have improved, you should continue with the basic dietary principles of Track 1. It provides the foundation for a whole-foods, fiber-rich diet that leads to long-term health. This eating program is rooted in the proven dietary patterns typical of the healthiest regions of the world, and it provides pleasures, tastes, and textures you can enjoy for a lifetime! You can continue using the meal plan and recipes for this plan for as long as you like, or you can make up your own meals based on the Track 1 Foundational Food Guide (see page 167). After 2 months on the program, you should check your progress by taking the GPS once more. If your symptoms have abated, it means this diet is working for you and you can stay on it indefinitely.

If you do *not* experience a reduction in your symptoms after 2 weeks on Track 1 and your GPS score does not change, or it unexpectedly worsens, we recommend that you transition to the Track 2 Exclusion Food Plan outlined in Chapter 9.

PERILOUS PICKS

Check labels for the following ingredients.[1,2] They are widespread in packaged foods and personal care products, including toothpastes, supplements, and medications.

- ✓ Artificial flavorings and colorings
- ✓ Artificial sweeteners, including acesulfame-K, aspartame, neotame, saccharin, and sucralose
- ✓ Benzoic acid, benzoyl peroxide, and sodium benzoate
- ✓ Brominated vegetable oil (BVO)
- ✓ Butylated hydroxyanisole (BHA)
- ✓ Butylated hydroxytoluene (BHT)
- ✓ Carrageenan
- ✓ Corn syrup, or high-fructose corn syrup
- ✓ Gums, including arabic, furcelleran, ghatti, guar, karaya, locust bean, tragacanth, and xanthan
- ✓ Monosodium glutamate (MSG), often found in hydrolyzed vegetable protein (HVP) or hydrolyzed plant protein (HPP)
- ✓ Novel sweeteners such as neotame, tagatose, etc.
- ✓ Nitrates and nitrites, including sodium nitrate, postassium nitrate, sodium nitrite, and potassium nitrite
- ✓ Olestra
- ✓ Parabens
- ✓ Partially hydrogenated oils (trans fats)
- ✓ Polyols or sugar alcohols, including erythritol, lactitol, hydrogenated starch hydrolysate, isomalt, maltitol, mannitol, sorbitol, and xylitol
- ✓ Potassium bromate
- ✓ Propyl gallate
- ✓ Sulfites, including sodium metabisulfite, potassium metabisulfate, sodium bisulfite, potassium bisulfite, sodium sulfite, sodium dithionite, sulfurous acid, and sulfur dioxide
- ✓ Titanium dioxide

You'll need a handful of tools to follow the Track 1 plan. They are:

- **The Track 1 Foundational Food Guide.** This food chart is based on the three Fs—the foods you should **favor,** those you should eat **few** of, and those you should **forget** while on the program (see page 170).
- **The Track 1 Seasonal Menu Plans.** The seasonal menu plans will

provide you with delicious meals you can eat while on Track 1 (see page 175).

- **The Track 1 Foundational Swift & Simple Food Charts.** In addition to delicious recipes, we have provided you with a number of meals that are quick and easy to prepare and that require no recipes at all. These meals are integrated into the meal plan. You can also options. These can be found with the recipes (see page 252).
- **Track 1 Foundational Recipes.** Kathie has combined her own extensive knowledge of preparing healthy, delicious, healing meals with that of a number of professional chefs she works with to bring you a set of mouthwatering recipes that not only will help heal your gut but also will surprise and delight your palate. These can all be found in the recipes section (page 237) or in the Swift & Simple Food Charts (starting on page 240).

In this chapter, we will explain how to use these tools to help heal your gut. But first read about Francine (on page 168), a woman with digestive health problems who found that her healing began when she reintroduced herself to her kitchen.

The Track 1 Foundational Food Guide

Like Francine, you will need to reestablish a relationship with your kitchen and learn to rely on healthy, whole foods to successfully follow this plan. The first step is understanding which foods you can safely eat, which you should forget about, and which you can eat in moderation. The Foundational Food Guide will help you learn which foods and beverages are nourishing to you and which are offensive to your GI tract. The core ingredients of eating for nutritional integrity have been integrated into this navigational instrument, and it can be used as a compass to lead you toward healthy eating.

We've ordered the foods in the Foundational Food Guide to emphasize a high-plant-to-animal (P:A) ratio. Vegetables and fruits come first because they rank highest in terms of foods you want to make sure you include in your diet. Herbs and spices are included next so you'll remember to use them liberally for their flavorful and medicinal benefits. And plant protein (found in legumes, nuts, and seeds) is situated ahead of animal protein and dairy products to prompt you to think about plant foods first.

FRANCINE'S STORY: A STRANGER TO HER KITCHEN

Kathie first met Francine when she came to our integrative/functional med-icine center a few years ago. Francine worked long hours, ate most meals out, rarely got more than 4 or 5 hours of sleep, and had been to numerous integrative medicine practitioners seeking help for her chronic digestive distress. Francine was 45 pounds overweight and had a history of creeping weight gain that started after a bout of a food-borne illness 10 years ago. She also believed that event was a tipping point in her health.

As we talked, Francine also revealed that she was taking 30 different dietary supplements—a different one had been prescribed by each of the practitioners she had been to over the past 2 years. One of her most dis-turbing symptoms was nausea, which led her to delay eating until late after-noon, at which point she would binge on refined carbohydrates like bread and pretzels. It was clear to me that this was likely aggravating the bloating, gas, and abdominal pain she experienced so frequently.

We talked about her history and lifestyle, and during the course of our conversation she realized that she was overly dependent on nutraceuti-cals to resolve her gut issues because, as a naturally minded woman, she did not want to take pharmaceuticals. Somehow, she thought that dietary supplements alone could solve her intestinal ills. During our meeting, Francine began to understand that she had put her hopes in "taking something" to cure her condition rather than "making something" to help her heal. Francine shared that she rarely went into her kitchen anymore, and she ignored her own intuition that preparing her own food was the pathway to better health.

I encouraged Francine to take a supplement retreat for at least 1 week and to reacquaint herself with her kitchen during that time. We talked about specific strategies and developed a nutritional plan for the week. This included a whole-foods menu and an organized plan for shopping and cooking simple meals, much like the ones provided in this chapter. I sug-gested that she hold a private "grand opening celebration" in her kitchen. As our consultation closed, she commented, "Kathie, I feel like this was an answered prayer. I have known in my gut for some time that I needed to return to my kitchen. This feels like a holy experience in reclaiming my health." I smiled and assured her that it was certainly the prelude to a holistic health journey that begins in the most integrative healing center available: our very own kitchens. Francine realized that she had been rely-ing on pills, potions, and practitioners' well-intended advice while disre-garding her own healing instincts, and that her true path to healing led through her kitchen.

Whole grain choices are included next, while undeserving refined grain products are eliminated. In addition to the foods on the "Forget" list, you will also want to forget or exclude any foods that you have allergies or intolerances toward, or that you determine to be "highly suspect" in aggravating your unique inside tract or in causing symptoms such as nasal congestion, headaches, or skin rashes, among others. Here is how to determine whether or not specific foods are contributing to your digestive disease.

3/3 Guideline for Determining an Adverse Food Reaction

To figure out if a food is causing problems, and assuming that it has not caused a serious adverse food reaction (such as anaphylaxis or breathing difficulties), you can do a food challenge. Consume the suspect food on three different occasions. If you experience symptoms within 3 days of consuming this food *and* the symptoms occur consistently on three separate occasions after eating it, the food you suspect may indeed be a problem for you.[3]

For example, let's say you eat eggs and find that you have an upset stomach or headache. The first time this happens, it doesn't automatically mean that this is a problem food for you.

If eating eggs results in the same symptoms on two separate occasions (allowing at least 1 week between tests), you should place them on the "Forget" list, as it's likely that they are contributing to your digestive problems. That doesn't necessarily mean you need to write off eggs forever. As your GI tract heals and your gut barrier function strengthens, you should find that you can tolerate foods that were once offensive to you. You can test eggs (egg yolks separately from egg whites) again after 3 to 4 weeks. When reintroducing these foods, you always want to test the food in the purest form possible. Test eggs alone, not by eating eggs included in a baked good. If the food still causes problems for you, eliminate it for 3 to 4 weeks. Reassess, and if it still causes symptoms after your food challenge, you may consider eating it only every once in a while or stay away from it for the long term.

It is also worth noting that many different factors influence adverse food reactions, such as the form of the food (raw versus cooked), the amount of food consumed (small amounts may not impact you as much as larger amounts do), what the food is combined with (for example, alcohol may incite an adverse reaction from an otherwise benign food), as well as other factors such as stress, health status, medications, and environmental factors (i.e. pollen) you may be taking, and more. Thus, a food and symptom journal is a very useful tool for tracking down adverse food reactions.

The Track 1 Foundational Food Guide

FOOD GROUP	FAVOR	FEW	FORGET
Vegetables	• All fresh, frozen, or fermented (e.g., sauerkraut) varieties • Sea vegetables (arame, wakame, kombu, etc.) • Starchy vegetables: corn, green peas, parsnips, potatoes, rutabagas, sweet potatoes, winter squash (acorn, buttercup, butternut, delicata, etc.) • 100% juices (fresh preferred)	—	• Those that are breaded, creamed, fried tempura-style, or overcooked
Fruits	• All fresh or frozen	• Dried, unsweetened, sulfite-free (cranberries, currants, dates, figs, prunes, raisins, etc.) • 100% juices • Concentrates (blueberry, Concord grape, cranberry, pomegranate, etc.) • Water-packed canned (BPA-free cans)	• Beverages • Canned in syrups • Jams and jellies, regular and sugar-free or artificially sweetened
Herbs and Spices	• Fresh or dried	—	• Mixes or seasonings with unacceptable food ingredients

(Continued)

The Track 1 Foundational Food Guide (cont.)

FOOD GROUP	FAVOR	FEW	FORGET
Legumes (plant protein)	• Beans, split peas, and lentils • Peanuts • Nonhydrogenated, unsweetened peanut butter • Soy (tofu, edamame, miso, tempeh)	—	• Beans, peas, lentils, peanuts, and soy foods with added sugars and other unacceptable ingredients • Highly processed soy foods or other vegetable protein products (soy hot dogs, soy chips, soy bacon, etc.) • Textured vegetable protein (TVP) and hydrolyzed vegetable protein (HVP) used for vegetarian meat substitutes, veggie burgers, etc.
Nuts and Seeds	• Nuts: almonds, Brazil nuts, cashews, hazelnuts (filberts), macadamias, pecans, pine nuts (pignolias), pistachios, walnuts, etc. • Seeds: chia, flax, pumpkin, sesame, sunflower, etc. • Nonhydrogenated, unsweetened nut and seed butters (almond, tahini, etc.)	—	• Nut and seed butters made with partially hydrogenated oils, peanut oil, or added sugars • Nut and seed products with unacceptable ingredients

(Continued)

The Track 1 Foundational Food Guide (cont.)

FOOD GROUP	FAVOR	FEW	FORGET
Whole Grains and Whole Grain Products	• Amaranth • Barley • Buckwheat • Corn, polenta • Millet • Oats, steel-cut and rolled • Quinoa • Rice (basmati, brown, black, Indian ricegrass, red, wild) • Rye • Sorghum • Teff • Triticale • Whole wheat • 100% whole grain products (bread, cereal, pasta, crackers, etc.) made from the grains above	—	• Refined grain products, such as low-fiber cereals (containing less than 5 g per serving), crackers, semolina pasta, white or wheat breads, and other grain products that do not have 100% whole grain listed as the primary ingredient
Animal Protein (pasture-raised, organic, wild caught)	• Eggs • Fish, wild caught (salmon, cod, halibut, etc.) or sustainably farmed (tilapia, oysters) • Poultry (chicken, turkey, duck without skin) • Shellfish (crab, lobster, shrimp) • Wild game	• Lean cuts of meat (beef, bison, lamb, pork) • Lean sausage, without nitrates (e.g., organic chicken sausage)	• Fatty cuts of meat (beef, pork, lamb) • Poultry with skin • Processed meat and poultry products (hot dogs, deli meats, canned meat products, bacon, ham, pepperoni, etc.)

(Continued)

The Track 1 Foundational Food Guide (cont.)

FOOD GROUP	FAVOR	FEW	FORGET
Dairy and Dairy-Free Alternatives (organic)	• Cultured dairy products: acidophilus milk, buttermilk, cheese, cottage cheese, kefir, sour cream, yogurt • Dairy-free alternatives: almond (or other nut), coconut, hempseed, oat, rice, and soy beverages, kefirs, yogurts	• Butter • Ghee • Milk (skim, low fat, whole)	• Cream • Frozen yogurt • Half-and-half • Ice cream • Margarine • Milk, condensed • Nondairy creamers • Sherbet • Whipped cream
Fats and Oils	• Extra-virgin olive oil	• Cold expeller-pressed oils: almond, canola, coconut, flaxseed, grape seed, palm, pumpkin, safflower, sesame, sunflower, and walnut	• Cottonseed oil • Lard • Peanut oil • Shortenings
Condiments/ Staples	• Arrowroot • Baking powder (aluminum-free) • Baking soda • Chutney • Cocoa powder • 100% pure flavor extracts (almond, orange, maple, etc.) • Horseradish • Ketchup • Mayonnaise • Mustard • Pesto • Sundried tomato paste • Vinegars (apple cider, balsamic, red wine, rice) • Wasabi powder	• High-sodium condiments: miso, soy sauce, tamari, Worcestershire sauce	• Any condiments/ staples with unacceptable ingredients

(Continued)

The Track 1 Foundational Food Guide (cont.)

FOOD GROUP	FAVOR	FEW	FORGET
Beverages	• Water • Coconut water • Coffee substitutes: grain beverages (barley, chicory, malted barley, rye) • Decaffeinated tea (black, green, white) • Herbal teas: chamomile, fennel, ginger, lavender, licorice, peppermint, etc.	• Red wine • Regular coffee and tea	• Energy drinks • Fruit beverages and juice drinks/ades • Sodas, regular and diet • Beverages with unacceptable ingredients
Sweets and Sweeteners	• Cocoa nibs • Dark chocolate, 70% or more	• Fruit sweeteners, 100% fruit juice concentrates • Maple syrup, 100% natural • Agave nectar • Blackstrap molasses • Brown rice syrup • Evaporated cane juice • Honey • Stevia	• Candy: regular, sugar-free, sugarless, or artificially sweetened • Desserts made with white sugars, refined flours, solid fats: cakes, cookies, doughnuts, pastries, pies, etc. • Sugar-free, artificially sweetened foods and sugarless gums • All sugar substitutes, artificial sweeteners, and sugar alcohols

The Track 1 Seasonal Menu Plans

Now that you know which foods to focus on and which to limit, the next step is to learn *what* to eat on the program. The Track 1 plan is a 7-day, seasonal approach to nourishment. We have provided you with rotational menus for Spring and Summer as well as for Fall and Winter. They include seasonal vegetarian and nonvegetarian options inspired by the healthiest diets in the world. Functional foods that have long track records of promoting digestive wellness, including dark greens, brassica vegetables, wild cold-water fish, legumes, and extra-virgin olive oil, as well as sensational spices like turmeric and healing herbs like parsley, are just some of the enticing ingredients to please your palate.

The first week you are on the program, just follow the menu that corresponds to the season you are currently in. Starting with the second week (and for as long as you stay on this plan), you can rotate the meals in any order you like. These flavorful menus contain many ingredients that you might not have purchased previously. Stocking your pantry and maintaining an inventory of "standard stock" items such as dried herbs and spices, beans and lentils, healthy oils, and a few other favorite staples is a time-saving and health-promoting practice that you will come to enjoy. Envision your pantry as your personal assistant to good health. To find out what to stock your pantry with, see the shopping lists starting on page 296. Keep your pantry stocked with these items and you'll have no trouble cooking up healthy meals any night of the week.

Even after you have stocked your pantry, it's likely you will need to shop more frequently to keep up with this meal plan. Don't be put off by this! Remember, it's essential that you reestablish your relationships with food, your kitchen, and your body if you want to heal your inside tract. That may mean reworking your personal schedule to secure more time for nourishing your body. If that's what it takes, we encourage you to do it. The healing benefits of using the freshest ingredients cannot be understated. What's more, you may discover (as so many do) that this approach to planning, shopping, and preparing your meals is likely to decrease your food costs, diminish your food waste, and prevent you from finding those ghastly, squishy, unidentifiable food objects (UFOs) decaying in your crisper.

Most of the recipes (which begin on page 252) take less than 30 minutes to prepare from start to finish. There's no need to buy fancy gizmos and gadgets to make these meals. Taking a minimalist approach in your healing center will actually maximize your efficiency. By outfitting your kitchen with a few essential culinary tools, you'll find you can shave precious minutes off meal preparation (see "Clean, Green, and Sustainable Kitchen Checklist" for recommendations).

Glass storage bowls are included on the kitchen minimalist list to ensure safe food storage. In addition, we recommend that you use refrigerated leftovers within 48 hours so that mold spores do not have a chance to proliferate, as they can be bothersome to a sensitive inside tract. If you need to store foods longer, go ahead and freeze them in freezer-safe glass containers.

All of the recipes and Swift & Simple Food Charts are in the recipes section beginning on page 240. The weekly menus are on page 178. Refer to the individual recipes for explicit instructions on how to make all of the meals in the menu plans.

Ready, Set . . . Shop, Chop, and Cook

You now have the tools and tactics you need in order to implement the Track 1 Foundational Food Plan. Your journey to improved gut health is about to begin in the kitchen, your center of health, healing, and culinary happiness. We hope you savor the experience and take some pleasure in this healing expedition, one nourishing bite at a time.

CLEAN, GREEN, AND SUSTAINABLE KITCHEN CHECKLIST

Following are a few essential cooking tools for your kitchen.
- ✓ Blender
- ✓ Cast-iron skillet, unseasoned
- ✓ Slow cooker
- ✓ Food processor
- ✓ Glass mixing bowls and bakeware
- ✓ Knives
- ✓ Mortar and pestle
- ✓ Pressure cooker
- ✓ Rice cooker (stainless steel)
- ✓ Stainless steel cookware
- ✓ Water filter (reverse osmosis, activated charcoal, or carbon)
- ✓ Wooden and stainless steel cooking utensils
- ✓ Wooden cutting board

Start using the following techniques as you "green" your kitchen:
- ✓ Avoid cookware with aluminum or nonstick surfaces; use cast iron and stainless steel for stove-top cooking.
- ✓ Eliminate soft plastic storage containers. Switch to glass for long-term water and food storage.
- ✓ Filter tap water for drinking and for use in cooking.
- ✓ Try using natural cleaning agents, including baking soda, hydrogen peroxide, lemon rind, and white vinegar.

To learn more about green cooking, check out the Environmental Working Group Web site (www.ewg.org) and Planet Green (www.planetgreen. discovery.com).

Track 1 Spring/Summer Menu Plan

	DAY 1	DAY 2	DAY 3
Breakfast	Poached Eggs with Herb Spread (page 253)	Berry Yogurt Parfait (page 254)	Morning Muesli (page 255)
Lunch	Black and Red Salad (page 259)	Shrimp Cashew Salad (Swift & Simple Salads, page 246)	Chickpea Avocado Salad (Swift & Simple Salads, page 246)
Dinner	Turkey Herb Burger (page 260) Gerardo's Gazpacho (page 260) Cabbage Salad (page 261)	Dilled Lemon Mustard Chicken (page 262) Summer Squash (page 262) Arugula salad	Macadamia Nut–Crusted Cod (page 263) Pineapple Black Rice (page 263) Steamed asparagus
Treats	–	Swift Energy Bar (page 272)	–

Track 1 Fall/Winter Menu Plan

	DAY 1	DAY 2	DAY 3
Breakfast	Walnut Raisin Steel-Cut Oats Power Porridge (Swift & Simple Power Porridges, page 242)	Southwestern Egg Wrap (page 268)	Sunrise Patty (page 268)
Lunch	Luscious Lentil Soup (page 274)	Salmon Barley Bowl (Swift & Simple Bowls, page 248)	Wild Rice Escarole Bowl (Swift & Simple Bowls, page 248)
Dinner	Mediterranean Turkey Meatballs with Whole Grain Pasta and Marinara Sauce (page 276) Sautéed Lacinato kale	Sage Roasted Chicken and Root Vegetables (page 276)	Vegetarian Black Bean Chili (page 277)
Snacks/ Treats	Lemon Ginger Cookie (page 271)	–	–

	DAY 4	DAY 5	DAY 6	DAY 7
	Herb Scramble (page 255)	Melon with Minted Yogurt (page 256)	Layers of Lox (page 257)	Lemon Cottage Cheese Pancakes (page 257)
	Curried Chicken Wrap (Swift & Simple Wraps, page 244)	White Bean Antipasto Salad (Swift & Simple Salads, page 246)	Turkey Avocado Crème Wrap (Swift & Simple Wraps, page 244)	Lentil Spinach Salad (Swift & Simple Salads, page 246)
	Broccoli Rabe and White Beans on Whole Grain Pasta (page 264) Greek Salad (page 264)	Grilled Wild Salmon (page 265) Green Beans with Slivered Almonds (page 266) Mesclun green salad	Lamb* or Beef* Vegetable Kabobs (page 266) Minted Brown Rice (page 267) Dandelion greens *Tofu or Tempeh (Veg Option)	Cilantro Cumin Tilapia (page 267) Baked Sweet Potato (page 291) Steamed broccoli
	—	Fruit Crisp (page 271)	—	Berry Delicious Slush (page 270)

	DAY 4	DAY 5	DAY 6	DAY 7
	Banana Sunflower Seed Log (page 269)	Almond Apple Amaranth Power Porridge (Swift & Simple Power Porridges, page 242)	Herb Scramble (page 255)	Layers of Lox (page 257)
	Soothing Chicken Soup (page 275)	Arugula Bulgur Bowl (Swift & Simple Bowls, page 248)	Turkey Avocado Crème Wrap (Swift & Simple Wraps, page 244)	Hummus Veggie Wrap (Swift & Simple Wraps, page 244)
	Citrus Salmon (page 278) Black rice Steamed asparagus	Lamb or Beet Vegetable Winter Stew (page 279)	Herbed White Fish (page 280) Roasted butternut squash Steamed green beans	Thai Shrimp and Vegetable Sauté (page 281) Brown rice Fresh pineapple
	—	—	Chocolate Cherry Chew (page 273)	—

CHAPTER 9

Track 2:
The Exclusion Food Plan

While the Track 1 Foundational Food Plan lays the groundwork for healthy eating, Track 2 entails a comprehensive elimination diet for a period of at least 2 weeks, followed by assessment and food reintroduction. This is why we call it "The Exclusion Food Plan." Your GPS score of 26 to 50 guided you to this pathway to personal healing. The purpose of Track 2 is to reduce the burden on your immune system and lessen your body's toxic load through the avoidance of foods that are sending "alarm and harm" messages with each bite that you take. These distress signals or adverse reactions to foods can result in a constellation of symptoms including headaches, behavioral changes, mouth sores, skin rashes, fluid retention, and other bothersome physical signs. Adverse food reactions can also contribute to an assortment of digestive disorders such as eosinophilic esophagitis, irritable bowel syndrome (IBS), inflammatory bowel disease (IBD), celiac disease, and more. The elimination diet outlined in this chapter offers hope and can spell relief for many health problems. It should be the first line of therapy for healing most moderate digestive disorders.

Unfortunately, elimination or exclusion diets are not widely accepted as a standard of care in conventional medicine today. This is largely because nutrition ranks very low on the totem pole of medical education and most doctors are unaware of this effective treatment. An elimination diet is an important tool for healing patients who have been from one doctor to another with a whole list of symptoms that have gone unresolved. If a drug showed as much promise as the elimination diet does for restoring a person's health, it would be the best-selling drug of all time. Recent guidelines published by an expert panel on food allergies and intolerances emphasize that the elimination diet is the gold standard of care.[1]

The specific details of the Track 2 Exclusion Food Plan are outlined on the next page. They include:

- **The Track 2 Exclusion Food Guide.** As with Track 1, we have laid out a food guide based on the three Fs (foods you should favor, foods you should eat few of, and foods you should forget), but as you will see, there are some additional considerations you need to make when undergoing an elimination diet like this. Everything will be explained in detail in the pages that follow.
- **The Track 2 Seasonal Menu Plans.** The seasonal menu plans for this track will provide you with delicious meals while helping you avoid the foods that most people find cause digestive distress.
- **The Track 2 Exclusion Swift & Simple Food Charts.** In addition to delicious recipes, we have provided you with a number of meals that are quick and easy to prepare and that require no recipes at all. These meals are integrated into the meal plan. You can also substitute any meal during the week for one of these quick-and-easy options. These can be found with the recipes (see pages 240–251).
- **The Track 2 Exclusion Recipes.** The recipes for this plan will delight your palate while avoiding the foods that may be contributing to your digestive troubles. Contrary to popular belief, you can make extraordinary meals while avoiding ingredients like gluten, dairy, and corn, to name a few common culprits. These recipes will teach you how to do this.

In a moment, we'll take a look at the particulars of the comprehensive elimination approach that will help you reclaim your health. But first, we want to tell the story of a man who was suffering from a long list of health problems and who found healing on the same kind of exclusion food plan (see page 192).

The Track 2 Exclusion Elimination Diet

In recent years, there's been a surge of adverse reactions to foods and a dramatic increase in food allergies and intolerances that cause digestive distress and a host of other systemic problems. We discussed these food sensitivities in Chapter 4 and explained some of the mechanisms by which they lead to digestive distress and other health problems. Track 2 is designed to eliminate some of the common food allergens that lead to gut

JIM'S STORY

Jim and his wife, Maggie, had decided to clean up their diets when they became pregnant with their first child. They became avid label readers; started to eat less animal fat by reducing their meat, milk, and cheese consumption; ate out less frequently; and even brown-bagged lunches to help ensure a higher intake of fruits and vegetables. In spite of these nutritional renovations, Jim continued to be plagued with chronic digestive, skin, and sinus problems for years. Their concerns grew about 5 years after their children were born, because one suffered from asthma while another had eczema and chronic ear infections. They felt that diet might be at the root of their health problems, but they couldn't pinpoint the problems in their diet. In spite of their efforts to eat well, Jim and his children did not feel well.

Kathie reviewed Jim's medical and dietary history and uncovered food-related clues from his childhood, including colic as a baby, chronic ear infections, skin rashes, and episodes of intermittent fevers. As a teenager, he suffered from acne, fatigue, chronic sinus infections, and—in his own words— "bowels that just weren't right." Jim had learned to live with these frustrating symptoms and had accepted that feeling lousy was "normal."

I explained to Jim and Maggie that a change in diet could make a big difference in Jim's chronic health problems, and I recommended that Jim begin the Track 2 Exclusion Food Plan. Maggie and Jim both wondered if this was something the whole family could follow, since they did not want to cook different meals for each person and believed in family mealtimes together. I explained to them that Track 2 was designed to be a healthy way of eating, even for children, as long as their energy needs for growth were met through the portions served. I suggested that we set up a separate appointment to review the children's health, with input from their pediatrician.

Jim and Maggie were excited about giving Track 2 a try and were curious as to what it entailed and what it *included*. I smiled, appreciating that people want to know *what they can eat*—not just what they need to exclude.

---

problems. The idea is to reduce the toxic and inflammatory load on your system, thereby giving your gut a chance to heal. Foods you will eliminate on Track 2 include:

- Corn
- Dairy
- Eggs
- Gluten (wheat, rye, barley, spelt, kamut, triticale)
- Peanuts

I explained the fundamentals of this plan and provided Jim and Maggie with the necessary tools for this dietary trial. I encouraged them to take some time to read over the materials and menus provided and assured them that even if it took a week or two to prepare for the journey, it was time well spent because planning and organizing are key to successful dietary change. I had no doubt that Track 2 was going to be helpful to Jim's inside tract, and I was also confident that it would be beneficial for the entire family.

I met with Jim and Maggie about 2 weeks after they started their Exclusive Food Plan. Jim's GPS score had already improved, and he related that he could not believe the difference in his bowels. He also noted that his energy was up a notch, even though he had previously thought his low energy levels were due to stress at work. We talked about some of the challenges they'd encountered, such as learning to avoid gluten and dairy favorites like bread, spaghetti, and ice cream, and I taught them some tricks for managing pizza night out with the kids. After strategizing and coming up with solutions to some of their problems, they agreed that the noticeable changes in Jim's energy and bowels were good signs and that they would continue on this plan for a few more weeks.

Two weeks later, Jim and Maggie returned for a follow-up visit. Jim's GPS continued to improve, and they were pleased to report that, in spite of a few hurdles, they were starting to see tremendous differences in Jim's energy and elimination patterns.

After 2 more weeks on the plan, they began to systematically reintroduce foods to see which were affecting Jim. They found that both dairy products and foods containing gluten caused severe distress when they were reintroduced. He was, however, okay with eggs and was now able to eat all of the fruits and vegetables in the "Few" category as often as he liked.

By our last consultation, Jim and Maggie had adapted to the change in diet and were enjoying the new foods and recipes so much that they didn't miss a thing! They also believed that this way of eating would eventually improve their children's health, and they had their pediatrician's blessing and watchful curiosity.

- Shellfish
- Alcohol
- Coffee (sorry!)

In addition to these foods, we also recommend that you eliminate the top four "FODMAPs" foods. If you've never heard of the term "FOD-MAPs," don't worry. It refers to certain carbohydrates that may be poorly absorbed when the gut is not in top-notch shape. We will explain more about the term, which foods these are, and precisely what you need to eliminate to avoid them (see page 189).

Understand that Track 2 does not attempt to eliminate *all* potential food allergens and intolerances, as this would make the plan unnecessarily restrictive. There are many different types of elimination diets used by dietitians, nutritionists, and integrative health practitioners, and the restrictions recommended by any given practitioner can range from the exclusion of one food (such as eggs), to a group of foods (such as dairy), to specific chemical constituents in foods (such as biogenic amines—histamines or tyramines, salicylates, etc.), to a mix of all of the above and even more. We created our elimination diet based on the best of science to date coupled with years of treating many patients with digestive disorders. For most of you, eliminating these foods is likely to reduce your symptoms. However, if you do not get better on this plan, you may require further dietary modifications. We will explain how to determine that in a moment.

Let's start by looking more carefully at the foods you are going to eliminate.

Foods to Eliminate on Track 2

Here is a review of some of the dietary ruffians that are removed from the Track 2 plan.

DAIRY

Adverse reactions to milk and milk products are quite common and can result in a number of symptoms in the gastrointestinal tract, including bloating, pain, gas, diarrhea, constipation, nausea, vomiting, and occasionally blood in the stool. Skin reactions such as eczema, hives, and tissue swelling, as well as respiratory tract symptoms such as nasal congestion or asthma also occur in some people when they consume milk and milk products. "Dairy exclusion" in Track 2 refers to the elimination of cow, goat, and sheep milk and their related products (cheese, yogurt, cottage cheese, cream, butter, etc.). There are a number of proteins in these milk products that can cause allergic reactions and inflame the gastrointestinal tract. Casein proteins represent the major proteins in dairy and are often the most problematic. The digestion of a particular type of casein protein (A1 beta-casein) has been shown to yield an opioid, narcoticlike product that has been associated with behavioral and autoimmune problems. In addition, intolerance to the chief carbohydrate in milk (lactose) can wreak havoc on your gut and contribute to your inside tract grief. This is due to a lack of the enzyme lactase, which is responsible for breaking down the lactose into a more digestible form. Those who are not lactose intolerant can be lactose sensitive, so even if you don't have a diagnosed milk allergy, it may still be a problem for you.

You may be wondering how you can live without your favorite cheese or glass of skim milk every morning. Don't fret! There are many delicious nondairy alternatives that you can enjoy, and they have been integrated into your Track 2 meal plan and recipes. As you try these new foods, remind your taste buds to be patient since some, like almond or hempseed beverages, may be unfamiliar to you. New tastes *can* be acquired, so give these new foods a number of tries and you will likely find that their flavors soon appeal to you. Remember the sage advice we give to our children when we are introducing them to new foods in their diets: Try it, you just might like it!

EGGS

These highly nutritious foods have golden yolks loaded with choline (a member of the B-vitamin family that's essential for neurological health), carotenoids like lutein and zeaxanthin (vital to your eye health), and a host of other nutritional jewels. Although eggs are the traditional symbol of fertility, they can also be food villains and provoke your inside tract. Eggs are one of the top eight food allergens. That is not to say that everyone is allergic to eggs, but many people are sensitive to them. The egg whites, which contain more of the proteins, may be more problematic than the yolks. However, there can be some cross-contamination between the white and the yolk, so we recommend eliminating all eggs and any egg ingredients lurking in your pantry or refrigerator. This includes baked goods and even some egg substitutes that are basically colored egg whites. While chicken eggs are most common in our culture, it's worth noting that eggs from many other species contain similar proteins. For this reason, all eggs are eliminated on Track 2, including the eggs of ducks, quail, and other birds.

WHEAT

Grains contain a number of proteins that can be responsible for adverse food reactions. Wheat is our most frequently consumed grain, and it is the primary ingredient in most breads, cereals, pastas, crackers, and other flour-based goodies. This "staff of life" may also irritate our inside tracts because wheat is rich in problematic proteins including gliadins and glutenins, which comprise the "gluten" complex. Wheat also contains high levels of fructans, which are in the FODMAPs family of foods discussed on page 189.

GLUTEN

On Track 2, you will also "forget" gluten. As you learned in Chapter 3, there are varying degrees of gluten sensitivity. The level of your sensitivity (assuming that you have one) will determine how harsh gluten's impact is on your inside tract. A gluten assault can cause your gut to become leaky, destroy the nutrient-absorbing carpet of villi in your small intestine, and disrupt your microflora. Individuals with celiac disease are especially susceptible to the ravages of gluten and must meticulously avoid it, because even minute amounts of this toxic protein can cause the body to turn on itself. If you have been diagnosed with celiac disease, we highly recommend that you work with a registered dietitian/licensed nutritionist, as every speck of gluten can jeopardize your health. In a personal consultation, one of these specialists can cover a number of different recommendations that are outside the scope of this book. An excellent, up-to-date guide for troubleshooting and thriving gluten-free is *Real Life with Celiac Disease* by Melinda Dennis, MS, RD, LDN, and Daniel Leffler, MD, MS.

However, even if you haven't been diagnosed with celiac disease, gluten may still be a problem for you. The tricky thing with gluten is that it can do its damage covertly and you might not even realize the harm it's causing until you eliminate it. This is why sensitivity to gluten is sometimes referred to as the "gluten syndrome or spectrum," because the outcome of its rampage on the inside tract varies from one individual to another. To preclude problems with gluten, we recommend that you eliminate it from your diet during this plan. The most common sources of gluten in your diet include wheat, rye, barley, kamut, spelt, triticale, and products made from any of these grains.

You may be thinking, "Oh dear, there goes that whole wheat bread I switched to in an effort to boost my fiber intake, and out go those whole rye crackers I thought were so good and that barley risotto I was eating to help lower my cholesterol." No worries! Eating gluten-free is an adventure that is well worth embarking on, as there are a number of whole grains and

GLUTEN IN DISGUISE

Gluten can be hidden in many processed food products. Your best insurance against consuming it is to avoid processed foods. However, now and then we all may rely on a packaged food such as a cereal, vegetable broth, nondairy beverage, condiment, or energy bar. Thus, it's smart to orient yourself to some of the places gluten can be hiding, since food manufacturers are not yet required to clearly label products that contain gluten. But keep a watch out for changes down the road, as more consumers have demanded that the government provide clarity and consistency on food labels when it comes to gluten. In the meantime, check the Gluten-Free Certification Organization Web site at www.gfco.org. This organization independently certifies products that meet the requirements of being gluten-free, defined as containing less than 20 parts per million (ppm) gluten in the product.

Gluten can be hidden in many food items, so check these and other products carefully before using them.

- ✓ **Baking powder:** Some brands do contain gluten, so look for those that are marked gluten-free.
- ✓ **Candy:** Wheat flour or starch may be used in the process of making candy or used as an ingredient.
- ✓ **Citric acid:** This can be fermented from wheat, corn, molasses, or beets.
- ✓ **Coffee:** Some flavored coffee drinks use wheat as a flavor carrier, but pure coffee is gluten-free.
- ✓ **Flavorings:** Natural flavorings are usually gluten-free, but some flavorings may contain wheat.
- ✓ **Miso:** This may be made from barley or rice koji that contains whole wheat flour.
- ✓ **Seitan:** This vegan meat alternative is pure wheat gluten.
- ✓ **Seasonings:** Packaged seasoning mixes usually contain wheat flour, and it may not be listed on the label.
- ✓ **Soba noodles:** These usually contain wheat. Look for 100 percent buckwheat noodles or rice noodles.
- ✓ **Soy sauce:** Contains wheat. Look for tamari that is labeled gluten-free.

Check www.celiac.com for a more extensive list of ingredients that may contain gluten.

starchy vegetables that do not contain these pesky proteins. The gluten-free grains in this plan include:

- Amaranth
- Buckwheat
- Millet
- Oats
- Quinoa

- Rice (all types)
- Sorghum
- Teff
- Wild rice

A quick word about oats, as they have been the topic of debate in the gluten-free-diet world for decades: Oats contain another protein, called avenin, that might also damage the villi in susceptible individuals. Some celiac-focused organizations call for the elimination of oats to be on the safe side. These days, though, you can easily obtain certified gluten-free oats from companies like Bob's Red Mill and Hodgson Mill. We recommend certified gluten-free oats in Track 2. So, yes, you can look forward to that morning bowl of oatmeal, which is rich in soluble fiber. However, as always, pay attention to your body's response. If you suspect that even gluten-free oats might be problematic, you can enjoy another morning option.

CORN

This plant, once revered by the native Pueblos and central to their "meaning of life,"[2] has been the subject of intense debate in recent years. Corn has been in the hot seat, nutritionally speaking, for various reasons—including its implication in adverse reactions and irritable bowel syndrome.[3] It has also been scrutinized and scorned as a crop that went from right to ruin due to genetic modification and extensive and inappropriate use as an animal feed staple, as well as for its insidious infiltration into our food supply in its fictitious form: high-fructose corn syrup (HFCS). Track 2 eliminates the major sources of corn, including the vegetable itself, cornmeal, corn syrup, corn oil, cornstarch, grits, hominy, maize, polenta, and succotash. It's been claimed by Michael Pollan that our entire food supply is contaminated with corn, but you can reduce your load by following this plan and scouting out the major sources of corn that could be contributing to your GI symptoms. If you suspect that you are highly sensitive to corn, you may want to obtain a comprehensive list of corn-containing products, available from the Web site www.cornallergens.com.

Peanuts

Although often referred to as a nut, peanuts are botanically unrelated to tree nuts. Peanuts belong to the legume family, along with peas, chickpeas, lentils, and other beans. Peanut allergies can be severe and sometimes life-threatening, especially in children, and any parent who has a child with a peanut allergy knows the due diligence one must take to ensure a peanut-free environment. Some adults may also experience respiratory or digestive problems with peanut consumption. Thus, we have eliminated peanuts from this food plan.

Shellfish

Fish and shellfish contain abundant amounts of many nutrients, including vitamin B_{12}, vitamin B_6, niacin, selenium, zinc, and iron. Yet, it has been our experience that crustaceans (which include crab, lobster, shrimp, and prawns) and mollusks or bivalves (which include clams, mussels, and scallops) might pose problems for some. Shellfish is considered one of the top eight food allergens and has therefore been eliminated from this plan. However, you can enjoy other species of fish unless you find you react adversely.

FODMAPs

FODMAPs is a novel dietary intervention that eliminates a group of carbohydrates and sugars that may be poorly absorbed and cause "functional gut symptoms"—primarily gas and bloat. FODMAPs is an acronym for Fermentable Oligo-, Di-, and Monosaccharides and Polyols.[4] While that may sound complicated, what it really refers to is a group of foods that contain easily fermentable, short-chain sugars that increase fluid delivery into your large bowel, resulting in gas, pain, bloat, and other troubling symptoms. Research indicates that reducing your intake of these foods often significantly improves digestive distress.

The FODMAPs include:

- **Lactose:** Dairy products such as milk, yogurt, cottage cheese, ice cream, etc.
- **Fructose:** High-fructose corn syrup (HFCS), agave, and honey; certain fresh fruits, such as apples, pears, peaches, mangoes, watermelon, and coconut; dried fruits; and fruit juices.

- **Fructans:** Wheat and rye; inulin and fructooligosaccharides added to food products as a fiber supplement; certain vegetables, such as artichokes, asparagus, beetroot, broccoli, Brussels sprouts, cabbage, chicory, garlic, leeks, okra, onions, radicchio, lettuce, shallots, and snow peas.
- **Galactans:** Chickpeas, lentils, kidney beans, and soy products; certain vegetables, such as broccoli.
- **Polyols:** Sweeteners such as xylitol, sorbitol, mannitol, maltitol, and isomalt found in sugar-free gums, mints, and candies; certain fruits, such as apples, apricots, blackberries, cherries, nectarines, peaches, pears, plums, prunes, and watermelon; certain vegetables, such as cauliflower, white button mushrooms, and snow peas.

Obviously, whole foods are prevalent in the diet, and for good reason: When your inside tract is in fine working order, eating these fruits, vegetables, and whole grains provides your friendly flora with valuable nutrients that they then ferment into beneficial substances. However, when your microflora are imbalanced, your gut microbes feast on these FODMAPs too aggressively. This out-of-control microbial feeding frenzy exceeds your tolerable threshold for the amount of FODMAPs your gut can handle—thus the gas, bloating, and cramping so common in people who have become sensitive to these foods.

Understand that this doesn't mean you need to eliminate *all* FODMAPs. Many of these foods, such as the cruciferous or brassica family of vegetables (broccoli, Brussels sprouts, cabbage, cauliflower, etc.) are vitally important to your health. That's why we recommend an approach similar to that of Dr. William Chey, co-editor-in-chief of the *American Journal of Gastroenterology* and professor of internal medicine at the University of Michigan Health System. Dr. Chey notes that, "paying attention to the total FODMAPs load in the diet often significantly improves GI symptoms."[5]

While on Track 2, we ask you to remove the FODMAPs foods that may be most problematic such as wheat, apples, pears, and raw onions. In addition, we strongly encourage you to consider the following:

1. **Remember that the dose is often the detriment.** The total amount of FODMAPs any one person can handle is extremely

individualized. We suggest you tailor your consumption of these foods based on your experiences with them. We recommend you use a journal to track your reactions to the foods you eat while on Track 2.

Carefully consider FODMAPs as you do this. Do you experience symptoms when eating foods from the previous list? If so, limit them. Choose Track 2 recipes that do not contain these foods.

2. **Eat ripe fruit.** Studies show that unripe fruit is more problematic than ripe fruit.
3. **Consider the preparation method.** Raw foods seem to be more problematic than cooked foods.
4. **Watch your total FODMAP load.** Eating a FODMAP-heavy meal may induce symptoms. Be sure not to overdo the amount of FODMAPs you consume at one time.

For most of you, simply following the Track 2 Meal Plan will suffice. However, if you continue to experience symptoms or notice that certain FODMAPs foods are contributing to your digestive distress, don't hesitate to tailor the plan to your needs by further limiting or even eliminating these foods.

Research will continue to determine which foods wreak the most havoc on an unconditioned GI tract. In the meantime, the guidelines above offer an intelligent and moderate approach to the treatment of FODMAPs.

COFFEE

Drinking coffee is an aromatic ritual, and we have heard more patients proclaim that they are willing to do anything to reclaim their health, but don't ask them to give up their coffee! Not everyone has an adverse reaction to coffee. In fact, research is brewing that indicates that moderate consumption of this energetic bean may be beneficial for people with Parkinson's disease and type 2 diabetes. But when it comes to our inside tracts, coffee—especially caffeinated coffee—may act as a gastric irritant and increase irritable bowel symptoms, so we recommend a coffee retreat, done sensibly. If you are used to drinking more than two cups of caffeinated coffee per day, gradually decrease your amount. You can substitute a cup of green tea for one of your cups of coffee on the first day, and then, over a period of a few days, continue to decrease the amount of coffee you consume until you are coffee-free.

ALCOHOL

Each of us may have a unique response to metabolizing alcohol. However, beer, wine, and distilled spirits are known irritants to the gastrointestinal tract, and therefore they are prohibited on Track 2. If you are someone who enjoys one or two alcoholic beverages daily, this warrants a major change in your habits.

Alcohol, coffee, diet sodas, and sugar-laden beverages are some of the most addictive substances, and removing them requires a serious commitment, an understanding of their hold on your health, and constant consciousness to maintain abstinence amid an alluring environment where these items are omnipresent. We know that you will do your best!

OTHER CONSIDERATIONS

Because your inside tract is one of a kind, it is important to keep a food journal and tailor the plan to your unique responses. While this is a comprehensive elimination food plan, there may be some food items that are problematic for you that we did not exclude. A core principle of our nutrition approach in this book is to pay attention to your body's distress signals and avoid any suspect foods that you believe you may be reacting adversely to.

We discussed the golden rule for determining an adverse reaction to food in Chapter 8, but it bears repeating here: If you suspect that you may be sensitive to a food not eliminated on this plan, try the suspect food three different times. If symptoms occur consistently each time you eat the food (within 3 days of ingesting it), it should be considered an adverse reaction and excluded from your diet for at least 2 weeks. For example, if you suspect tomatoes or tomato products, don't forgo these nutrient-dense foods until you have tested them. Eat tomatoes on three separate occasions. If you consistently experience symptoms within 3 days of consuming tomatoes, then eliminate them for 2 weeks. Most foods can be removed temporarily while your gut restores itself, and then they can be safely reintroduced after a time. To do this, follow the reintroduction guidelines on page 208.

Don't hesitate to adjust your food plan as necessary to maximize your healing. Stay tuned in to the way you respond to fat, fiber, chocolate, acidic foods, herbal teas, and other foods to identify whether or not they are problems for you. Remember, you are the chief pilot of your nutritive care.

Don't hesitate to make some "course corrections" if your dietary data dictates a food or menu modification.

The Exclusion Elimination Diet Time Frame

Now let's walk through the elimination diet process and look at how Track 2 works. You will stay on this track for a minimum of 2 weeks. At the end of 2 weeks, you should take the GPS again and reassess your condition. If your symptoms have improved after 2 weeks on this plan, you can start reintroducing the foods you eliminated by following the step-by-step reintroduction process outlined on page 208.

If you have not experienced a reduction in your symptoms at the end of 2 weeks, we recommend that you continue on the Track 2 plan for 2 more weeks. At this 4-week interval, take the GPS again and reassess your symptoms once more. Most people will improve after 4 weeks on Track 2. However, in the unlikely event that your symptoms have not improved, continue on Track 2 for 4 more weeks, as it may take this much time for your inside tract to heal. Staying on Track 2 for 8 weeks is not unusual for someone who has chronic health problems related to food sensitivities. So stick with it!

After 8 weeks have passed, take your GPS once more and reassess your condition. If you have improved, it is time to start the reintroduction process. On the other hand, if you continue having gastrointestinal symptoms including pain, significant mucus discharge, or blood in your stool, we recommend that you consult with your medical provider and discuss a transition to the Track 3 Specific Food Plan, which is outlined in Chapter 10.

To help you keep all of this clear, see the Track 2 Exclusive Food Plan Map. It outlines each step of the process and describes what to do at each point.

Expectations and Common Concerns While on Track 2

Most people begin to feel better after the first week on an elimination diet. However, it is not unusual to experience some unwanted symptoms on Days 2 through 5, as your body slowly clears itself of the foods responsible for causing troubles in your digestive tract. The reality is, you may actually feel worse before you feel better.

Track 2 Exclusion Food Plan Map

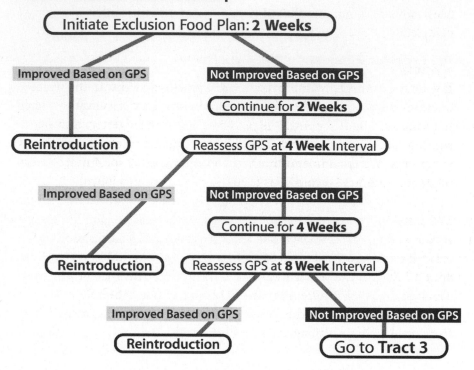

DAYS 2 THROUGH 5
You may experience increased fatigue, muscle aches, joint pains, and cravings, and you may experience changes in bowel function as your body withdraws from the dietary injuries that were once a part of your typical day. Stick with it, and these symptoms will soon pass.

DAYS 6 THROUGH 10
You should start to feel better if the offending foods have been eliminated from your diet.

DAYS 11 THROUGH 14
If your food triggers have been eliminated, your symptoms should continue to improve.

DAYS 15 THROUGH 28

Most of your symptoms should have improved significantly or resolved completely after 4 weeks.

4 WEEKS

If your symptoms have improved, you are now ready to begin the reintroduction process outlined on page 208. However, if your symptoms have not improved by this point, it is possible that you inadvertently are consuming food triggers or that there are other agents responsible for your symptoms. We recommend that you continue Track 2 for 4 more weeks while continuing to record your foods and reactions in a journal.

8 WEEKS

If your symptoms have improved after the additional 4 weeks on Track 2, it is time to start the reintroduction process (see page 208). However, if your symptoms have not improved, we recommend that you initiate Track 3, which is a more selective elimination diet to be followed for a period of just 14 days. At this point, we also recommend that you seek help from a medical practitioner.

The Track 2 Exclusion Food Guide

Despite the limitations outlined above, the Track 2 Exclusion Food Guide includes many delicious foods that you *can eat!* The guide is structured in the Favor, Few, and Forget (three Fs) format. "Favor" means including the foods listed because they will support your health and healing; "Few" means limiting certain foods that, when eaten too frequently, may contribute to symptoms; and "Forget" means excluding potentially irritating foods that contribute to adverse reactions and ill health. Although you will be excluding certain foods in Track 2, there is more than enough choice to make this eating plan fun and delicious.

The guide has been organized by food groups in the order that you should focus on them. Maximize your plant-based choices, especially vegetables, fruits, herbs, and spices. Enjoy other "Favor" foods in moderation. Just because animal protein, nuts, seeds, and other foods are included in the "Favor" column doesn't mean that you should eat excessive amounts of them. Pay attention to the foods highlighted in the "Few" column, and make sure you limit your intake of them. But be sure to keep an especially close eye on FODMAPs that might provoke symptoms if you consume too many of them at one time. Also, watch other items in the "Few" category, because when consumed too frequently (more than two or three times per week), they may contribute to health problems.

We recommend that you allow yourself adequate time to study the food guide before you embark on this plan. Beliefs, attitudes, and your understanding of this program will influence your success in transforming your diet and your health. I (Kathie) believe this based on decades of experience as a nutrition counselor. There is fascinating research confirming that how you feel about a diet or health program is a key factor in its efficacy. Your gut feelings, beliefs, sense of confidence, and can-do attitude are all important to your healing journey. Study the chart that starts below, then review the menu plan. Once you feel comfortable with this information, begin down your path toward optimal digestive function.

Track 2 Exclusion Food Guide

FOOD GROUP	FAVOR	FEW	FORGET
Vegetables	• Fresh or frozen, except those on the Forget list	• FODMAPs: artichokes (globe and Jerusalem), asparagus, beetroot, broccoli, Brussels sprouts, button mushrooms, cabbage, cauliflower, garlic, leek, okra, onions, radicchio, shallots, snow peas • 100% vegetable or tomato juice (fresh preferred)	• Corn • All breaded, creamed, fried, overcooked • Tempura-style • Any known to aggravate your symptoms

(Continued)

Track 2 Exclusion Food Guide (cont.)

FOOD GROUP	FAVOR	FEW	FORGET
Fruits	• Fresh or frozen (unsweetened), except those on the Forget list	• FODMAPs: apricots, blackberries, cherries, coconuts, mangoes, nectarines, peaches, plums, prunes, watermelons • Canned, water-packed • 100% juices or concentrates (use for marinades)	• Apples, applesauce, apple butter, and apple cider • Dried (dates, figs, prunes, etc.) • Beverages • Canned in syrups • Pears, pear nectar, and pear preserves • Any known to aggravate symptoms
Herbs and Spices	• Fresh or dried		• Mixes or seasonings with unacceptable food ingredients
Legumes (vegetable protein)	—	• FODMAPs: baked beans, bean sprouts, black-eyed peas, broad beans (fava beans), garbanzo beans (chickpeas), kidney beans, lentils, navy beans, peas, split peas • Soybeans (edamame, tofu, miso, tempeh)	• Highly processed soy foods or other vegetable protein products (soy hot dogs, soy chips, soy bacon, garbanzo bean chips) • Highly processed vegetable protein alternatives (textured vegetable protein/TVP, hydrolyzed vegetable protein/ HVP, Quorn, seitan) • Peanuts and all peanut products (peanut butter, peanut oil)

(Continued)

Track 2 Exclusion Food Guide (cont.)

FOOD GROUP	FAVOR	FEW	FORGET
Nuts and Seeds	—	• Nuts: almonds, Brazil nuts, cashews, hazelnuts (filberts), macadamias, pecans, pine nuts (pignolias), pistachios, walnuts • Seeds: chia, flax, pumpkin, sesame, sunflower, etc. • Nonhydrogenated, unsweetened nut and seed butters (almond, tahini, etc.) • Nut and seed beverages, homemade or plain, unsweetened, with no carrageenan/ gums	• Nut and seed butters made with partially hydrogenated or peanut oils • Nut and seed products with unacceptable food ingredients
Whole Grains	• Amaranth • Buckwheat • Millet • Oats, certified gluten-free • Quinoa • Rice (basmati, black, brown, Indian ricegrass, red, wild) • Sorghum • Teff • 100% whole grain gluten-free, yeast-free products made with the grains listed above	—	• Cornmeal, polenta, and corn-containing grain products (cereals, pastas, etc.) • Gluten-containing grains and grain products: barley, kamut, rye, spelt, triticale, wheat (see "Gluten in Disguise" on page 197) • Gluten-free grain products that contain yeast or other unacceptable food ingredients

(Continued)

Track 2 Exclusion Food Guide (cont.)

FOOD GROUP	FAVOR	FEW	FORGET
Animal Protein (pasture-raised; organic; wild caught)	• Fish, wild-caught (salmon, cod, halibut), or sustainably farmed (tilapia) • Lox, wild-caught salmon (nitrate-free and naturally smoked) • Poultry (chicken, duck, turkey) without skin • Wild game	• Lean cuts of meat, (beef, bison, lamb, pork)	• Eggs (whole, yolks, whites, powdered), egg substitutes, and egg-containing food products • Fatty cuts of meat (beef, pork, lamb) • Poultry with skin • Processed or aged fish, meat, and poultry products (hot dogs, deli meats, canned meat products) • Shellfish (crab, lobster, shrimp), mollusks (clams, mussels, oysters), and imitation crab or fish products

(Continued)

Track 2 Exclusion Food Guide (cont.)

FOOD GROUP	FAVOR	FEW	FORGET
Dairy and Dairy-Free Alternatives	• Almond, hemp, or rice non-dairy beverages, plain and unsweetened	• FODMAPs • Coconut: flesh, kefir, milk, water • Yogurt, plain soy • Kefir, plain, unsweetened	• Butter • Buttermilk • Cheese, all types, including cottage cheese, cream cheese, and cheese curds • Cream • Custard • Ghee • Half-and-half • Ice cream • Margarine • Milk (whole, low-fat, skim, evaporated, condensed) • Sherbet • Sour cream • Whey, whey protein powder • Whipped cream
Fats and Oils	• Extra-virgin olive oil	• Cold, expeller-pressed oils: almond, canola, flaxseed, grape seed, palm, pumpkin, safflower, sesame, sunflower, and walnut • Coconut oil	• Peanut oil • Cottonseed oil • Lard • Shortening, all types

(Continued)

Track 2 Exclusion Food Guide (cont.)

FOOD GROUP	FAVOR	FEW	FORGET
Condiments	• Arrowroot • Baking powder (aluminum-free) • Baking soda • Cocoa powder • 100% pure flavor extracts (almond, orange, maple, etc.) • Horseradish • Mustard, organic, and dry mustard powder • Wasabi powder (without artificial coloring)	HIGH SODIUM: • Sea salt • Miso, gluten-free • Soy sauce, gluten-free • Tamari, gluten-free FODMAPs: • Chutney • 100% fruit preserves (no apple or pear) • Ketchup (organic, no high-fructose corn syrup) • Sun-dried tomato paste	• Malt vinegar • Mayonnaise • Pesto • Yeast: baker's, brewer's, nutritional, torula • Yeast extracts • Condiments with gluten and other unacceptable ingredients
Beverages	• Water • Decaffeinated tea (black, green, white) • Herbal teas: chamomille, fennel, ginger, lavender, licorice, peppermint (avoid peppermint if you find it exacerbates GERD)		• Apple cider • Caffeinated beverages (coffee, tea, energy drinks) • Chicory-based coffee substitute beverages • Carbonated beverages • Fruit beverages and juice drinks/ades • Sodas, regular and diet • Beverages with unacceptable food ingredients

(Continued)

Track 2 Exclusion Food Guide (cont.)			
FOOD GROUP	**FAVOR**	**FEW**	**FORGET**
Sweets and Sweeteners	—	• Dark chocolate, 70% or more (dairy-free) • Maple syrup, 100% natural • Blackstrap molasses • Brown rice syrup • Stevia FODMAPs: • Agave • Honey • Fruit sweeteners, 100% fruit juice concentrates, except apple and pear	• Artificial sweeteners, all types • Candy, regular and sugar-free • Milk chocolate • Desserts (cakes, cookies, doughnuts, pastries, pies) made with refined flours, gluten-containing flours, and other unacceptable food ingredients • Sugar (white, brown, evaporated cane juice) • Sugar-free foods and gums

The Track 2 Seasonal Menu Plans

Your Track 2 Seasonal Menu Plan "translates" the food guide into meal-by-meal dining so that you don't have to worry about what to eat for breakfast, lunch, or dinner. All you have to do is follow the menus, which have been designed with ease and feasibility in mind. The Track 2 menus contain a delicious array of meals that are based on the elimination guidelines in this chapter. This allows you to begin the process of healing, secure in the knowledge that you don't have to know every trivial detail about gluten or FODMAPs foods to be able to consume a diet that will help optimize your health.

For the first 7 days of Track 2, you can simply follow the menu plan for the season you are currently in with full confidence that your nutritional needs are being met. During the second week, you can stick to the menu plan as outlined or you can mix and match recipes any way you wish. If you need to stay on Track 2 for more than 2 weeks, you may want to develop some of your own recipes based on the Track 2 Exclusion Food Guide (see page 195). Feel free to do that, but just be sure you watch the three Fs and make sure you track your symptoms in a journal to remain mindful of any potentially harmful agents in your diet.

You may be wondering how food can taste good when many former staple ingredients like wheat, flour, cheese, eggs, and corn are no longer in your pantry or refrigerator. What you will discover is that the Track 2 recipes have been created with both familiar ingredients and a few new ones for you to try. We know that changing your food habits and shifting your dietary compass in the direction of healthy everyday foods—plus a few foods that may not be as familiar to you, like amaranth, quinoa, or teff—can be a bit unnerving. For that reason, we have kept these unfamiliar foods to a minimum in the menus. However, we encourage you to try them with an open mind.

For some of you, this may be the first time that you have the comfort of actually knowing what you will be eating for dinner the next evening. Meals shouldn't just "happen" anymore—they should be anticipated, planned for, and thoughtfully prepared in your own home. The days of missed breakfasts, hurried lunches, dinner dilemmas, and eating out more than eating at home are in the past because you are committed to healing. So get comfortable and cozy up to these Track 2 menus. They will rev up your digestive juices and motivate you to get healthy in the kitchen, one meal at a time!

All of the recipes and Swift & Simple Food Charts are in the recipes section beginning on page 240. Refer to the individual recipes for explicit instructions on how to make all of the following meals.

Track 2 Spring/Summer Menu Plan

	DAY 1	DAY 2	DAY 3	
Breakfast	Blueberry Mint Smoothie (Swift & Simple Smoothies, page 240)	Scrambled Tofu with Spinach and Olive Tapenade (page 282)	Raspberry Quinoa Power Porridge (Swift & Simple Power Porridges, page 242)	
Lunch	Black and Red Salad (page 259)	Wild Salmon and Bok Choy Salad (Swift & Simple Salads, page 246)	Lentil Spinach Salad (Swift & Simple Salads, page 246)	
Dinner	Turkey Herb Burger (page 262) Parslied Red Potatoes (page 283) Spinach salad	Dilled Lemon Mustard Chicken Breast (page 262) Summer Squash (page 262) Arugula salad	Macadamia Nut–Crusted Cod (page 263) Pineapple Black Rice (page 263) Red leaf lettuce salad	
SNACKS/ TREATS	–	Lemon Ginger Cookie (page 271)	–	

Track 2 Fall/Winter Menu Plan

	DAY 1	DAY 2	DAY 3	
BREAKFAST	Banana Buckwheat Power Porridge (Swift & Simple Power Porridges, page 242)	Autumn Spiced Soy Yogurt Parfait (page 284)	Morning Millet Power Porridge with Pink Grapefruit (Swift & Simple Power Porridges, page 242)	
LUNCH	Luscious Lentil Soup (page 274)	Salmon Quinoa Bowl (Swift & Simple Bowls, page 248)	Tofu Veggie Wrap (Swift & Simple Wraps, page 244)	
DINNER	Mediterranean Turkey Meatballs with Gluten-Free Pasta and Marinara sauce (page 276) Sauteed Lacinato kale	Sage Roasted Chicken and Root Vegetables (page 276)	White Bean Minestrone Soup (page 285)	
SNACKS/ TREATS	–	–	–	

DAY 4	DAY 5	DAY 6	DAY 7
Strawberry Kiwi Smoothie (Swift & Simple Smoothies, page 240)	Cinnamon Blueberry Steel-Cut Oats Power Porridge (Swift & Simple Power Porridges, page 242)	Raspberry Cucumber Smoothie (Swift & Simple Smoothies, page 242)	Layers of Lox (page 257)
Curried Chicken Wrap (Swift & Simple Wraps, page 244)	White Bean Antipasto Salad (Swift & Simple Salads, page 246)	Turkey Avocado Crème Wrap (Swift & Simple Wraps, page 244)	Tofu Veggie Wrap (Swift & Simple Wraps, page 244)
Mediterranean Turkey Meatballs with Gluten-Free Pasta and Marinara Sauce (page 276) Romaine lettuce salad	Grilled Wild Salmon (page 265) Green Beans with Slivered Almonds (page 266) Mesclun green salad	Lamb* or Beef* Vegetable Kabobs (page 266) Minted Brown Rice (page 267) *Tofu or Tempeh (Veg Option)	Cilantro Cumin Tilapia (page 267) Baked Sweet Potato (page 291) Rainbow swiss chard
–	–	–	–

DAY 4	DAY 5	DAY 6	DAY 7
Berry Almond Smoothie (Swift & Simple Smoothies, page 240)	Strawberry Amaranth Power Porridge (Swift & Simple Power Porridges, page 242)	Pumpkin Orange Smoothie (Swift & Simple Smoothies, page 240)	Layers of Lox (page 257) Clementine wedges
Soothing Chicken Soup (page 275)	Adzuki Millet Bowl (Swift & Simple Bowls, page 248)	Turkey Avocado Crème Wrap (Swift & Simple Wraps, page 244)	Hummus Veggie Wrap (Swift & Simple Wraps, page 244)
Citrus Salmon (page 278) Black rice Steamed asparagus	Lamb or Beef Vegetable Winter Stew (page 279)	Herbed White Fish (page 280) Roasted butternut squash Steamed green beans	Thai Chicken* Sauté (page 286) Gingered rice *Tofu
–	–	–	–

Troubleshooting: Challenges and Solutions

Change can be difficult, so it's natural that some challenges may surface while you are on Track 2. We've anticipated some hurdles you may face and provided a few additional tips to help you troubleshoot issues as they arise.

Are More Modifications Necessary?

A one-size-fits-all approach is rarely useful for managing gut symptoms, and it is important to note that in addition to eliminating potentially offensive foods during this plan, you can also make other changes that may have an impact on your improvement. These include modifying your meal frequency, meal size, and fiber or fat intake. During this phase, a journal can provide valuable information regarding your inside tract's response to specific foods and to other influences, such as meal timing, food forms (raw versus cooked), food combinations, and meal composi-tion. For example, you may notice that you do not tolerate higher-fat items such as salad dressings, avocados, nuts, seeds, or nut butters. If that's the case, try diluting the salad dressings with a bit more water or freshly squeezed lemon or lime juice (they will still taste great!) and reducing or eliminating the other healthy fat items to see if this makes a difference in your symptoms. You're the pilot in the cockpit, and a journal can be a "personal instrument panel" during this phase. Your journal is there to help you detect turbulence in your inside tract. It can also be invaluable in identifying environmental and lifestyle factors, such as sleep deprivation, stress, or toxic relationships that influence how you digest your life. Follow the clues it provides and make the adjustments necessary to find balance and health once more.

How Do I Handle the Addictive Nature of Favorite Foods?

Cutting out sugar, coffee, and alcohol requires a major attitude adjustment due to the addictive nature of these substances and the influence they have over our minds and moods. Mind-body techniques can be especially help-ful when withdrawal symptoms surface. Use the techniques in Chapter 5 (see page 101) and try positive affirmations such as "Feeling fully is healing wholly." I (Kathie) have found these techniques to be helpful to many of my patients. Having a "conversation with your symptoms" can also be useful. Try writing a short story about them or just reflecting on their role in healing your inside tract. The memorable United Kingdom poster from World War II with the message "Keep calm and carry on" offers a witty reminder that you are on the right track and should reinforce your resolve to continue on the highway to healing.

Taking It to Extremes: Orthorexia and Food Vetting

Orthorexia is a term first coined by Dr. Steven Bratman to denote disordered eating that is characterized by an extreme fixation on healthy eating.[6] "Food vetting" describes some consumers' constant need for assurance that they are eating the right things, that their food is safe, and that they are not ingesting pesticides or anything else that will someday prove harmful.[7] Note the two phrases in these definitions that signify imbalance: "extreme fixation" and "constant need for assurance." An elimination trial often does entail that you pay considerable attention to your food choices, and we certainly endorse safe, clean eating by avoiding the perilous picks outlined in Chapter 8 (see page 165). However, it is very important that you approach your Track 2 Exclusion Food Plan as a pathway to healing, not a route to extremism. For more than 2 decades, we have been coaching and counseling individuals suffering from chronic health problems and searching for dietary solutions like the ones in this book. We are also aware that the wise eater embraces the art of nourishment while acknowledging the difference between extreme fixation and making conscious choices for healing. As always, attempt to achieve balance in all things.

Are There Too Many Restrictions?

The Track 2 plan is a *comprehensive* elimination program and involves the exclusion of multiple foods from your diet. This is *not* a diet for life, unlike the Foundational Food Plan outlined in Chapter 8. Track 2 is a "therapeutic" food trial that is designed for the management of symptoms related to food allergies and intolerances. This plan can be personalized further, if desired. For example, after reading this chapter, you may decide that you want to start by eliminating a single food or food group, such as dairy products or gluten-containing foods. You can use the Track 2 Exclusion Food Guide (see page 167) as your compass by focusing on the "Forget" list for dairy and gluten and removing these possible triggers from your everyday diet. Meanwhile, you can gradually work on intelligently transforming your diet to be more in line with the core nutritional factors discussed in Chapter 4. Whether you do the full exclusion or not, we advise you to follow the steps at the end of this chapter to reintroduce foods after the recommended trial is over. An elimination diet is not a way to eat for life. It is a time to reduce the burden on your body and allow it to heal, and it's a way to look for triggers that impact your gut. Once you've done that, it's important to eat a wide range of foods for life.

What If I Experience Weight Changes?

The Track 2 Exclusion Food Plan is not a weight-loss diet, but you may experience some changes in your body weight. This can be caused by the loss of fluid in your tissues due to the removal of trigger foods that were causing water retention. It may also be due to a shift in the microflora that can occur with changes in diet. On the other hand, you might, unexpectedly, experience a slight weight gain while on this plan. This may be due to improved absorption of nutrients as your gut heals. If undesirable weight changes occur, we recommend that you consult with a registered dietitian or licensed nutritionist who can assess your history and guide you accordingly. A skilled practitioner will consider multiple factors that may have influenced a change in your body weight, including caloric intake, physical activity, stress, sleep patterns, medications, and other lifestyle-related influences on energy metabolism. A professional can provide personal recommendations for you.

Ready, Set, Reintroduce . . .

After you have completed Track 2 as previously outlined, retaken the GPS, and recorded your body's response to this elimination phase, the next step in identifying adverse food reactions is food reintroduction. This is a very important step in determining which foods are responsible for your symptoms. You, like many others, may feel so much better after completing this plan that you may not want to challenge your body by reintroducing the eliminated foods, but it's important that you do so. This step is *the* litmus test of legitimacy that specific foods—not other factors—are the causative agents in your digestive health problem. No test currently available is as useful in identifying food sensitivities as the elimination diet and reintroduction process. But the only way it fully works is if you test the foods you may be sensitive to by reintegrating them systematically. Reintroduction is also essential so that you do not continue unnecessarily restricting foods that are not contributing to symptoms or are not detrimental to your health.

The process of food reintroduction that we recommend, which takes you through a set of sequential food challenges, has been adapted from the work of Dr. Janice Vickerstaff Joneja, an internationally recognized food allergy expert. Here are the steps for food reintroduction.

1. Plan ahead for this test period, which can take 3 to 4 weeks or longer. Try to lighten your schedule and commitments during this time, in the event that you have symptoms that make you feel unwell.
2. *Do not* test any food that has ever caused a severe or anaphylactic reaction. If you suspect that you may have a severe reaction, you should discuss this with your physician before proceeding.
3. Refer to the Food Reintroduction Chart at www.theinsidetract.org; it outlines the order of foods that you will test and you can record the results of each food challenge (i.e., Pass or Fail). If you have avoided other foods in addition to those excluded from the Exclusion Food Plan while on Track 2, you can add those foods to your reintroduction chart. (Add foods that have a greater likelihood of causing a reaction closer to the end of the sequence.)
4. Test the food in a pure form so that you can be certain of your results. For example, if you are testing dairy, use milk as your test food, not cereal with milk. To test eggs, use a hard-boiled egg as your test food, rather than egg salad. Test the egg white and the egg yolk separately. To test wheat, use puffed wheat as your test food, not macaroni and cheese. The same goes for all of the other foods you have eliminated.
5. Perform an initial oral screening challenge by placing the test food in your mouth and allowing it to rest there for a few minutes. Remove the food—do not swallow it—and observe any local irritation, inflammation, or other systemic symptoms such as a rash, itching, nasal discharge, etc. These can occur up to 30 minutes after you have placed the food in your mouth.

    a. If symptoms do appear during the oral screening, do not reintroduce the test food. Note your reaction on your Food Reintroduction Chart by recording it simply as "Fail." Continue to avoid the food and then retest it at a later date, well after your body has adjusted to all of the other foods you've reintroduced.

    b. If no symptoms appear and the oral screening is negative, you can proceed to Step 6.

6. Consume the test food at least three times on Day 1 at approximately 4-hour intervals, and monitor for the development of symptoms as outlined here:

    a. Eat a small quantity (about 2 tablespoons) of the test food between breakfast and lunch.

    b. If no symptoms occur, wait 4 hours and consume double the quantity (about ¼ cup) of the same test food eaten in the morning.

    c. Wait 4 hours, monitor yourself, and if no symptoms occur, consume double the quantity of the test food (about ½ cup) eaten in the afternoon.

7. If the test food *does not* cause a reaction on Day 1 of reintroduction, continue to monitor for symptoms and delayed reactions on Day 2 and Day 3. Do not consume the test food you have been avoiding on Day 2 and Day 3. Record your results on the Food Reintroduction Chart. You will then continue testing the next food in the sequence following these same guidelines until you have completed the reintroduction process with each new food having been tested 3 days apart.

    a. If you are *unclear* whether symptoms you're experiencing are due to the food or some other lifestyle factor, such as stress, or if the reaction you experience is extremely mild, consume the same test food again on Day 4, but in larger quantities than on Day 1. Repeat the process of eating it at 4-hour intervals with increasing amounts at each interval.

    b. If no symptoms develop, consider the food safe, record it as "Pass," and proceed with testing the next food in the sequence.

    c. If the test food *does cause* symptoms, eliminate the
       problem food and retest in 3 months.

8. Test the next food in the sequence 48 hours after any symptoms
     have disappeared.

9. Continue testing all the foods in this step-by-step manner until
     you complete the reintroduction process with each new food hav-
     ing been tested 3 days apart.

Closing Thoughts: Track 2 Exclusion Food Plan

After completing this elimination and reintroduction process, you will
have learned which foods support your health and identified the food culprits responsible for undermining your health and diminishing your vitality. You may have one or two foods or a group of foods, such as the top
FODMAPs foods or gluten-containing foods, that failed the reintroduction test. Continue to eliminate them for at least 6 months while your
inside tract heals. Some individuals come to the concrete conclusion that
they are better off with dairy, gluten, or some other food group perma-
nently eliminated.

If you do uncover that some of these foods are disturbing to your inside
tract and overall health, we encourage you to explore other whole-food
resources to expand your dietary choices. Kathie created one such gluten-
and dairy-free resource with a team of the country's best whole-foods
chefs. It is called My Foundation Diet (www.myfoundationdiet.com) and
includes both semivegetarian (high plant-to-animal ratio) and vegetarian
versions. It outlines the specifics on this dietary approach that, for many,
is the long-term key to their health and healing.

The Track 2 Exclusion Food Plan, along with the other lifestyle measures you have been experimenting with, will serve you well on your
health journey. It will help you stay on a more nourishing path to maintain
a dynamic, high-functioning inside tract. We encourage you to continue
to experiment with new recipes using seasonal, whole foods; gut-friendly
ingredients; and smart cooking methods. And we hope you continue to
savor time in your kitchen, your center of healing and good gut health!

CHAPTER 10

Track 3:
The Specific Food Plan

The Track 3 Specific Food Plan is a short-term dietary intervention intended for those who scored 51 and above on the GPS or whose symptoms did not markedly improve or fully resolve on the Track 2 Exclusive Food Plan. It is a 2-week, limited-ingredient "specific" diet that is anti-inflammatory in nature and lower in fiber—especially the insoluble fibers found in the husks of grains, nuts, and seeds, which can irritate the inside tract.

It is important to note a few essential facts about the Track 3 plan.

- ☐ This track is more restrictive than either of the previous tracks. This is because it is intended for people with moderate to severe digestive disorders. This track is most likely to be effective if you are following it in conjunction with the guidance of a physician and/or a registered dietitian or licensed nutritionist who is experienced in holistic approaches to healing digestive disease.
- ☐ It is intended to be used as a short-term dietary trial for a period of 2 weeks. It is *not* a long-term dietary solution. You will evaluate your response to this intervention at the end of 2 weeks using the GPS.
- ☐ It is based on foods that are least likely to cause an adverse reaction. This will give your gut the best chance to heal. Since adverse food reactions are highly individual, we recommend that you avoid any item in this food plan that you know is offensive to you and substitute another item. For example, if you do not tolerate spinach, you can substitute Swiss chard.
- ☐ This plan should be followed at a time when you can prepare and eat most or all of your meals at home.
- ☐ It includes a 7-day, grain-free menu that incorporates easily digested, specific healing foods such as cooked vegetables, fruit,

fish, poultry, lean meat, healthy oils, decaffeinated green tea, and some herbs and spices.

☐ This track obviously excludes many food items, including beans, soy foods, nuts, and seeds, and it lacks the abundant variety of fruits and vegetables available in the Track 1 and Track 2 plans. However, digestive-friendly vegetables do comprise a major portion of your food intake on this track.

This chapter includes:

☐ **The Track 3 Specific Food Guide.** Because this is an ingredient-limited diet, this guide simply lists the foods to include in your diet. You should eliminate everything not in the guide.

☐ **The Track 3 Specific Menu Plan.** While it's not seasonal (due to the specificity of the foods required), we have provided a 7-day meal plan for you to follow while on Track 3.

☐ **The Track 3 Specific Recipes.** The recipes to go along with this meal plan can be found in the recipes section (see page 287).

Track 3: How to Use the Specific Food Plan

When you begin Track 3, you need to follow the food plan outlined in this chapter as carefully as possible. Whether you landed here directly from the GPS or you moved to this plan because you did not see an improvement in your symptoms after completing Track 2, it's likely that you have significant digestive health issues that may require a more restrictive meal plan. To best resolve them using this dietary plan, it's important that you adhere to it for 2 full weeks.

After you have completed 2 weeks on Track 3, reassess your condition using the GPS. We also recommend that you review your journals to see if you discovered any significant factors that contributed to a reduction in your symptoms while on this track. You should also be attentive to rare cases where your symptoms flare up while on this plan. After your reassessment and review of your symptoms, if you are still experiencing distress and the Track 3 food plan has not helped you as much as you anticipated, we recommend that you consult with a physician or gastroenterologist as

MADELINE'S STORY

Madeline was referred to Kathie from a GI clinic in Boston. She was suffering from ulcerative colitis, and despite efforts made to heal her battered bowel, Madeline had not improved and was facing impending surgery.

Her gastroenterologist recommended that she consult with me due to my experience in integrative and functional nutrition therapy. I reviewed Madeline's medical history along with the volume of medical information provided, including laboratory tests and diagnostics. But it wasn't until I reviewed her detailed food records that I uncovered why her inflammatory condition was raging out of control: Her diet was filled with high-fiber whole grains like whole wheat cereal and bread; high-fat dairy products such as full-fat yogurt, cheddar cheese, and butter; lots of red meat; and two highballs every night.

She shared that the dietitian at the GI clinic had tried to motivate her to change her diet, but she just wasn't ready. Madeline shared her frustrations and fears with me, and we shared some tissues as her story unfolded. We discussed our partnership in her healing process and then moved on to the business of cleaning up her diet, starting by putting her on the Track 3 Specific Food Plan.

Madeline mastered the details of the short-term Track 3 plan and began to show improvement. Her GI doc agreed that we should continue with the dietary interventions that I developed. Madeline graduated to the Track 2 Exclusive Food plan with some minor modifications that I recommended. After 4 months, Madeline's condition had improved significantly. She continued to rebuild her strength, energy, and inside tract while also transforming her kitchen in the process. Madeline maintained a dairy- and gluten-free, semivegetarian diet for many months, which helped to keep her inflammation at bay. Even after she graduated from Track 2, she continued to eat in a way that promoted healing. The fire that once was raging within Madeline's inside tract was now slowly being extinguished.

well as with a registered dietitian or licensed nutritionist who can assess your personal history and guide you appropriately.

If your GPS score does improve (and it is likely that it will), you can gradually expand your food options using the Track 3 reintroduction process at the end of this chapter. Note that this reintroduction system is specific to this track and is different from the one outlined in Track 2. On page 216, you will find a week-by-week reintroduction roadmap to help you navigate toward your next phase in healing.

Before we get to that, let's review the food guide and meal plans for this track.

The Track 3 Specific Food Guide

Rather than building this food guide on the three Fs (favor, few, and forget), as we did in previous plans, we have simply listed the foods you *should* include in your diet during Track 3. Everything not on this list should be avoided for the duration of this track.

Track 3 is organized based on the following food groups: vegetables, fruits, herbs and spices, animal protein, oils, condiments, nutritional extras, and beverages. The foods in the "Specific Foods" column are the items that will make up your diet during this short-term elimination experiment designed to foster the healing of your inside tract. See page 216 for the food guide and the specific foods that are included in your healing foods menu.

The Track 3 Specific Menu Plan

We have included a 7-day Track 3 menu plan and recipes based on the Track 3 Specific Food Guide. The menu plan includes foods that are simply prepared and lightly seasoned. You will find smoothies, broths, soups, vegetables, fruit, fish, and poultry. Some recipes include some extra-virgin olive oil and a few herbs and spices, including ginger, the soothing, anti-inflammatory spice. This is not a menu plan for the gourmand, but rather a specific food plan that will guide you toward healing when your gut is inflamed. In the process of eating these specific foods, you will find this meal plan to be an easy, convenient, and powerful ally in soothing your inside tract.

There are a few things to keep in mind while you're on this meal plan.

☐ **Be flexible.** The menu plan does allow for flexibility in exchanging food items. If you prefer a smoothie for dinner or want to swap a dinner meal for lunch or a lunch for breakfast, feel free. Don't be

Track 3 Specific Food Guide

FOOD GROUP	SPECIFIC FOODS
Vegetables	• Fresh or frozen: beetroot, bok choy, butternut squash, carrots, celeriac (celery root), collard greens, cucumbers, green beans, kale, parsley, parsnips, potatoes (Yukon gold), shiitake mushrooms, spinach, sweet potatoes, Swiss chard, turnips, yellow squash, zucchini • Sea vegetable: kombu • Dried: shredded burdock root • Canned: organic pumpkin *Note: Steam vegetables to retain nutrients and drizzle them with some extra-virgin olive oil. Slow cookers and pressure cookers can also be helpful; soups can be frozen for later use.*
Fruits	• Bananas • Avocados • Citrus: lemons, orange zest *Note: Use ripe, not under- or overripe fruit. Use freshly squeezed lemon juice on your vegetables as tolerated.*
Herbs and Spices	• Fresh and/or dried bay leaf, burdock root, curry powder, ginger, mint, nutmeg *Note: Avoid any herb or spice that you feel you do not tolerate.*
Animal Protein	• Wild cold-water fish: cod, sablefish or black cod, salmon, Pacific sardines, skipjack tuna • Organic turkey and chicken, without skin *Note: Use simple preparation methods, such as baking or roasting poultry and steaming, poaching, or baking fish.*
Oils	• Extra-virgin olive oil
Condiments	• Sea salt (optional) • Maple syrup, 100% natural (optional)
Nutritional Extras	• Balanced omega oil (such as a 3-6-9 liquid blend) • Brown rice protein powder, organic fruit and vegetable powder
Beverages	• Water • Decaffeinated green tea • Herbal teas • Inside Tract Vegetable Broth (see page 287)

concerned that you are upsetting the balance, as the most important element is adhering to the specific food items allowed and avoiding other items that are not included in the menu plan.

☐ **Plan ahead.** Think about preparing ahead and freezing some items, such as the soups and broths. These can be prepared on the days that you have a bit more energy to devote to cooking. You can roast a turkey breast or chicken and have it available for another meal the next day, if you desire.

☐ **Eliminate additional foods as needed.** If there are any foods included in this food plan that you do not eat because you already know that they cause adverse reactions, do not consume them. You can substitute one of the other suggested menu items in the plan. For example, if you do not eat or tolerate fish, then substitute turkey or chicken, instead. Don't be concerned if you are repeating foods, since this is expected with a specific "few foods" or limited-ingredient diet.

☐ **Practice mindful eating.** Eat mindfully, at an unhurried pace, and remember to chew thoroughly. This will activate the flow of saliva that is essential for digestion. (For more on this, see Chapter 4.)

☐ **Eat just enough.** Consume enough so that you feel just right or "gently satisfied." Don't under- or overfeed your inside tract during this period. Feel free to increase or decrease the recipe portions to suit your body's needs. Double the amount of soup, make an extra smoothie, or have a bit more protein if you are still hungry. Find an amount that is just right to satisfy your hunger.

☐ **Stay well hydrated.** Be sure to drink fluids throughout the day, including water (it's especially refreshing flavored with a ginger slice or mint leaves), herbal teas, or decaffeinated green tea.

☐ **Keep a journal.** Be sure to faithfully update your journal while you are on Track 3 to keep yourself aware of how your body is responding to this specific plan.

☐ **A word on fiber.** Because high-fiber or "high-residue" diets—especially the insoluble fiber found in the husks and hulls of plant foods—may initially aggravate an inside tract that is already inflamed, and because of the higher fiber content of plant foods such as legumes, nuts, and seeds, the Specific Food Plan is not a vegetarian plan. To avoid further inflaming your already suffering gut, we have capped the fiber intake in this track. In Chapter 4, you learned how crucial fiber is for GI health. The goal is to eventually increase your inside tract's tolerance of this vital substance by eating diverse sources of prebiotic soluble fiber to nourish your good gut bacteria and produce beneficial short-chain fatty acids. You will eventually be on that path, but for now, limit your fiber intake and stick to forms that are soothing, such as cooked versus raw vegetables and some fruits.

☐ **Vegetarian options:** If you are a vegetarian, you can substitute very well cooked, simply prepared legumes (beans, peas, lentils, and organic soy foods) for the animal protein in the food guide. Be sure to monitor your response.

Track 3 Menu Plan

	DAY 1	**DAY 2**	**DAY 3**	
Breakfast	Inside Tract Smoothie* (page 287)	Inside Tract Smoothie (page 287)	Inside Tract Smoothie (page 287)	
Lunch	Herbed Wild Cod (page 280) Steamed spinach Inside Tract Vegetable Broth (page 287)	Creamy Greens Soup (page 288) Baked chicken	Canned skipjack tuna Baked Sweet Potato (page 291) Inside Tract Vegetable Broth (page 287)	
Dinner	Turkey Herb Burger (page 260) Steamed yellow squash	Baked fish Steamed bok choy	Roasted turkey breast Steamed spinach	
Snacks	Inside Tract Smoothie (page 287) Cucumber Avocado Mint Soup (page 290)	Inside Tract Smoothie (page 287)	Inside Tract Smoothie (page 287)	

*A medical food can be used in the Nutri-Smoothie or on its own mixed with water to provide a range of gut-healing nutrients as outlined in the supplement chapter. (See "Medical Foods" on page 146 for more information about these products.)

All of the recipes are in the recipes section beginning on page 252. Refer to the individual recipes for explicit instructions on how to make all of the meals below.

Track 3 Reintroduction Roadmap

Assuming your GPS score improves and you experience a reduction in digestive symptoms after 2 weeks on Track 3, follow these guidelines to systematically reintroduce foods into your diet.

	DAY 4	DAY 5	DAY 6	DAY 7
	Inside Tract Smoothie (page 287)	Inside Tract Smoothie (page 287)	Inside Tract Smoothie (page 287)	Inside Tract Smoothie (page 287)
	Carrot Squash Soup (page 289) Canned Pacific sardines	Baked chicken Steamed bok choy Inside Tract Vegetable Broth (page 287)	Pumpkin Bisque (page 289) Turkey Burger Steamed spinach	Canned Pacific sardines Steamed yellow squash Inside Tract Vegetable Broth (page 287)
	Baked chicken Steamed Swiss chard	Herbed Wild Cod (page 280) Steamed zucchini squash	Grilled wild salmon Steamed green beans	Baked chicken Steamed collard greens
	Inside Tract Smoothie (page 287)	Inside Tract Smoothie (page 287) Cucumber Avocado Mint Soup (page 290)	Inside Tract Smoothie (page 287)	Inside Tract Smoothie (page 287)

General Reintroduction Guidelines

☐ Do not reintroduce any food to which you have had a severe adverse reaction in the past.

☐ Record your responses to each reintroduced item suggested on the Food Reintroduction Chart on our Web site, www.theinsidetract.org. That way, you have a record of foods that support your healing and foods that contribute to your health problems.

☐ Reintroduce foods into your diet in the order indicated below. If you have an adverse reaction to a food, eliminate it, wait for the reaction to subside before you proceed to the next food, and then try it again after you finish the complete reintroduction process outlined below.

☐ Be patient and try to enjoy this digestive experiment. It is going to help you figure out what is best for your inside tract and your overall health in the long haul.

Reintroduction Week by Week

☐ **Week 1: Brown rice.** You may be looking for those grains that you have missed. Brown rice contains some valuable functional components for your inside tract. Start by eating ¼ cup of steamed brown rice up to three times on Day 1 of your reintroduction process. Monitor your response for the next 3 days. If you tolerated the brown rice well, you can consider it safe to include and enjoy it in your meal plan. Do not add any other foods back until the start of Week 2.

☐ **Weeks 2 through 4: Vegetables.** You will now begin the sequential addition of more cooked vegetables into your meal plan. Begin with one new vegetable at a time, allowing at least 2 days between new additions, as tolerated. Continue with the addition of vegetables until you are tolerating approximately 4 cups per day.

☐ **Weeks 4 through 6: Fruits.** At this stage, you can begin to integrate some other fruits into your meal plan, avoiding the higher FODMAPs foods. (See the Track 2 grid starting on page 196 to determine what foods are appropriate for you to add at this point.)

Start with one serving (one small piece, or approximately ½ cup) per day. Allow 2 days between new additions, as tolerated. Limit your fruit intake to two servings per day, including any fruit used in your smoothie. Your inside tract should be adapting to the gradual increase in fiber.

☐ **Weeks 6 through 8: Nuts, seeds, fats, and oils.** You can now begin introducing some other healthy oils and natural nut or seed butters into your menu plan. Start slowly, with the addition of 1 tablespoon per day of almond butter or ½ cup of Homemade Nut or Seed Milk (almond; see page 252). If tolerated, you can gradually increase the variety of nut and seed butters (sunflower seed butter, cashew butter, etc.—but not peanut butter). Allow 2 days between new additions. Be sure to notice the impact of this increase in the fat content of your diet, as everyone has a unique fat budget that is best not only for their arteries but also for their inside tracts.

☐ **Weeks 8 through 10: Herbs and spices.** At this time, you can begin to boost other herbs and spices in your diet. Start with the flavors that you missed the most! Like the other additions, go slowly when introducing them back into your diet.

☐ **Weeks 10 through 12: Legumes.** Now try introducing small amounts of very well-cooked beans, peas, and lentils into your diet. Start with ¼ cup of hummus, and if that's tolerated, try introducing some well-cooked adzuki beans or lentils a few days later. Feel free to use canned beans, but be sure to choose a brand that is not loaded with sodium.

☐ **Weeks 12 through 14: Gluten-free whole grains.** You can now try introducing other gluten-free whole grains in addition to brown rice. Start with one or two per week in small amounts. For example, have a small serving of cooked millet (½ cup), and if that's tolerated, after 3 or 4 days, you can try ½ cup of well-cooked buckwheat groats (kasha). Rinsing and soaking the grains prior to cooking may help your body tolerate them better.

☐ **Weeks 14 through 16: More gluten-free whole grains.** Continue adding gluten-free whole grains during this time. For example, try adding some quinoa to your diet. Again, start with a ½-cup serving and, if that's tolerated, advance to other grains like amaranth and then teff 3 or 4 days later, if desired.

☐ **Weeks 16 through 18: More gluten-free whole grains.** Continue to introduce other nutrient-rich, gluten-free options, such as certified gluten-free oats. Keep in mind that the number of gluten-free grains that you introduce is up to you and should be based on your desire for and tolerance of these whole grains. Remember that a low- or no-grain diet may be indicated for continued healing if, upon reintroduction, your symptoms are aggravated.

☐ **Weeks 18 through 20: Take the GPS and move to Track 2.** Take the GPS again. By now it should have improved. Assuming it has, you can now move on to Track 2 (Chapter 9) and follow the instructions for completing that diet plan.

A Nourishing Voyage

Managing chronic gastrointestinal symptoms requires understanding, commitment, knowledge, skills (in the kitchen), and a megadose of resolve. As you move forward in healing, it's important that you continue to pay attention to your diet and lifestyle-related factors, such as your sleep habits, stress levels, physical activity, and the relationships that have an impact on your gut. This quest is aimed at improving your overall quality of life so that you may be able to enjoy the gift of each and every beautiful day. We hope that your nutritional journey using *The Inside Tract* has been a nourishing voyage and a well-deserved passage to optimal health and healing. May your diet continue to provide you with a wealth of whole foods that will serve to nourish and sustain your inside tract.

CHAPTER 11

Putting It All Together: Case Histories

It is much more important to know what sort of patient has a disease than what sort of a disease a patient has.
—Sir William Osler

An illness is like a journey into a far country; it sifts all one's experience and removes it to a point so remote that it appears like a vision.
—Sholem Asch

As we have shown throughout this book, the gut is a conduit to health and vitality—the highway to healing or the pathway to pathology. It truly is the "inner tube" of life.

Over the course of the last few chapters, we have discussed the importance of nutrition, supplementation, stress reduction, and other lifestyle changes, as well as how balancing your mind, body, and spirit is essential to promoting and maintaining good gut health. We have provided you with a self-help guide to help you overcome your digestive symptoms and detailed our Inside Tract Prescription to Wellness.

All of this is intended to be self-navigated, unless your symptoms are so severe that you require medical supervision. That said, we also know that one size does not fit all and that the program will require a personalized approach for some.

In this chapter, we will present you with a series of compelling stories from Gerry's practice that illustrate the principles of this program. You will read stories from people who suffered from the most common digestive tract illnesses, and you'll learn how each healed his or her own gut and found the inside "tract" to health. Some of these cases required medical supervision; others were self-navigated through good gut guidance. We hope they inspire you and serve as models for how much healing you can achieve by following the holistic, integrative approach in this book.

MEGHAN'S STORY

A Matter of Life and Death

Meghan was a 47-year-old mother of two. Only a few months before she came to see me, she had been a vibrant and thriving woman at the very pinnacle of her career. While driving home one evening I got a phone call from a friend who was on staff at Johns Hopkins. She asked me to intervene because this wonderful woman was "disappearing before their very eyes."

In a very short amount of time and with no explanation, Meghan had dropped from 135 pounds (her normal and healthy weight) to 85 pounds. She was literally starving to death for no apparent reason. She had not changed anything in her diet or lifestyle. Seemingly out of the blue she had developed loose stools and a variety of food intolerances.

Needless to say, she was terrified. She could not understand why she was deteriorating so rapidly and she was desperate for answers. Finding them was a matter of life and death.

Meghan's Inside Tract to Wellness

When Meghan was admitted to the Johns Hopkins Hospital, her malnutrition was life threatening. Her serum albumin was 2.3 g/dL, predicting high morbidity and mortality from malnutrition. Meghan was sliding fast.

We immediately hospitalized her for total parenteral nutrition infusion (a process by which a person is fed intravenously, thus bypassing the digestive system). Though for many people such drastic measures aren't necessary, in Meghan's case this intervention was critical if we were going to save her life.

Meghan had been suffering from Sjögren's syndrome, an autoimmune disorder that can foster small intestinal bacterial overgrowth (SIBO). The SIBO precluded her from properly absorbing much of the nutrients she had been eating. I have rarely seen anyone with a case of SIBO as profound as what we found in Meghan.

Over time, we were able to completely eliminate her SIBO using herbal therapies, and her nutritional status began to stabilize as well. She was placed on a Track 3 diet, given the severity of her disease. She gained weight steadily, and when she was up to about 114 pounds, I judged that it was time to wean her off the intravenous nutrition therapy we had her on.

At that point, I suggested our Track 2 program because it would eliminate FODMAPs that could potentially contribute toward the overgrowth of bad bugs in her small intestine. I knew Meghan would likely have to stay on such a diet for an extended period of time due to her health problems and the possibility that her Sjögren's syndrome could lead to a recurrence of the SIBO that she suffered from.

She tolerated her diet very well and steadily gained more weight. We began incorporating medical foods (functional foods in a powder form) that provided additional nutrients to help her rebuild her intestinal lining, which had been damaged over the course of her illness. Slowly and systematically, Meghan improved through the entire treatment protocol. After several months, we transitioned her onto a long-term Track 1 program of whole, healthy foods.

Meghan continued to gain weight, and her symptoms of SIBO and malabsorption abated. The last time I saw Meghan, she was back up to a healthy weight (131 pounds), and she looked vibrant and full of energy again.

While Meghan's treatment was far from simple, it nonetheless shows how powerful dietary and lifestyle interventions can be. By giving her the nutritional support she needed, adding the appropriate supplements, and slowly eliminating the bad bugs that were literally stealing her life away from her, we helped save Meghan's life.

Testimonial by Meghan

My odyssey started in January of 2008, when I began wasting away due to excessive weight loss and malnutrition. For months, multiple doctors were unable to diagnose or treat my problem.

Then came my answer—that miracle connection people make once in their lifetime if they are immensely lucky. I was referred to Dr. Gerard Mullin at Johns Hopkins in Baltimore, Maryland. My referring physician called him the "House" of Johns Hopkins—like that character in the medical detective television series who specializes in figuring out cases other people can't.

The day I met Dr. Mullin was the day that I got my life back.

(Continued)

Meghan's Story (cont.)

He mapped out a plan of testing to find the root cause of my problem instead of jumping to simply treat the symptoms.

Dr. Mullin left nothing unexplored when trying to find the medical cause for my condition, and he worked with me to discover the best solutions for my care. He is an extraordinary doctor and never once did he make me feel that *any* question, big or small, was unimportant. Bottom line: Dr. Mullin made me feel as if my health was his top priority.

I am forever grateful that I was that "one in a million" person who was fortunate enough to be cared for by Dr. Gerard Mullin. His wisdom and patience while working with my condition saved my life.

Tasha's Story

Coming from Moscow for a Miracle

It was the end of August of 2006 when Tasha and her husband, Sergey, were anxiously waiting in the exam room at the Johns Hopkins Clinic at Green Spring Station in Lutherville, Maryland. They were there to meet the physician for whom they had traveled over 5,000 miles to see. They were hoping for a miracle.

Tasha was a 29-year-old vibrant and energetic attorney. She had worked in Moscow and lived a full and satisfying life with her husband until their fortunes suddenly reversed. An undercooked hamburger that they had shared was the turning point. They both developed chills and diarrhea the morning after eating that meal. While Sergey fully recovered, Tasha's health spiraled down. Her illness progressed and her abdominal pain became incapacitating, making sleep very difficult.

Tasha's quality of life was poor, and she was forced to leave her job. She was now an attorney on disability. Despite seeing doctors in Russia and Germany, she could find neither answers nor solutions, only a steady worsening of her overall health. She was losing weight, energy, and stamina, and she was becoming weak. Both Tasha and her husband were looking for answers while their lives were being turned upside down. As I entered the room, I was struck by a warm greeting from a couple of visibly worn and exhausted travelers. This moment touched my soul.

Tasha had been told by many specialists that all she had was a garden-variety case of IBS, but none of their treatments seemed to work.

One of my favorite television shows when I was growing up was *Quincy*. The show was about a medical examiner who was notorious for his endless investigations and thinking outside the box until the medical mystery he was working on had been solved. Being an "outside the box" analyst has been my style as a practitioner for over a decade, as I evolved into an integrative medical detective.

Tasha's situation—development of IBS following a food-related infection while traveling—is quite common. As much as 25 percent of IBS can be attributed to an enteric infection. The fact that she had been raised in Russia, had lost about 13 pounds, suffered from around-the-clock diarrhea, had eosinophils present in her stool, and had low levels of intestinal secretory IgA antibody raised a red flag in my mind, signaling a parasite. Yet all of her conventional stool testing failed to disclose any problems.

Tasha's Inside Tract to Wellness

Following a hunch, I sent Tasha to the Jetti Katz Tropical Medicine Lab in New York City to be tested for parasites. The Jetti Katz Lab is world-renowned for discovering the presence of parasites that conventional medical testing fails to disclose. There they collect stool specimens fresh and analyze them right away. This was the key that unlocked the mystery of Tasha's illness. She was infected with the parasite *Giardia lamblia*, and it was contributing to her fatigue, exhaustion, malabsorption of nutrients, weight loss, disability, and poor quality of life.

Once we "cleaned up her gut" by eliminating the pathogens, restored her proper balance of intestinal flora with probiotics, placed her on a modified Track 2 diet, and got her some cognitive behavioral therapy to help her retrain her thinking patterns, Tasha's health returned. This was the beginning of her road to recovery. It gave her a second chance at a healthy and productive life with her beloved and devoted husband, and it allowed her to resume her career as a lawyer.

As I had the pleasure of watching her heal, it was so clear to me that Sergey's love and devotion were crucial for Tasha's success. As Bernie Siegel wrote in his book *Love, Medicine, and Miracles,* "one of the greatest healers is unconditional love." Outcome studies have consistently shown that people who are supported during their lives, in health and in illness, do better than those who are socially isolated. In this case, Tasha found her miracle through faith, love, and an integrative approach to her problem.

CAROLYN'S STORY

Bad Bugs in the Gut

It was at the height of the 2008 presidential campaign when Carolyn and her husband showed up in my clinic at Johns Hopkins. Carolyn worked on Capitol Hill, and as her work began to intensify, she fell ill. Diarrhea, fatigue, and bloating were keeping her from performing her job, and that was not something she could allow to happen in the middle of one of the most important presidential races in history.

It took some investigative work, but together Carolyn and I, along with her loving husband (with whom she obviously enjoyed a very full life), were able to track down the true source of her imbalance. What we found didn't surprise me, but Carolyn was rather shocked.

Carolyn's Inside Tract to Wellness

When she came into my office, Carolyn was a young woman who did Pilates regularly, had a wonderful career, enjoyed a happy marriage, and who by all accounts seemed to live a healthy life. But somehow her appearance lacked the vibrancy one would expect to see in a woman in the prime of her life. She was visibly fatigued, and her stress level was palpable the moment she walked in the room.

In situations like this one, I strongly believe that the best way to begin treatment is to develop a strong connection with the patient. In a world where HMOs dominate billing practices and doctors are forced to limit to mere minutes the amount of time they spend with patients, the whole idea of "bedside manner" has virtually gone out the window. This is a shame, because being a healer is much more than simply being a medical technician. As I took the time and spent the necessary energy to truly listen to Carolyn and assure her and her husband that I understood their concerns, that I truly cared, and that I would do everything I could to help them find an answer to Carolyn's health problems, I could see some of their tension melt away.

Early on, I suspected that Carolyn had stress-related irritable bowel and SIBO. After her tests for celiac disease came back negative, I then ordered a lactulose hydrogen breath test to see if we could substantiate a SIBO diagnosis. She ingested 10 grams of lactulose and produced abnormal amounts of breath hydrogen from the immediate fermentation of the sugar by misplaced bacteria in her upper digestive tract. SIBO was now confirmed.

Our first priority: Eliminate the bacterial overgrowth in her small intestine. Given the degree of the symptoms she was experiencing, I knew that following a classic Track 2 diet along with our lifestyle program would achieve this, so that was the course we took as a team.

A course of antibiotics failed to clear her SIBO, so I treated her condition with a combination of essential aromatic oils and an antimicrobial herbal formula. She followed the Track 2 diet, eliminating sugars, legumes, and FODMAPs to help starve out the bacteria in her upper digestive tract.

Several weeks after she began this treatment protocol, Carolyn came back for a follow-up visit. When she walked into my office, I asked her if she had just returned from vacation—that's how relaxed and vibrant she looked. In fact, she'd taken the train from Union Station in Washington, DC, to Baltimore so she could meet me in the clinic after a long day at work!

We repeated the lactulose hydrogen breath test, and it showed that her SIBO had completely cleared up. In Carolyn's case, the Track 2 dietary interventions, supplementation, and lifestyle strategy worked!

Carolyn safely transitioned to a Track 1 whole-foods, broad-based diet.

Testimonial by Carolyn

After struggling with intestinal issues for many years, I became desperate to ascertain the root cause of my health issues. God lead me to Dr. Gerard Mullin at Johns Hopkins; he is the only physician I have ever seen who conducted a thorough, no-holds-barred examination of my health. One of the things I appreciate and admire most about Dr. Mullin is his willingness to think outside the box when treating a patient. His approach worked wonders, and over the past year, when some of my symptoms started to return, I simply followed his method to return my body to health.

ELLEN'S STORY

Willing to Travel Anywhere—Desperate for Help

Ellen was only 30 years old but had already suffered a lifetime's worth of trauma and abuse. She drove from Indiana to Baltimore to find solutions to the many years of digestive symptoms that she had suffered from since she was a teenager.

(Continued)

Ellen's Story (cont.)

She had seen many doctors over the years—many of whom had labeled her as having a bad case of IBS—and she had tried a variety of medications that did not help her. She was tired of feeling "labeled" and was sick of the seemingly copycat diagnoses and approaches these doctors all seemed to take. Ellen was looking for a fresh start and a new life.

She came into my office in May of 2009 with poor appetite, weight loss, anxiety, depression, heartburn, indigestion, nausea, vomiting, abdominal pain, abdominal swelling, constipation, and diarrhea. She also noted periods of cold sensitivity and recurrent headaches.

In probing into her history, I discovered that Ellen was in the process of filing for divorce after a failed marriage and that she had been traumatized by the experience. She appeared to be in pain both physically and emotionally. I suspected we would need to help her balance her whole self in order to help her heal.

Ellen's Inside Tract to Wellness

One of her physicians in Indiana had diagnosed Ellen with gastroparesis. However, the medications the doctor prescribed—Reglan and Erythromycin—were ineffective, and Ellen had developed a sensitivity to them.

My instincts told me that Ellen was really suffering from a series of traumatic events in her life (most recently, her divorce) that led her to develop a severe functional gastrointestinal disorder. So we had a long discussion regarding some possible approaches that would help her improve her condition by balancing her mind-body connection.

First and foremost, I encouraged Ellen to continue going to psychotherapy (something she had been engaged in for several months but had considered dropping). I also suggested that she consider practicing either meditation, yoga, or breath work daily. Ellen stated that she was committed to work through her trauma and apply one of these mind-body techniques to help resolve her emotional and digestive problems.

In order to help stabilize her emotions faster, Ellen and I agreed to try some supplements that would help balance her brain chemistry. Since Ellen has some difficulties winding down at night, I suggested she try a melatonin-based product to help restore her normal sleep patterns. I also recommended 5-HTP—the precursor to serotonin—to help with her depression.

I encouraged Ellen to explore acupuncture, given the literature showing that it enhances gastric motility. In one study, electroacupuncture outper-formed Reglan—the typical medication given for treating motility problems.[1] We also discussed other possible options for improving her gastric motility. For example, I recommended 20 milligrams of domperidone four times a day, as it has been shown to be useful in promoting gastric motility.[2]

Ellen's diet was also in need of an overhaul. She relied on fast foods and snacks as calorie sources, and that was a real source for concern, given her condition. I suggested a modified Track 3 diet with small, fre-quent meals to stabilize her condition. I suspected that she would be able to transition to Track 2, and eventually even Track 1.

Given her symptoms of bloating and underlying gastroparesis, we tested Ellen for SIBO using the lactulose hydrogen breath test. Her results showed bacterial overgrowth, so I started her on an herbal regimen to eliminate the bad bugs from her small intestine and to restore proper gut ecology.

In addition to all of this, Ellen was also suffering from GERD. We dis-cussed having her take the herb licorice root in a deglycyrrhizinated form to help with her heartburn. I also added gingerroot to her list of supplements to improve her gastroparesis and dyspepsia.

Ellen was very concerned that none of this would work and that she would need a gastric pacemaker, as one of her previous physicians had suggested. I strongly suspected that this wouldn't be the case, and the pacemaker indeed turned out to be unnecessary. Over a period of months, Ellen rebalanced her emotions and watched many of her gut symptoms completely resolve. In the end, she found a new life, renewed health, and freedom from digestive disorders that had plagued her for so long.

Testimonial by Ellen

For more than 13 years, I knew something was wrong with my body. My chronic, debilitating symptoms brought me to a place where I felt my life wasn't worth living. Naturally, I turned to medical professionals for guid-ance. One misdiagnosis followed another. I was even told that it was all in my head.

Immediately, I knew Dr. Mullin was different. He entertained my ques-tions, empathized with me, and was willing to find the answers to things he did not instantly know. Together, we tailored a holistic treatment plan for my situation. Through strict adherence to the plan and with Dr. Mullin's ongoing support, I was able to take back the reins of my life.

JUNE'S STORY

Praying for a Miracle

It was late afternoon, and I was on my way to a reception honoring the career of a physician at Johns Hopkins when I received a "cry for help." The message came from a lady who worked in human resources at Johns Hopkins. Her daughter was becoming seriously ill and needed assistance. At the time, I pondered how odd it was that this woman worked in the very building in which I was about to attend that reception. I suggested we meet after the reception to discuss how I could help her daughter.

June was only 30 years old, but her life was becoming a living purgatory that she could never have imagined. June was chronically ill from left-sided ulcerative colitis and had essentially no quality of life. She had been diagnosed 5 years before our first encounter and had been placed on aggressive medications, including immunosuppressives. Her disease "spun out of control" shortly after that.

My first encounter with June included her mother, Frances, and her husband, Bill, who worked for the Department of Defense. They gathered in my office to tell June's dramatic story. The session was intense.

June was a master's-level second-grade teacher in the Howard County, Maryland, school system. Her work was challenging, as it demanded very high energy, which June could barely muster. She was running to the bathroom up to 15 times per day. Her exhaustion, in conjunction with the energy she was pouring into her new marriage with Bill, was too much. June was desperate to survive day to day without taking sick leave from work, and she was going downhill fast. Frances recalled how she would watch her daughter cry in pain while she struggled to make it through each and every day. This gut-wrenching story nearly moved me to tears.

June's Inside Tract to Wellness

In assessing June's case, I performed a colonoscopy. It revealed that she had active colitis that was limited to the rectum and sigmoid colon, hence left-sided distribution of disease. This meant that her disease had not progressed in extent or severity. This was good news for June! Special stool testing showed that June was deficient in short-chain fatty acids. Knowing that June was already on aggressive medication for her disease, I suggested a few measures.

First, I placed June on a Track 2 dietary program, as the foundation of

this diet is anti-inflammatory. Because of her short-chain fatty acid deficiency, her stool butyrate levels were low, so I prescribed butyrate in enema
form to administer rectally every evening. Since the majority of her active
disease was within the reach of an enema, I was hopeful that this medication could provide her with some immediate relief. We also discussed nutritional supplements that might be beneficial, including curcumin and
essential fatty acids.

Six weeks after placing her on this program, June and her family came to
visit me. She looked renewed and invigorated. Her symptoms were minor,
her GPS score was down from 61 to 10, and she had her life back. We were
able to successfully wean her off the corticosteroids that she had been taking to control her symptoms for the previous 2 years, and we continued to
refine her program by assigning a few additional medications and probiotics as adjuncts to her treatment. At the time of this writing, June is thriving
and has more vitality than she has felt in years.

Testimonial by June

When I was first diagnosed with ulcerative colitis, I was able to keep it
under control with small amounts of medicine. The condition was affecting
every area of my life. I was newly married, and the first years of our marriage were spent mostly in the bathroom and at doctor visits.

I felt defeated and upset. Time went by and I continued to be sick every
day. I left my first consult with Dr. Mullin feeling something I hadn't felt in
a long time: hope. He said that there were still a lot of things that hadn't
been tried, and he immediately began reevaluating me to see what was
going on. From that point on, I began to make a fast recovery and I have
been symptom-free ever since. Dr. Mullin's compassion for his patients is
insurmountable. His knowledge and patient care is unmatched. I'm so
thankful to God for placing Dr. Mullin in my path. I firmly believe my faith in
God is what healed me, but God used Dr. Mullin as the main instrument in
my healing.

Your Digestive Journey: The Path Ahead

Optimizing your digestive health requires that you have the necessary
tools: awareness of your body and its needs, nutritional knowledge, support from friends and family, time to relax and take care of yourself, and

an understanding of this fascinating and intricate inner tube of life that is so central to your health and well-being.

As you move forward on your journey toward digestive health and vitality, it is helpful to keep in mind the following:

You are unique. Your genetics, biochemical makeup and lifestyle all impact your digestive integrity and your response to dietary interventions, therapeutic supplementation, or other healing modalities. Practice self-observation and you will continue to learn what works best for you and feels best to your inside tract.

Your food is medicine. Your diet provides the bioactive raw materials that support the amazing architecture of your inside tract. Your food choices matter. With each nourishing meal, you have an opportunity to: *Eat, digest, absorb, and be healthy.*

Your lifestyle matters. Restorative sleep; movement and exercise; a non-toxic environment; healthy relationships; mindfulness; and relaxation practices are all essential nourishment for your inside tract. Self-care requires reflection: Be willing to examine the lifestyle habits that influence your digestion, and ultimately your health, and change them as needed.

You have learned that your inside tract is sensitive and vulnerable. It can be impacted by toxins (negative thoughts, unsafe chemicals), allergens and intolerances, pathogens, and imbalances in nutrients resulting from poor diet. But your digestive tract is constantly renewing, rebuilding, and recreating itself. And through this book, we hope you have discovered strategies that you can incorporate into your life to keep you on the path to health and healing.

Your inside tract is resilient. It is responsive. It is intelligent.

We hope that these stories inspire you to take charge of your own gut health and seek out ways to heal. For many, a full recovery is within reach simply by following the steps in this book. It is our greatest hope that you can take advantage of this plan and discover the inside "tract" to health and wellness for yourself. Good luck on the journey.

APPENDIX

Recipes

Welcome to your cookbook for good gut health. In this section, you will find:

- All of the recipes for Tracks 1, 2, and 3 organized according to meal (breakfast, lunch, dinner, desserts, and snacks)
- The Swift & Simple Food Charts that provide you with easy, no-recipe solutions to your daily meal choices

The recipes you will find here are uncomplicated and do not include lengthy lists of ingredients or complex instructions. Despite their simplicity, these foods are full of flavor. They will allow you to enjoy the taste of wholesome meals while providing your inside tract the nourishment it needs to heal.

Review the recipes with your inside tract and body in mind. Feel free to omit a particular ingredient if you have already determined it exacerbates your gut symptoms. For example, if soy foods are antagonistic, simply substitute another protein option such as lentils, black beans, or perhaps a piece of wild cod or salmon in place of the tofu or edamame in any given recipe.

You may also substitute one recipe for another or change the order of your meals throughout the day. The essential point is that you stick to menus in your particular track. We outlined what meals go with which tracks in the meal plans in Chapters 8–10. However, we have also identified which recipes are associated with each track in the recipes themselves, so there should be no confusion about what you can eat and what you should stay away from.

We encourage you to embrace the seasons and take advantage of local produce picks and fresh market items as they become available in your area. This may mean making some minor substitutions in a recipe. Feel free to do this as well, as long as the alternative item is not in the Forget category of the food guide that goes along with the track to which you have been assigned.

These recipes will provide you delicious meal options while you are on the program. But as you proceed down your path to good gut health, don't be afraid to experiment in the kitchen. Alter these recipes to your tastes or even develop your own. Remember, your kitchen is your laboratory of learning to discover the great tastes that soothe your inside tract. It is the inner sanctum of your home that will heal and nourish your inner tube of life.

Enjoy!

Swift & Simple Food Charts

The Swift & Simple Food Charts are shortcuts to creating easy and delicious meals in a fuss-free, no-recipe-required way. They are intended to help you throw together nutritious, delicious meals in an effortless manner. Some of these meal ideas have been integrated into the seasonal menus. These "diagrams for delicious dining" also include some additional "Anytime" suggestions for your enjoyment.

The Swift & Simple Food Charts include tempting food templates for smoothies, power porridges, wraps, salads, salad dressings, and back-to-basics bowls. All you have to do is start with the first ingredient listed and read from left to right in each block to create a whole food feast. For example, a power porridge can be created starting with amaranth, adding the correct amount of liquid and cooking it for the time indicated, and then tossing in those flavorful additions such as almonds, apples, and a touch of allspice (refer to the relevant power porridge recipe on pages 242–243). The other charts work much the same way.

You can even mix and match most food items in these charts, and adjust the fruits and veggies based on your local produce picks. However, make sure you are mindful of the grain/liquid/cooking time instructions, as these are not subject to change.

All of these interesting combinations have been balanced to your taste buds to spell "yum!" to your inside tract.

Swift & Simple Smoothies (Serves 1)

NAME/SEASON	TRACK	LIQUID	FRUIT/VEGGIES
Berry Almond Spring/Summer	Track 1	Almond beverage, ½ cup + plain yogurt, 1 cup	Mixed berries, 1½ cups
Tropical Spring/Summer	Track 1	Coconut milk, ½ cup + plain yogurt, 1 cup	Banana, ½ frozen Mango, 1 cup
Autumn Spice Fall/Winter	Track 1	Rice beverage, ½ cup + plain yogurt, 1 cup	Apple, 1 cup Pumpkin puree, ½ cup
Pear Ginger Fall/Winter	Track 1	Water, ½ cup + plain yogurt, 1 cup	Pear, 1 cup
Chocolate Dream Anytime	Track 1	Hazelnut beverage, ½ cup + plain yogurt, 1 cup	Banana, ½ frozen
Blueberry Mint Spring/Summer	Track 2	Water, 1 cup	Blueberries, ½–1 cup Watercress, ½ cup chopped
Strawberry Kiwi Spring/Summer	Track 2	Almond beverage, unsweetened, 1 cup	Strawberries and kiwi, ½–1 cup Spinach, raw, 1 cup chopped
Raspberry Cucumber Spring/Summer	Track 2	Soy beverage, plain, unsweetened, 1 cup	Raspberries, ½–1 cup Cucumber, 1 whole
Berry Almond Fall/Winter	Track 2	Water, 1 cup	Mixed berries, ½–1 cup Sweet potato, ½ cup cooked
Pumpkin Orange Fall/Winter	Track 2	Hempseed beverage, unsweetened, 1 cup	Orange slices, ½–1 cup

SWIFT & SIMPLE NOTES

- **Sweet tastings:** If your taste buds are thirsting for more sweet, you can increase the spices or add a splash of a pure organic flavor extract (for example, vanilla, maple, or peppermint), 100 percent fruit juice (for example, pomegranate, acai, or mango), or 100 percent maple syrup. But remember, you're trying to take your taste buds on a sweet retreat, so use as little as possible of these sweet additions.
- **Liquid:** Feel free to add more liquid or ice depending on how thick or thin you like the consistency of your smoothie.
- **Freezing bananas:** Peel and halve those ripe bananas you have hanging around. Wrap them in waxed paper and store in the freezer for a naturally sweet addition to any smoothie!

NUTS/SEEDS	SPICE (TO TASTE)	NUTRI-BOOSTS (OPTIONAL)
Almond butter, 1 Tbsp.	Cinnamon	Whey protein powder, 1 scoop
Macadamia nut butter, 1 Tbsp.	Nutmeg	Tofu, silken, 4 ounces
Walnuts, 2 Tbsp.	Allspice	Hempseed protein, 1 scoop
Tahini, 1 Tbsp.	Ginger	Avocado, ¼ cup
Dates, 2 Tbsp. chopped Peanut butter, 1 Tbsp.	Cocoa powder, 1 tsp.	Coconut, raw or shredded, 1 Tbsp.
Cashew nut butter, 1 Tbsp.	Mint, 8 leaves finely chopped	Brown rice protein powder, 1 scoop
Flaxseed, ground, 1 Tbsp.	Allspice or nutmeg	Hempseed protein powder, 1 scoop
Pecan nut butter, 1 Tbsp.	Cinnamon	Yogurt, soy 1 cup (omit ½ cup liquid)
Almond butter, 1 Tbsp.	Ginger	Brown rice protein powder, 1 scoop
Pumpkin puree, ½ cup Walnut butter, 1 Tbsp.	Cloves	Fruit and veggie powder, 1 scoop

- **Fruit and veggie powders:** The green/red/blue concoctions of fruit and veggie extracts can be added to your smoothies as a nutri-boost, but they are no substitute for the whole food package you obtain by using Mother Nature's fresh or frozen picks.
- **Homemade nut and seed milks:** Try making your own fresh nut and seed milks (page 252). However, if you do decide to purchase nondairy beverages, be sure to choose plain, unsweetened ones, and be aware that many nondairy beverages have added gums that might be good for some inside tracts and not so great for others.
- **Experiment:** Feel free to create your personal favorite smoothies using the categories of Liquid, Fruit/Veggies, Nuts/Seeds, Spice, and Nutri-Boosts and estimated portions as your guide, to ensure a beverage that provides a perfect balance of flavor and nutrition.

Swift & Simple Power Porridges

NAME/SEASON	GRAIN	TRACK	LIQUID (water or Inside Tract Vegetable Broth recipe)
Walnut Raisin Steel-Cut Oats Fall/Winter	Steel-cut oats, 1 cup	Track 1	3 cups
Almond Apple Amaranth Fall/Winter	Amaranth, 1 cup	Track 1	3 cups
Banana Pecan Buckwheat Anytime	Buckwheat groats, 1 cup	Track 1	2–2½ cups
Apricot Teff Anytime	Teff, 1 cup	Track 1	2½–3 cups
Raspberry Quinoa Spring/Summer	Quinoa, 1 cup dry	Track 2	2 cups
Cinnamon Blueberry Steel-Cut Oats Spring/Summer	Steel-cut oats, gluten-free, 1 cup dry	Track 2	3 cups
Banana Buckwheat Fall/Winter	Buckwheat, 1 cup dry	Track 2	2 cups
Morning Millet Fall/Winter	Millet, 1 cup dry	Track 2	3 cups
Strawberry Amaranth Fall/Winter	Amaranth, 1 cup dry	Track 2	3 cups

COOKING TIME	NUTS/SEEDS	FRUIT	SPICE/HERB (⅛ tsp. or to taste)
30 minutes	Walnuts, 1–2 Tbsp.	Raisins, 2 Tbsp.	Pumpkin pie spice
20–25 minutes	Almonds, 1–2 Tbsp.	Apple, ½	Allspice
15–20 minutes	Pecans, 1–2 Tbsp.	Banana, ½ small	Ginger
10–20 minutes	Cashews, 1–2 Tbsp.	Apricots, 1 small	Garam masala
10–15 minutes	N/A	Raspberries, ½ cup	Cloves
30 minutes	N/A	Blueberries, ½ cup	Cinnamon
15 minutes	N/A	Banana, ½ small	Ginger
20–30 minutes	N/A	Pink grapefruit (on the side)	Cinnamon
20–25 minutes	N/A	Strawberries, ½ cup	Allspice

Swift & Simple Wraps

NAME/SEASON	TRACK	PROTEIN
Curried Chicken Spring/Summer	Track 1	Grilled chicken, 3 ounces
Spring Summer	Track 2	
Turkey Avocado Crème Spring/Summer; Fall/Winter	Track 1	Roast turkey breast, 3 ounces
Spring/Summer; Fall/Winter	Track 2	
Hummus Veggie Fall/Winter	Track 1	Hummus, ⅓ cup
Fall/Winter	Track 2	
Wild Salmon Cucumber Dill Spring/Summer	Tracks 1, 2	Wild salmon, 4 ounces
Tofu Veggie Spring/Summer	Tracks 1, 2	Tofu, baked, 4 ounces

SWIFT & SIMPLE NOTES

- **Dressings:** Refer to the "Swift & Simple Dressings Chart," page 250, for dressing for each of these.
- **Keep it local:** Vary veggies and fruits with season/availability at local markets.

FRUIT/VEGETABLE/HERB (1-INCH THICKNESS IN WRAP)	SALAD DRESSING (1 TBSP.)	WRAP (ONE 6-INCH OR TWO 3-INCH WRAPS)
Red leaf lettuce Cilantro	Curried Avocado Crème	Whole or sprouted grain tortilla Brown rice tortilla
Basil leaves Sunflower sprouts	Curried Avocado Crème	Whole or sprouted grain tortilla Brown rice tortilla
Arugula Tomato	Cilantro Cumin	Whole or sprouted grain tortilla Brown rice wrap
Spinach Cucumber	Dilled Lemon Mustard	Brown rice tortilla, Boston lettuce, or savoy cabbage leaves
Arugula Red pepper Grated carrots	Lime Miso	Brown rice tortilla, Boston lettuce, or savoy cabbage leaves

Swift & Simple Salads

NAME/SEASON	TRACK	GREENS AND OTHER VEGGIES/HERBS
Shrimp Cashew Spring/Summer	Track 1	Bok choy, chopped 2 cups Carrots Thai basil
Chickpea Avocado Spring/Summer	Track 1	Red leaf lettuce, 2 cups Celery Tomato
White Bean Antipasto Spring/Summer	Tracks 1, 2	Romaine lettuce, 2 cups Artichoke hearts, canned Roasted red peppers Green beans, steamed
Lentil Spinach Spring/Summer	Tracks 1, 2	Spinach, 2 cups Tomato
Sardine Arugula Anytime	Tracks 1, 2	Arugula, 2 cups Kalamata olives Oregano
Sunflower Mesclun Anytime	Track 1	Mesclun greens, 2 cups Cucumber
Wild Salmon and Bok Choy Salad Spring/Summer	Track 2	Bok choy, 1 cup Carrots Thai basil
Lentil Spinach Salad Spring/Summer	Track 2	Spinach, 1 cup Tomato

SWIFT & SIMPLE NOTES

- **Dressings:** Refer to the "Swift & Simple Dressings Chart," page 250, for dressing for each of these.
- **Keep it local:** Vary veggies and fruits with season/availability at local markets.

PROTEIN	NUTS/SEEDS (2–3 TBSP.)	SALAD DRESSING (1 TBSP.)
Shrimp, 3–5 large	Cashews	Lime Miso
Chickpeas, ½ cup	Avocado (healthy fat)	Cilantro Cumin
White beans, ½ cup	Almonds	Herbal Essence
Lentils, ½ cup cooked	Walnuts	Dilled Lemon Mustard
Sardines, 4 ounces	Pumpkin seeds	Dilled Lemon Mustard
Goat or sheep cheese, 2 ounces	Sunflower seeds	Herbal Essence
Wild salmon, 4 ounces	Cashews	Lime Miso
Lentils, ½ cup cooked	Walnuts	Dilled Lemon Mustard

Swift & Simple Basics Bowls
(Makes 2 servings—one for now and one for later!)

NAME/SEASON	TRACK	GRAIN (½ CUP DRY)	LIQUID	COOKING TIME
Salmon Barley Fall/Winter	Track 1	Barley, unpearled, ½ cup	Water, 1½ cups	1 hour 15 minutes
Wild Rice Escarole Fall/Winter	Track 1	Wild rice, ½ cup	Water, 1½ cups	50–60 minutes
Arugula Bulgur Fall/Winter	Track 1	Whole wheat bulgur, ½ cup	Water, 1 cup	15 minutes
Black Bean Quinoa Fall/Winter	Track 1	Red quinoa, ½ cup	Water, 1 cup	15 minutes
Basmati Rice and Edamame Fall/Winter	Track 1	Brown basmati rice, ½ cup	Water, 1½ cups	35–40 minutes
Salmon Quinoa Fall/Winter	Track 2	Quinoa, ½ cup	Water, 1 cup	15 minutes
Adzuki Millet Fall/Winter	Track 2	Millet, ½ cup	Water, 1½ cups	20 minutes
Edamame Black Rice Fall/Winter	Track 2	Black rice, ½ cup	Water, 1 cup	30 minutes

SWIFT & SIMPLE NOTES

- **Dressings:** Refer to the "Swift & Simple Dressings Chart," page 250, for dressing for each of these.
- **Keep it local:** Vary veggies and fruits with season/availability at local markets.
- **Herbs:** Vary herbs and spices according to your taste preferences and tolerance. (If you do not tolerate a particular spice, omit it and substitute one you tolerate; if you prefer rosemary to oregano, use rosemary!)
- **Use medicinal ingredients:** Kombu (kelp) strips, bay leaf, fennel, and epazote (a wild herb) may help decrease gaseous factors in beans, so experiment with these flavorful and medicinal ingredients.

PROTEIN	GREENS + OTHER VEGGIES (3 CUPS)	HERB/SPICE OR DRESSING (⅛ TSP. OR TO TASTE)
Wild salmon, 8 ounces, canned or leftover	Collard greens Cauliflower Garlic and onions	Bay leaf
Seeds: pumpkin, sunflower, ½ cup	Escarole Red pepper Garlic and onions	Basil
Adzuki beans, 1 cup	Arugula Carrots Garlic and onions	Garam masala
Black beans, one 15-ounce can	Parsley Tomato Garlic and scallions	Cilantro Cumin Dressing
Edamame, 1 cup	Spinach Shiitake mushrooms Garlic and onions	Lime Miso Dressing
Wild salmon, 8 ounces, canned or leftover	Kale Shiitake mushrooms	Curry powder
Adzuki beans, 1 cup + Kombu (kelp), 5-inch strip	Swiss chard Carrots	Garam masala
Edamame, 1 cup	Bok choy Celery	Ginger and red-pepper flakes

Swift & Simple Dressings

These dressings can be used in Track 1 & Track 2.

DRESSING NAME	LIQUID	OIL
Cilantro Cumin	¼ cup freshly squeezed lime juice 2 Tbsp. water	½ cup extra-virgin olive oil
Curried Avocado Crème	¼ cup freshly squeezed lime juice ¼ cup water	1 Tbsp. extra-virgin olive oil
Dilled Lemon Mustard	¼ cup freshly squeezed lemon juice ¼ cup water	½ cup extra-virgin olive oil
Herbal Essence	¼ cup freshly squeezed lemon juice ¼ cup water	½ cup extra-virgin olive oil
Lime Miso	2 Tbsp. miso ¼ cup freshly squeezed lime juice 2 Tbsp. sesame tahini ¼ cup water	¼ cup grape seed oil

SWIFT & SIMPLE NOTES

- **Tip:** ¼ cup freshly squeezed lemon or lime juice = approximately 1 lemon or lime
- **Prepare in advance:** Make a batch of these dressings and store in airtight glass jars to use on salads, wraps, entrees, basics bowls, etc.
- **Oil:** You can decrease the oil and substitute Inside Tract Vegetable Broth or water if you are more sensitive to fat-based ingredients.

HERB	SPICE	NOTES
2 Tbsp. fresh cilantro, chopped, or 2 tsp. dried cilantro	1 tsp. grated orange peel, organic ¼ tsp. ground cumin Sea salt and freshly ground pepper, optional to taste	Whisk all ingredients in a small bowl until well blended.
1 avocado, peeled and chopped	½ tsp. curry powder Sea salt and freshly ground pepper, optional to taste	Puree in a food processor or blender until smooth.
2 Tbsp. fresh dill, finely chopped, or 2 tsp. dried dill	2 tsp. mustard powder Sea salt and freshly ground pepper, optional to taste	Whisk until well blended.
2 Tbsp. fresh parsley, finely chopped, or 2 tsp. dried parsley	½ tsp. ground turmeric Sea salt and freshly ground pepper, optional to taste	Combine in a food processor or blender.
1 Tbsp. fresh ginger, minced, or 1 tsp. dried ginger powder	Freshly ground pepper, optional to taste	Whisk until well blended.

Track 1 Spring/Summer—Breakfast

Homemade Nut or Seed Milk

—*Leslie Cerier, author of* **Gluten-Free Recipes for the Conscious Cook**

TRACKS 1 & 2

Leslie and I teach whole-food, gluten-free workshops at Kripalu Center for Yoga and Health. It's fun to dabble in making your own nut or seed milks. You will have a nondairy beverage that is free of gums and ingredients like carrageenan that might be bothersome to your gut!

PREP TIME: 20 MINUTES | **SOAK TIME:** OVERNIGHT | **COOK TIME:** NONE | **MAKES:** 4 CUPS

> 1 cup raw almonds (with skins)
> 4 cups filtered water

Combine the almonds and 1½ cups of water (not from the 4 cups filtered water) and soak for at least 12 hours or overnight. Drain the almonds, discarding their soaking water, then rinse and drain well.

Put the almonds and the filtered water in a blender. Blend until smooth, or until the water looks like milk.

Pour the mixture through a fine-mesh sieve, pressing the almond meal with the back of a spoon to get every last drop of almond milk. (You can also strain the milk using a cheesecloth or a nut milk bag; be sure to squeeze to get every last drop of milk.) Discard the almond meal.

Store in an airtight container in the refrigerator for up to 5 days.

PER CUP OF NUTS OR SEEDS (VOLUME PRIOR TO SOAKING)	WATER (CUPS)
Almonds	4
Brazil nuts	2½
Cashews	3½
Coconut, unsweetened, shredded	2
Hazelnuts	2½
Hempseeds	3
Sesame seeds	6
Sunflower seeds	6

Note: For a thicker, creamier milk, you can use less liquid. You can also add 100% organic flavor extracts, maple syrup, molasses, or honey for a touch of sweetness.

Poached Eggs with Herb Spread

TRACK 1 SPRING/SUMMER

Egg yolks are one of the best sources of the essential nutrient choline, important for the neurological system. Partnering them with this green herb spread makes a powerful anti-inflammatory wake-up call.

PREP TIME: 5 MINUTES | **COOK TIME:** 5 MINUTES | **MAKES:** 1–2 SERVINGS

> 2 eggs
> 2 slices whole grain toast
> Herb Spread (page 254), to taste

Heat water in a shallow saucepan until almost boiling. Crack the eggs in a small cup, one at a time, and add gently to the water. Turn off the heat, cover, and let sit for 4 minutes. Using a slotted spoon, lift the eggs out of the water. Place on the toast and drizzle with Herb Spread.

Herb Spread

TRACK 1, TRACK 2, & TRACK 3

PREP TIME: 5 MINUTES | **COOK TIME:** NONE | **MAKES:** ½ CUP

¼ cup fresh herbs, loosely packed (dill, parsley, basil, tarragon,
   or cilantro), chopped
¼ cup extra-virgin olive oil
2 tablespoons freshly squeezed lemon juice
½ teaspoon ground turmeric

Place all of the ingredients in a blender or small food processor and process until well blended. If not using immediately, transfer to an airtight container and refrigerate for up to 3 days.

Berry Yogurt Parfait

TRACK 1 SPRING/SUMMER

Seeds are a delicious and nutritious addition to this berry yogurt parfait. Flaxseed, chia seeds, and hempseeds provide essential fatty acids. Pumpkin seeds pack in zinc, and sunflower seeds offer a hefty dose of antioxidant vitamin E.

PREP TIME: 5 MINUTES | **COOK TIME:** NONE | **MAKES:** 2 SERVINGS

1 cup fresh or frozen berries (blueberries, blackberries,
   cherries, raspberries)
1 cup plain yogurt (cow, goat, or sheep milk)
¼ cup chopped nuts (almonds, walnuts, pecans)
2 teaspoons ground seeds (chia, flax, hemp, pumpkin, or
   sunflower)

Crush the berries slightly with the side of a spoon to release the juices.
   In two 8-ounce glasses, layer the ingredients beginning with the berries: ¼ cup berries, ¼ cup yogurt, 1 tablespoon nuts, and ½ teaspoon seeds. Repeat the layers.

Morning Muesli

TRACK 1 SPRING/SUMMER

The addition of one apple in your Morning Muesli packs your breakfast with dietary fiber, vitamin C, and antioxidants including flavonoids and phenols. Try quinoa flakes along with certified gluten-free oats for a Track 2 Morning Muesli that is gluten-free.

PREP TIME: 5 MINUTES | **SOAK TIME:** OVERNIGHT | **COOK TIME:** NONE | **MAKES:** 8 (½-CUP) SERVINGS

> 2 cups rolled oats
> 3 tablespoons seeds (sunflower or pumpkin)
> 3 tablespoons nuts, chopped (walnuts or pecans)
> 3 tablespoons dried fruit (raisins, currants, blueberries, or cranberries)
> 1 apple, grated or finely chopped
> 3 cups homemade almond or other nut/seed beverage (page 252)

Combine the oats, seeds, nuts, dried fruit, and apple in a large bowl. Heat the almond beverage on low heat until it comes to a gentle boil. Pour over the dry mixture, mixing lightly. Cover and refrigerate overnight. Serve cold or heated, if desired.

Herb Scramble

—Caroline Nation, chef and founder of MyFoodMyHealth.com

TRACK 1 SPRING/SUMMER

This is a high-protein kickoff to the day and can be enjoyed with your favorite herbs. The scramble is also delicious with chives, dill, basil, or cilantro. Blanching the herbs for 1 minute keeps them bright green.

PREP TIME: 10 MINUTES | **COOK TIME:** 5 MINUTES | **MAKES:** 2 SERVINGS

¼ cup parsley or mixture of fresh herbs, finely chopped and
   minced
4 eggs
Pinch of sea salt
Freshly ground black pepper
1½ teaspoons extra-virgin olive oil

Bring a medium pot of water to a boil over high heat. Add the parsley or herb mixture and cook for 1 minute, then drain and rinse under cold water.

Whisk the eggs in a medium bowl. Add the parsley, sea salt, and several grinds of pepper and whisk to combine.

Warm the oil in a cast-iron skillet over medium heat. Pour in the eggs and stir gently and constantly, for 2 to 3 minutes, or until the eggs form large curds and are cooked to your preference. Serve immediately.

Melon with Minted Yogurt

TRACK 1 SPRING/SUMMER

Cantaloupe and honeydew melon are sources of vitamin C, vitamin A, and beta-carotene. The addition of antispasmodic mint leaves creates a GI-calming breakfast loaded with antioxidants and phytonutrients.

PREP TIME: 5 MINUTES | **COOK TIME:** NONE | **MAKES:** 2 SERVINGS

2 cups plain yogurt (cow, goat, or sheep milk)
¼ cup fresh mint leaves, chopped
2 teaspoons honey
½ honeydew or cantaloupe melon, seeded and cut into chunks

Mix the yogurt, mint, and honey. Pour over the melon chunks and enjoy.

Layers of Lox

TRACK 1 SPRING/SUMMER & TRACK 2

Just a drizzle of the dressing to the omega-3-rich wild salmon adds phyto-nutrients including phenolic acids from the dill and antioxidants including vitamin C, carotenoids, flavonoids, and phenols from the lemon.

PREP TIME: 5 MINUTES | **COOK TIME:** NONE | **MAKES:** 2 SERVINGS

> 4 ounces wild caught lox, nitrate free and naturally smoked
> 1 small English cucumber, thinly sliced
> 1 tomato, thinly sliced
> 2 tablespoons Dilled Lemon Mustard Dressing (page 250)

Place the salmon, cucumber, and tomato in stacks and drizzle with the dressing.

Lemon Cottage Cheese Pancakes

—Myra Kornfeld, chef at MyFoodMyHealth.com

TRACK 1 SPRING/SUMMER

Alkalinizing lemons are digestive aids, and the pectin in the citrus peel enhances the body's natural detoxification process. When choosing a lemon, look for a fresh lemon with a full, bright yellow color.

PREP TIME: 10 MINUTES | **COOK TIME:** 12–15 MINUTES | **MAKES:** 9–10 PANCAKES

> 1 cup whole wheat pastry flour
> ½ teaspoon baking powder
> ¼ teaspoon baking soda
> ¼ teaspoon sea salt
> ½ cup 2% cottage cheese, small curd
> 1 egg
> Grated zest of 1 lemon

2 tablespoons freshly squeezed lemon juice
1 tablespoon melted butter
½ cup water

In a medium bowl, whisk together the flour, baking powder, baking soda, and salt.

In another bowl, whisk together the cottage cheese, egg, lemon zest, lemon juice, butter, and water. Stir into the dry ingredients and mix well.

Preheat a cast-iron griddle and lightly grease with butter or oil. Ladle ⅓ cup of the batter onto the griddle and cook until the top bubbles. Flip and cook until golden and cooked throughout. Continue with the remaining batter.

Serve hot with fresh fruit and/or a drizzle of 100% maple syrup.

Track 1 Spring/Summer—Lunch

Black and Red Salad

TRACK 1 SPRING/SUMMER & TRACK 2 (OMIT SHALLOTS)

Quinoa is a quintessential gluten-free grain source of dietary fiber, manganese, magnesium, and lignans and offers a protein and calcium boost.

PREP TIME: 15 MINUTES | **COOK TIME:** 25 MINUTES | **MAKES:** 6 (½-CUP) SERVINGS

> ½ cup red quinoa
> 1 15-ounce can black beans, drained and rinsed
> 2 plum tomatoes, diced
> ½ small bunch parsley, coarsely chopped
> ¼ cup kalamata olives, diced
> 2 scallions, white and green parts, thinly sliced
> 2 cloves garlic, finely chopped
> 1 medium cucumber, peeled, seeded, and diced
> ¼ cup Cilantro Cumin Dressing (page 250)

Rinse the quinoa well in cool water and drain in a fine-mesh strainer. Place the quinoa in a small pot with 2 cups water. Bring to a boil, stir to combine, turn down the heat, and cover with a tight-fitting lid. Simmer for 15 minutes, or until the water is absorbed and the quinoa is cooked. Do not disturb the steam holes that form as the quinoa cooks. Remove from the heat and let sit an additional 10 minutes. Transfer the quinoa to a large bowl and toss gently. Cover and chill in the refrigerator while preparing the remaining ingredients.

Combine the beans, tomatoes, parsley, olives, scallions, garlic, and cucumber with the dressing. Add to the quinoa and mix thoroughly. Serve.

Track 1 Spring/Summer—Dinner

Turkey Herb Burger

TRACK 1 SPRING/SUMMER, TRACK 2, & TRACK 3 (SPICES AS TOLERATED)

In these burgers, lean turkey is mixed with herbs that offer healing properties, including chives that stimulate digestion. For a quick meal, the burgers can be frozen and reheated, or try one at breakfast for a morning protein lift along with a splash of one of the dressings or salsa.

PREP TIME: 10 MINUTES | **COOK TIME:** 12 MINUTES | **MAKES:** 4 SERVINGS

> 1 pound ground turkey, 93% lean
> ¼ cup fresh basil, finely chopped
> ¼ cup fresh mint, finely chopped
> ¼ cup fresh chives, finely chopped
> 1 teaspoon dried sage
> Sea salt
> Freshly ground black pepper

In a large bowl, combine the turkey, basil, mint, chives, and sage. Add salt and pepper to taste. Mix gently and form into 4 patties. Heat a cast-iron skillet or grill pan brushed with oil. Brown the burgers for 6 minutes on each side, or until cooked through.

Gerardo's Gazpacho

TRACK 1 SPRING/SUMMER

The apple cider vinegar and mint in this recipe perk up the flavor and stimulate digestion. And gazpacho consumption may cool down inflammation.

PREP TIME: 30 MINUTES | **CHILL TIME:** 2 HOURS | **COOK TIME:** NONE |
MAKES: 8 (1 CUP) SERVINGS

1½ pounds tomatoes (5 medium), chopped
1 medium English cucumber, seeded and diced
¼ cup diced red onion
1 yellow bell pepper, diced
1 tablespoon freshly squeezed lime juice
3 cups low-sodium vegetable or tomato juice
¼ cup apple cider vinegar
2 tablespoons fresh mint, finely chopped
2 tablespoons fresh parsley, finely chopped

Combine the tomatoes, cucumber, onion, and pepper in a large bowl. Add the lime juice, vegetable or tomato juice, vinegar, mint, and parsley. Mix well and chill at least 2 hours before serving. The longer gazpacho sits, the more the flavors develop.

Cabbage Salad

TRACK 1 SPRING/SUMMER

Red and green cabbage partner with other antioxidant- and polyphenol-rich ingredients in this raw salad with a caraway crunch for digestive harmony.

PREP TIME: 15 MINUTES | **COOK TIME:** NONE | **MAKES:** 6 (½-CUP) SERVINGS

1 cup shredded Chinese (Napa) or green cabbage
1 cup shredded red cabbage
2 large carrots, shredded
⅓ cup scallion greens, thinly sliced
1 green apple, chopped
1 tablespoon caraway seeds
¼ cup Lime Miso Dressing (page 250)

In a large bowl, combine the cabbages, carrots, scallions, apple, and caraway seeds. Pour the dressing over the slaw and toss well.

Dilled Lemon Mustard Chicken Breasts

TRACK 1 SPRING/SUMMER & TRACK 2

Dill and lemon combine to offer a fresh and digestive-soothing marinade for a quick summer dinner.

PREP TIME: 1 HOUR TO MARINATE | **COOK TIME:** 10 MINUTES | **MAKES:** 4 SERVINGS

⅔ cup Dilled Lemon Mustard Dressing (page 250)
4 chicken breasts, boneless and skinless

Marinate the chicken breasts in the dressing. Cover and refrigerate for 1 hour.

Preheat an outdoor grill or grill pan. Grill the chicken for 4 to 5 minutes per side, depending on the thickness, or until the chicken is cooked through and the juices run clear.

Summer Squash

TRACK 1 SPRING/SUMMER & TRACK 2

Both zucchini and yellow summer squash offer manganese, vitamin C, the antioxidant lutein, and dietary fiber to your day. Try finding fresh, local sources of these vegetables.

PREP TIME: 5 MINUTES | **COOK TIME:** 6 MINUTES | **MAKES:** 2 SERVINGS

2 zucchini
1 yellow summer squash
⅓ cup Dilled Lemon Mustard Dressing (page 250)

Cut the zucchini and squash lengthwise to ¼" thickness. Drizzle with the dressing. Grill for 3 minutes per side.

Macadamia Nut–Crusted Cod

TRACK 1 SPRING/SUMMER & TRACK 2

Macadamia nuts contain antioxidants, vitamin E, and oleic acid. Although very high in fat, when eaten in moderation they promote heart health, protect cell membranes from free radical damage, and stimulate the liver.

PREP TIME: 15 MINUTES | **COOK TIME:** 20 MINUTES | **MAKES:** 4 SERVINGS

⅓ cup macadamia nuts
2 teaspoons shredded coconut, unsweetened
1 tablespoon parsley, minced
1 tablespoon freshly squeezed lime juice
1 teaspoon Chinese five-spice seasoning powder
1 pound wild cod, cut into 4-ounce portions

Preheat the oven to 350°F. Brush an ovenproof dish with a small amount of olive oil. Place the macadamia nuts in a food processor and grind until coarse. Add the coconut, parsley, lime juice, and spice blend. Pulse until blended. Brush the cod with a small amount of olive oil using a pastry brush. Press the nut mixture onto the top surface of the cod to adhere. Transfer to the prepared dish. Bake for 20 minutes, or until the fish flakes.

Pineapple Black Rice

TRACK 1 SPRING/SUMMER & TRACK 2

Bromelain in the pineapple stimulates digestion and provides a beautiful color combination with the high-antioxidant, high-flavor black rice.

PREP TIME: 3 MINUTES | **COOK TIME:** 30 MINUTES | **MAKES:** 4 SERVINGS

1 cup black rice
1¾ cups water
1 cup diced fresh pineapple

Combine the rice and water and bring to a boil. Cover and reduce the heat to a simmer for 30 minutes. Remove from the heat and fluff with a fork. Add the pineapple and serve.

Broccoli Rabe and White Beans on Whole Grain Pasta

TRACK 1 SPRING/SUMMER

Broccoli rabe contains vitamin K, vitamin C, vitamin A, and dietary fiber, and is rich in antioxidants. This bitter brassica promotes heart health, intestinal health, and improves natural detoxification.

PREP TIME: 10 MINUTES | **COOK TIME:** 10 MINUTES | **MAKES:** 4 SERVINGS

> 1 pound whole grain pasta
> 1 pound broccoli rabe, cleaned and chopped
> 2 tablespoons olive oil
> 2 cloves garlic, thinly sliced
> 1 medium shallot, thinly sliced
> 1 can (15 ounces) white beans, drained
> ⅛ teaspoon red-pepper flakes

Cook the pasta according to package directions. While the pasta is cooking, steam the broccoli rabe for 2 to 3 minutes, or until tender. Plunge the broccoli rabe into an ice water bath to stop the cooking and retain the bright green color. Drain after a few minutes.

Add the oil, garlic, and shallot to a medium pan and cook over medium heat until golden brown. Add the beans, broccoli rabe, and pepper flakes. Toss gently to mix. Remove from the heat and pour over the cooked pasta.

Greek Salad

TRACK 1 SPRING/SUMMER & TRACK 2 (OMIT FETA CHEESE)

Basil and oregano team up to infuse flavor and medicinal benefits to this traditional Greek salad, also rich in lycopenes from the tomatoes.

PREP TIME: 10 MINUTES | **COOK TIME:** NONE | **MAKES:** 2 SERVINGS

> 2 medium cucumbers, diced
> 3 ripe tomatoes, diced

¼ cup basil, thinly sliced
¼ cup oregano, finely chopped
2 tablespoons halved kalamata olives
2 tablespoons feta cheese
1 tablespoon extra-virgin olive oil
1 tablespoon red wine vinegar
Freshly ground black pepper

Add the cucumbers, tomatoes, basil, oregano, olives, and feta to a salad bowl. Mix together the oil and vinegar, then toss with the salad. Add pepper to taste.

Grilled Wild Salmon

Ginger and citrus impart flavor to, and enhance the anti-inflammatory index of, this quick and easy wild salmon. You can also enjoy any extra for your breakfast the next morning.

TRACK 1 SPRING/SUMMER & TRACK 2

PREP TIME: 30 MINUTES TO MARINATE | **COOK TIME:** 8–10 MINUTES |
MAKES: 4 SERVINGS

¼ cup fresh orange juice
¼ cup tamari, gluten-free
1 tablespoon organic Dijon mustard
3 teaspoons fresh ginger, peeled and grated, or 1 teaspoon dried
4 (6-ounce) wild salmon fillets

Whisk together the orange juice, tamari, Dijon mustard, and ginger. Set aside one-third of the marinade. Add the remaining marinade to the salmon, cover, and refrigerator for at least 30 minutes.

Prepare an outdoor grill or grill pan. Grill the salmon fillets for 4 to 5 minutes per side, depending on the thickness, or until the fish is cooked through and flaky. Drizzle the remaining marinade over the cooked salmon to serve.

Green Beans with Slivered Almonds

TRACK 1 SPRING/SUMMER & TRACK 2

Green beans up your intake of beta-carotene, vitamin C, and dietary fiber. The crunchy almonds add healthy monounsaturated fats.

PREP TIME: 8 MINUTES | **COOK TIME:** 5–8 MINUTES | **MAKES:** 4 SERVINGS

> 1 pound green beans
> ¼ cup slivered almonds

Fill the bottom of a steamer pot with 2" of water. Steam the green beans for 5 minutes, or until al dente. Sprinkle with the almonds.

Lamb or Beef Vegetable Kebabs

TRACK 1 SPRING/SUMMER

These delicious oregano-scented kebabs can easily be made with 1 pound of extra-firm tofu or tempeh for a vegetarian twist.

PREP TIME: 10 MINUTES + 1 HOUR TO MARINATE | **COOK TIME:** 15 MINUTES | **MAKES:** 4 SERVINGS

> ½ cup freshly squeezed lemon juice
> 2 tablespoons dried oregano
> ¼ cup extra-virgin olive oil
> 1 pound lean lamb or beef, trimmed of fat and cut into 1" cubes
> 16 cherry tomatoes
> 1 large green bell pepper, cut into 1" pieces
> 1 large red bell pepper, cut into 1" pieces
> 1 large onion, cut into 1" pieces

In a small bowl, combine the lemon juice, oregano, and oil. Set aside ¼ cup, cover, and refrigerate. Pour the remaining marinade over the lamb or beef cubes and marinate for at least 1 hour, or overnight. Preheat a grill. Drain the marinade. Using metal or soaked wooden skewers, alternately thread the meat cubes and the vegetables. Grill the kebabs, uncovered, over medium heat for 3 minutes per side. Baste with the reserved marinade. Grill for 8 to 10 minutes longer, or until the meat is done, turning and basting frequently.

Serve with Minted Brown Rice (below) and steamed dandelion greens.

Minted Brown Rice

TRACK 1 SPRING/SUMMER & TRACK 2

Fresh mint enhances the cooling and calming properties of this gluten-free pantry staple.

PREP TIME: 5 MINUTES | **COOK TIME:** 30 MINUTES | **MAKES:** 6 SERVINGS

> 2 cups basmati brown rice
> 4 cups water
> ¼ cup fresh mint, chopped

Rinse the rice in a mesh colander. Place the rice in a medium saucepan. Add the water and cook, covered, over medium heat for 25 to 30 minutes, or until the rice is cooked. Add the mint and toss gently.

Cilantro Cumin Tilapia

TRACK 1 SPRING/SUMMER & TRACK 2

Cilantro, featured in the dressing, is a cooling and detoxifying herb. When purchasing these leaves of the coriander plant, choose a bunch that looks very fresh and has a pleasant aroma.

PREP TIME: 5 MINUTES + 1 HOUR TO MARINATE | **COOK TIME:** 15 MINUTES | **MAKES:** 4 SERVINGS

> 4 (6-ounce) tilapia fillets
> ¾ cup Cilantro Cumin Dressing (page 250)

Preheat the oven at 350°F. Place the fish in a baking dish and pour two-thirds of the dressing over the fish. Cover and refrigerate for 1 hour.

Bake for 12 to 15 minutes, or until flaky and moist on the inside. Remove the fish from the baking dish, discard the liquid, and use the remaining one-third of the dressing as a drizzle over each serving.

Track 1 Fall/Winter—Breakfast

Southwestern Egg Wrap

TRACK 1 FALL/WINTER

Going green in the morning ensures your day will begin with vitamins, minerals, and phytonutrients to provide your body with antioxidant protection and promote health.

PREP TIME: 10 MINUTES | **COOK TIME:** 10 MINUTES | **MAKES:** 2 SERVINGS

> 4 eggs
> 2 sprouted corn tortillas
> ¼ cup prepared salsa
> ¼ cup greens of your choice (spinach, watercress, arugula, parsley)

Place the eggs in a saucepan and cover with cold water. Bring to a boil, turn off the heat, and let sit for 10 minutes. Rinse the eggs in cold water, then peel and slice. Lay the tortillas flat and layer with the sliced eggs, salsa, and greens. Roll to enclose.

Sunrise Patty

TRACK 1 FALL/WINTER

Sweet potato and oats are combined with the zip of curry, sweet red bell peppers, and parsley to stimulate digestion and healing. These patties can be made ahead and frozen for later use.

PREP TIME: 15 MINUTES | **FREEZE TIME:** 15 MINUTES | **COOK TIME:** 10 MINUTES + TIME TO BAKE SWEET POTATO (50–60 MINUTES) | **MAKES:** 4 SERVINGS

> 1 large sweet potato, baked
> ⅔ cup rolled oats
> 1 egg

2 tablespoons fresh parsley, finely chopped
2 tablespoons red bell pepper, finely chopped
1 teaspoon curry powder
¼ cup sunflower seeds
2 teaspoons olive oil

Peel the baked sweet potato and mash with a fork until small chunks remain. Add the oats, egg, parsley, pepper, and curry and combine. Stir in the seeds. Shape the dough into 4 patties and place in the freezer for 15 minutes. Add the oil to a large skillet and heat over medium heat. Cook each patty for 2 to 3 minutes on each side, or until cooked through.

Banana Sunflower Seed Log

TRACK 1 FALL/WINTER

Sunflower seed butter is a tasty, nutrient-dense addition to the fruit log that provides protein, B vitamins, vitamin E, and a load of magnificent minerals including magnesium, calcium, potassium, and selenium.

PREP TIME: 3 MINUTES | **COOK TIME:** NONE | **MAKES:** 2 SERVINGS

2 small bananas
2 tablespoons natural sunflower seed butter
1 tablespoon coconut flakes

Peel and slice the bananas lengthwise. Spread with the butter and sprinkle with the coconut.

Track 1 Desserts/Treats

Homemade Coconut Milk

TRACK 1

Make your own coconut milk without gums or carrageenan. Place in an airtight jar and store in the refrigerator for up to 5 days.

PREP TIME: 1 MINUTE | **COOK TIME:** NONE | **MAKES:** 1 CUP

> 1 tablespoon creamed coconut (I used Let's Do Organic
>   Creamed Coconut)
> 1 cup hot water

Add the creamed coconut and water to a blender and process until smooth.

Berry Delicious Slush

TRACK 1

This berry slush infused with mint or lavender leaves is a nutritious, sweet, and soothing warm-weather treat for any time of the day.

PREP TIME: 5 MINUTES | **COOK TIME:** NONE | **MAKES:** 4 SERVINGS

> 1 cup Homemade Coconut Milk
> 1 cup fresh or frozen berries (raspberries, strawberries, or
>   blueberries)
> 2 frozen bananas
> 2 tablespoons 100% frozen juice concentrate
> 2 teaspoons dried mint or lavender leaves

Place all the ingredients in a blender and process until smooth. Serve immediately or freeze for later enjoyment.

Fruit Crisp

TRACK 1

You can use gluten-free oats in this recipe for a delicious crisp that is a traditional fall/winter favorite. It makes a yummy breakfast, too!

PREP TIME: 15 MINUTES | **COOK TIME:** 45 MINUTES | **MAKES:** 12 SERVINGS

> 7 apples, unpeeled, cored, and sliced
> 4 teaspoons freshly squeezed lemon juice
> 2½ teaspoons pumpkin pie spice
> ¾ cup maple syrup
> 1½ cups rolled oats
> 6 tablespoons brown rice flour
> 6 tablespoons organic butter, softened

Preheat oven to 375°F. Place the apples in a 9" × 13" × 2" glass baking dish. Sprinkle the lemon juice and 1 teaspoon of the pumpkin pie spice over the apples. In a medium bowl, add the maple syrup, oats, flour, butter, and the remaining 1½ teaspoons pumpkin pie spice. Stir until well blended. Spoon the mixture evenly over the apples. Bake for 45 minutes. Serve warm or cold.

Lemon Ginger Cookie

TRACKS 1 & 2

Make a batch of these lemon ginger gems that use delicious almond meal instead of flour as a base.

PREP TIME: 5 MINUTES | **COOK TIME:** 8–10 MINUTES | **MAKES:** 2 DOZEN

> 2½ cups almond meal/flour
> 1 teaspoon baking soda
> 2 tablespoons ground ginger
> ¼ cup grape seed oil
> ½ cup maple syrup
> 1 tablespoon lemon zest

Preheat the oven to 350°F. In a large bowl, combine the almond meal, baking soda, and ginger. In a medium bowl, combine the oil, syrup, and zest. Add to the dry ingredients and mix until well blended. Scoop 1 tablespoon of the dough onto a parchment-lined baking sheet. Bake for 8 to 10 minutes, or until the tops start to crack.

Swift Energy Bar

TRACK 1

Commercial energy bars abound, but it's far more fun and economical to create your own. You can vary the types of nuts, seeds, and dried fruit to include your favorites, so don't be afraid to make some substitutions.

PREP TIME: 10 MINUTES | **CHILL TIME:** 30 MINUTES | **COOK TIME:** 3 MINUTES | **MAKES:** 16 BARS

> 1 cup Crunchy Flax cereal
> ¼ cup chia seeds, ground
> ½ cup pumpkin seeds
> ½ cup sunflower seeds
> ½ cup chopped pecans
> ½ cup slivered or chopped almonds
> ½ cup dried fruit (no added sugar)
> ½ cup water
> 1 cup cashew nut butter
> ½ cup maple syrup

In a large bowl, combine the cereal, seeds, nuts, and dried fruit. Set aside. In a 3-quart saucepan, combine ¼ cup of the water, the nut butter, and maple syrup. Cook over medium heat, stirring constantly, until well blended. Add the remaining ¼ cup water and keep stirring to maintain consistency, as the mixture has a tendency to thicken quickly. Remove from the heat and immediately stir in the dry ingredients until mixed. Press the dough into an 8" × 8" baking dish. Store in the refrigerator for at least 30 minutes. Cut into 16 bars.

Chocolate Cherry Chews

TRACK 1

The combination of prunes, cocoa powder, and tart cherry juice packs some antioxidant, anti-inflammatory potential in these sweet gems that are also stimulating to the bowel.

PREP TIME: 5 MINUTES │ **CHILL TIME:** 30 MINUTES │ **COOK TIME:** NONE │
MAKES: 12 CHEWS

¼ cup tart cherry juice
1 tablespoon cocoa powder
½ cup prunes, pitted
½ cup dates, pitted
½ cup almond meal
1 teaspoon orange zest

In a small saucepan over medium heat, add the cherry juice. Stir in the cocoa powder and whisk until smooth.

Place the prunes and dates in a food processor and pulse for 30 seconds, or until a thick puree consistency. Add the almond meal, zest, and cocoa-cherry juice to the puree and pulse to combine. Transfer the mixture to a bowl and place in the freezer for 30 minutes. Remove from the freezer, and roll into twelve 1" balls. Coat with additional almond meal, if desired.

Track 1 Fall/Winter—Lunch

Luscious Lentil Soup

TRACK 1 FALL/WINTER & TRACK 2

Lentils offer folate, iron, zinc, and selenium and pack in a hefty dose of dietary fiber. They're complemented by quinoa, vegetables, and the aromatic and anti-inflammatory spice, garam masala.

PREP TIME: 15 MINUTES | **COOK TIME:** 40 MINUTES | **MAKES:** 8 (12-OUNCE) SERVINGS

> 8 cups Inside Tract Vegetable Broth (page 287), or commercial low-sodium, gluten-free vegetable broth
> 3 large carrots, washed and sliced
> 2 ribs celery, diced
> ¼ fennel bulb, chopped
> 3 cloves garlic, minced
> 2 teaspoons garam masala
> 1½ cups red lentils, rinsed
> ⅓ cup quinoa
> 2 tablespoons tomato paste
> 1 bay leaf

Add all the ingredients to a 6- to 8-quart pot and bring to a boil. Cook for 5 minutes, stirring occasionally. Reduce the heat to low, cover, and cook over low heat for 30 minutes, or until the lentils and quinoa are tender. Discard the bay leaf and serve.

Soothing Chicken Soup

TRACK 1 FALL/WINTER & TRACK 2

The bay leaves in this soothing soup add not only flavor but also medicinal properties from anti-inflammatory and antioxidant compounds. The dried leaves have traditionally been used to relax digestive organs.

PREP TIME: 20 MINUTES | **CHILL TIME:** OVERNIGHT | **COOK TIME:** 2½–3 HOURS | **MAKES:** 12 (12-OUNCE) SERVINGS

1 (3–4-pound) whole chicken, cleaned, with giblets and liver removed
4 quarts cold water
3 ribs celery with leaves, chopped
3 large carrots, sliced
½ fennel bulb, chopped
1 medium sweet potato, peeled and diced
3 cups escarole, chopped
2 bay leaves
2 teaspoons turmeric
¼ cup fresh parsley, chopped, or 1 tablespoon dried
¼ cup fresh dill, chopped, or 1 tablespoon dried
¼ cup fresh tarragon, chopped, or 1 tablespoon dried
Sea salt
Freshly ground black pepper

Place the chicken into a large pot and cover with the water. Bring to a gentle boil and skim off any scum that rises to the top. Turn down the heat and add the vegetables, bay leaves, and herbs. Season to taste with salt and pepper. Simmer on low for at least 2 hours, or until the chicken is tender. When simmering, the surface of the liquid should tremble slightly.

Remove the chicken from the broth, debone it, and return it to the pot. Continue to simmer for at least 30 minutes longer. Chill the soup overnight. Remove the solidified fat layer with a spoon and discard. Remove the bay leaves. To serve, reheat the soup and enjoy.

Track 1 Fall/Winter—Dinner

Mediterranean Turkey Meatballs with Whole Grain Pasta and Marinara Sauce

TRACK 1 FALL/WINTER & TRACK 2 (WITH GLUTEN-FREE PASTA)

Warming oregano has traditionally been used to treat gastrointestinal disorders. The relative of basil has antimicrobial and antibacterial properties, while the flaxseed gel makes for a naturally delicious egg substitute.

PREP TIME: 15 MINUTES | **COOK TIME:** 35 MINUTES | **MAKES:** 6 SERVINGS

> 1 tablespoon flaxseed, ground
> ¼ cup water
> 1 pound ground turkey, 94% lean
> ¼ cup fresh basil, chopped, or 1 tablespoon dried
> 3 teaspoons fresh oregano, finely chopped, or 1 teaspoon dried
> 1 teaspoon crushed rosemary
> Pinch of sea salt
> 1 pound whole grain pasta
> 1½–2 cups prepared marinara sauce

Preheat the oven to 350°F. In a large bowl, mix the flaxseed with water and whisk until slightly thickened into a gel. Add the turkey, herbs, and salt. Gently combine and form into 1" meatballs. Place on a lightly oiled baking sheet. Bake for 35 minutes, or until no longer pink.

Meanwhile, cook the pasta according to the package directions. Serve the meatballs over the pasta and top with the marinara sauce.

Sage Roasted Chicken and Root Vegetables

TRACK 1 FALL/WINTER & TRACK 2

The extremely nutritious sweet potato combines with other root vegetables and is a delightful complement to this sage-and-lemon-scented roasted chicken.

PREP TIME: 20 MINUTES | **COOK TIME:** 2½–3 HOURS | **MAKES:** 8 SERVINGS

> 2 lemons, thinly sliced
> 6 fresh sage leaves
> 1 (6-pound) chicken
> 4 teaspoons olive oil
> 1 teaspoon freshly ground black pepper
> 1½ cups 1" chunks parsnips, washed and trimmed
> 1½ cups 1" chunks carrots, washed and trimmed
> 1 cup 1" chunks turnips, washed and trimmed
> 2 medium sweet potatoes, washed, trimmed, and cut into
>   1" chunks

Preheat the oven to 325°F. Place 6 lemon slices and the sage leaves under the skin of the chicken. Put the remaining lemon slices in the cavity. Tie the legs together with twine and tuck the wings under. Brush 2 teaspoons of the oil over the chicken and sprinkle with the pepper. Place the chicken in a roasting pan. Roast in the lower third of the oven for 1½ to 2 hours.

Toss the parsnips, carrots, turnips, and potatoes with the remaining 2 teaspoons oil. Brush a baking sheet with olive oil and place the vegetables in a single layer. Roast with the chicken, stirring occasionally, for 45 minutes, or until the vegetables are tender and the internal temperature of the chicken reaches 180°F on a meat thermometer.

Remove the chicken and vegetables from the oven. Carefully remove the skin from the chicken. Discard the lemons from the cavity. Slice the chicken and serve with the vegetables.

Vegetarian Black Bean Chili

TRACK 1 FALL/WINTER

The many spices in this black bean chili, infused with cocoa and cinnamon, combine to create warmth and offer digestion-stimulating properties.

PREP TIME: 15 MINUTES | **COOK TIME:** 30 MINUTES | **MAKES:** 4 SERVINGS

> 2 tablespoons olive oil
> ½ onion, chopped

1⅔ cups coarsely chopped red bell peppers (about 2 medium)
2–3 cloves garlic, chopped
2 tablespoons chili powder
2 teaspoons cinnamon
2 teaspoons unsweetened cocoa powder
1½ teaspoons ground cumin
½ teaspoon cayenne pepper
2 cans (15 ounces each) black beans, drained
1 can (16 ounces) tomato sauce
1 medium avocado, chopped
1 cup cilantro, chopped

Heat the oil in a large pot over medium-high heat. Add the onion, bell peppers, and garlic and cook for 10 minutes, or until the vegetables soften. Mix in the chili powder, cinnamon, cocoa powder, cumin, and cayenne. Stir and cook for 2 minutes. Mix in the beans and tomato sauce. Bring the chili to a boil, stirring occasionally. Reduce the heat to medium-low and simmer, stirring occasionally, for 15 minutes, or until the flavors blend and the chili thickens.

Ladle the chili into bowls. Top with chopped cilantro and avocado.

Citrus Salmon

TRACK 1 FALL/WINTER

The trio of citrus juices and the herbs marinating this heart-healthy wild salmon provide a healing tonic for the digestive system.

PREP TIME: 10 MINUTES + 1 HOUR TO MARINATE | **COOK TIME:** 30 MINUTES |
MAKES: 4 SERVINGS

¼ cup orange juice
¼ cup freshly squeezed lemon juice
¼ cup freshly squeezed lime juice
1 tablespoon fresh ginger, peeled and chopped
1 tablespoon fresh mint, chopped
1 tablespoon fresh basil, chopped
4 (6-ounce) wild salmon fillets, center-cut pieces

In a food processor or blender, combine the juices, ginger, mint, and basil. Puree until smooth. Set aside ¼ cup of the marinade. Arrange the salmon in a shallow baking dish and pour the remaining marinade on top. Cover and chill in the refrigerator for 1 hour.

Preheat the oven to 350°F. Discard the marinade from the baking dish and bake the salmon for 25 to 30 minutes, or until cooked through. Pour the reserved marinade over the salmon and serve.

Lamb or Beef Vegetable Winter Stew

TRACK 1 FALL/WINTER
& TRACK 2 (OMIT RED WINE AND INCREASE VEGETABLE BROTH TO 2 CUPS)

Soothing fennel improves circulation and accelerates the digestion of fatty foods. It contains antimicrobial oils, similar to antibacterial garlic, which is known for its detoxifying effects and digestive healing attributes.

PREP TIME: 20 MINUTES | **COOK TIME:** 2 HOURS | **MAKES:** 4 SERVINGS

1½ pounds boneless lean lamb or beef stew meat,
    cut into 1" cubes
½ teaspoon freshly ground black pepper
1 tablespoon olive oil
1 cup 1" chunks onions
1 cup 1" chunks fennel
1 cup 1" chunks carrots
1 medium sweet potato, cut into 1" chunks
2 cloves garlic, chopped
1 tablespoon curry powder
1 cup red wine
1 cup vegetable broth
1 can (14½ ounces) diced tomatoes

Season the meat with pepper. In a Dutch oven, heat the oil over medium heat and brown the meat on all sides. Transfer to a dish and set aside. Add the onions, fennel, carrots, potato, garlic and curry powder to the Dutch oven. Cook for 10 minutes. Add the wine, broth, and tomatoes with juice. Bring to a boil, then lower the heat to a simmer. Stir in the meat and simmer for 1½ hours, stirring occasionally.

Herbed White Fish

TRACK 1 FALL/WINTER, TRACK 2, & TRACK 3

Parsley, lemon, and warming spices impart rich flavor and added nutrition to the protein-and-mineral-packed white fish.

PREP TIME: 15 MINUTES | **COOK TIME:** 20 MINUTES | **MAKES:** 4 SERVINGS

> ¼ cup Inside Tract Vegetable Broth (page 287), or commercial
>   low-sodium, gluten-free vegetable broth
> 2 tablespoons freshly squeezed lemon juice
> 2 tablespoons fresh parsley, chopped
> 1 teaspoon organic seafood seasoning (optional Track 3)
> Sea salt
> Freshly ground black pepper
> 4 (6-ounce) white fish fillets (wild cod or sole)

Preheat the oven to 350°F. Add the broth, lemon juice, parsley, and seafood seasoning in a small mixing bowl and blend. Add salt and pepper to taste. Place the fish in a baking dish and pour the mixture over the fish. Cover and bake for 18 to 20 minutes, or until the fish flakes. Serve, pouring the seasoning mixture over the fish.

Thai Shrimp and Vegetable Sauté

TRACK 1 FALL/WINTER

Broccoli, queen of the brassicas, adds protective phytonutrients that aid in liver detoxification. But be sure to cook until just al dente, as overcooking depletes these valuable compounds.

PREP TIME: 20 MINUTES | **COOK TIME:** 40 MINUTES | **MAKES:** 4 SERVINGS

>   1 cup brown rice
>   1 pound large shrimp, peeled and deveined
>   2 tablespoons freshly squeezed lime juice
>   Sea salt
>   Freshly ground black pepper
>   2 tablespoons coconut oil
>   1 bunch broccoli, florets and stems cut into ½" pieces
>   1 medium yellow bell pepper, seeded and cut into 1" pieces
>   2 cups cherry tomatoes, halved
>   1 cup shiitake mushrooms, sliced
>   1 teaspoon red-pepper flakes
>   ½ cup Lime Miso Dressing (page 250)

Cook the rice according to package directions.

Meanwhile, rub the shrimp with the lime juice, salt, and black pepper. Heat 1 tablespoon of the oil over medium heat in a stainless steel skillet Add the broccoli, bell pepper, tomatoes, and mushrooms and cook until just al dente. Remove the vegetables. Add the remaining 1 tablespoon oil to the skillet and add the shrimp. Cook for 2 to 3 minutes, turn the shrimp over, and cook until pink. Return the vegetables to the skillet and toss in the pepper flakes and dressing until blended. Serve with the rice.

Track 2 Spring/Summer—Breakfast

Scrambled Tofu with Spinach and Olive Tapenade

—Myra Kornfeld, chef at MyFoodMyHealth.com

TRACK 1 & TRACK 2 SPRING/SUMMER

Cooling tofu contains protein, omega-3 fatty acids, and isoflavones, and is enlivened with the anti-inflammatory spice turmeric and olive tapenade.

PREP TIME: 10 MINUTES | **COOK TIME:** 15 MINUTES | **MAKES:** 4 SERVINGS

> 1 pound fresh spinach
> 2 tablespoons extra-virgin olive oil
> 1 red bell pepper, diced
> 1 can (14½ ounces) diced tomatoes
> 2 scallions, cut into 1" pieces
> 1 pound soft or firm tofu, rinsed, patted dry, and loosely
>   crumbled
> ¼ teaspoon turmeric
> Sea salt
> Freshly ground black pepper
> 2 tablespoons prepared olive tapenade

Remove the stems from the spinach and wash thoroughly. Wilt the spinach in a medium skillet over medium heat, stirring frequently or tossing with tongs to push the uncooked leaves to the bottom of the pot. You don't have to add water to the pot, because the water clinging to the leaves from washing is enough to cook them. Cook until the leaves have wilted and shrunken and are bright green. Remove the spinach to a strainer and press to squeeze out the extra water. Chop roughly.

Wipe out the skillet, add the oil, and heat over medium heat. Add the bell pepper and cook for 5 minutes, or until softened. Add the tomatoes and scallions and cook for 3 or 4 minutes, or until the tomatoes have reduced and thickened a bit. Add the tofu and turmeric and a sprinkling of salt and pepper. Cook for 5 minutes to let the tofu absorb the juices. Break up any chunks with a wooden spoon. Stir in the olive tapenade, then stir in the spinach to heat through. Serve immediately.

Track 2 Spring/Summer—Dinner

Parslied Red Potatoes

TRACK 1, TRACK 2 SPRING/SUMMER, & TRACK 3

Parsley, an antioxidant-rich member of the carrot family, contains carotenoids, vitamin K, vitamin C, and iron to stimulate the bowel and reduce inflammation.

PREP TIME: 10 MINUTES | **COOK TIME:** 10 MINUTES | **MAKES:** 4 SERVINGS

> 1¼ pounds red potatoes, cut into quarters
> 1½ tablespoons fresh parsley, minced
> 1 teaspoon lemon zest
> 1 teaspoon olive oil

Place the potatoes in a large saucepan and cover with water. Bring to a boil, reduce the heat, and cook for 7 to 10 minutes, or until tender. Drain.

While the potatoes are cooking, mix together the parsley, lemon zest, and oil. Drizzle over the warm potatoes.

Serve with spinach salad.

Sardine Arugula Salad: See Track 2 Swift & Simple Salads chart (page 242), and as a side salad, omit the protein.

Sunflower Mesclun Salad: See Track 2 Swift & Simple Salads chart (page 246), and as a side salad, omit the protein.

Track 2 Fall/Winter—Breakfast

Autumn Spiced Soy Yogurt Parfait

TRACK 1 & TRACK 2 FALL/WINTER

Spice up your morning with this grab 'n' go high-protein, flavorful breakfast.

PREP TIME: 5 MINUTES | **COOK TIME:** NONE | **MAKES:** 2 SERVINGS

    1 teaspoon organic pumpkin pie spice
    1 cup plain yogurt (soy)
    ½ cup gluten-free muesli or granola
    1 cup frozen mixed berries

Add the pumpkin pie spice to the yogurt and stir until blended. In two 8-ounce glasses, layer the ingredients beginning with the granola: 1 tablespoon granola, ¼ cup yogurt, and ¼ cup berries. Repeat the layers.

Track 2 Fall/Winter—Dinner

White Bean Minestrone Soup

TRACK 1 & TRACK 2 FALL/WINTER

Basil, a member of the mint family, is known for its digestive healing characteristics. It not only stimulates digestion but also can help relieve flatulence, stomach cramps, nausea, and constipation.

PREP TIME: 20 MINUTES | **COOK TIME:** 40 MINUTES | **MAKES:** 6 (1½-CUP) SERVINGS

> 6 cups Inside Tract Vegetable Broth (page 287), or commercial low-sodium, gluten-free vegetable broth
> 2 carrots, peeled and cut into ½"-thick rounds
> 2 ribs celery, cut into ½" pieces
> 1 cup baby portobello mushrooms, quartered
> 3 small zucchini, halved lengthwise, cut into ½" pieces
> 1 can (15 ounces) cannellini beans, drained
> 1 can (14½ ounces) chopped tomatoes
> 1 teaspoon dried basil
> 1 teaspoon crushed dried rosemary
> Sea salt to taste
> Freshly ground black pepper to taste
> 2 cups chopped escarole
> Fresh basil

Add all the ingredients except the escarole to a 6- to 8-quart pot. Increase the heat to high and bring the soup to a boil. Reduce the heat to medium-low, partially cover the pot and simmer for 30 minutes. Stir in the escarole and simmer 5 minutes longer. Sprinkle with fresh basil and ladle the warm soup into 6 bowls.

Thai Chicken Sauté

TRACK 1 & TRACK 2 FALL/WINTER

Fermented miso is health promoting and contains beneficial bacteria to aid digestion.

PREP TIME: 20 MINUTES | **COOK TIME:** 40 MINUTES | **MAKES:** 4 SERVINGS

> 1 cup brown rice
> 2 tablespoons coconut oil
> 1 bunch broccoli, florets and stems cut into ½" pieces
> 1 medium yellow bell pepper, seeded and cut into 1" pieces
> 2 cups cherry tomatoes, halved
> 1 cup shiitake mushrooms, sliced
> 2 boneless chicken breasts, cut into 1" pieces
> 1 teaspoon red-pepper flakes
> ½ cup Lime Miso Dressing (page 250)

Cook the brown rice according to package directions.

Heat 1 tablespoon of the oil over medium heat in a stainless steel skillet. Add the broccoli, bell pepper, tomatoes, and mushrooms and cook until al dente. Remove the vegetables and add the remaining 1 tablespoon oil to the skillet. Add the chicken and cook for 3 minutes. Turn the chicken over and cook for 3 minutes longer, or until done. Return the vegetables to the skillet and toss in the pepper flakes and dressing until well blended. Serve with the rice.

Track 3

Inside Tract Smoothie

The folate-packed spinach and prebiotic banana stimulate good gut bacteria growth and activity in this soothing, nutrient-dense smoothie. Feel free to add spices and herbs such as ginger, mint, cinnamon, and a splash of maple syrup if your taste buds desire.

PREP TIME: 5 MINUTES | **COOK TIME:** 2 MINUTES | **MAKES:** 1 SERVING

    8 ounces chilled water
    ½ small banana, frozen
    1 cup steamed spinach leaves (around 2 cups raw)
    1 scoop organic brown rice protein powder
    1 scoop organic vegetable and fruit powder
    2 teaspoons balanced 3-6-9 liquid oil
    Spices and herbs such as ginger, mint, and cinnamon, as
        tolerated (optional)
    Splash of 100% maple syrup, as little as possible (optional)

Mix all the ingredients in a high-speed blender and process until smooth. Serve immediately.

Inside Tract Vegetable Broth

Celeriac contains antioxidants, and when combined with other healing vegetables—like shiitake mushrooms, purifying burdock root, and kombu—this cleansing broth becomes a warm and satisfying beverage that can also be incorporated in soups, stews, dressings, and marinades.

PREP TIME: 30 MINUTES | **COOK TIME:** 2–3 HOURS | **MAKES:** 6–7 QUARTS (24–28 CUPS)

    4 carrots, unpeeled, cut into thirds
    1 small celeriac (celery root), quartered

10 whole shiitake mushrooms, trimmed
4 parsnips, with skins on, cut into thirds
1 turnip, cut into thirds
2 medium beets, trimmed and cut in half
2 sweet potatoes with skins on, cut into thirds
½ bunch fresh flat-leaf parsley
1 (8") strip of kombu
2 bay leaves
1 tablespoon shredded burdock root
1 piece (1") fresh ginger, sliced

Rinse the vegetables well, including the kombu. In a 10-quart or larger pot, combine all the ingredients. Fill the pot to 2" below the rim with water, cover, and bring to a boil. Remove the lid, decrease the heat to low, and simmer for at least 2 hours. As the stock simmers, some of the water will evaporate. Add more water if the vegetables begin to peek out. Strain the stock using a large coarse-mesh strainer (remember to use a heat-resistant container underneath). Save the vegetables for another use (puree and freeze in ice cube trays to add to sauces or other soups) or serve with the broth.

Cool to room temperature before refrigerating or freezing.

Creamy Greens Soup

Dark greens are emerald jewels rich in B vitamins, vitamin C, magnesium, and iron, while curry powder—the combination of coriander, cumin, fenugreek, and turmeric—contributes anti-inflammatory digestive benefits.

PREP TIME: 10 MINUTES | **COOK TIME:** 40 MINUTES | **MAKES:** 10 CUPS

4 cups chopped dark greens (spinach, bok choy, lacinato kale)
2 cups peeled and diced sweet potato or Yukon gold potatoes
8 cups Inside Tract Vegetable Broth (page 287), or commercial
   low-sodium, gluten-free vegetable broth
1 teaspoon curry powder
Pinch of sea salt (optional)

In a 6- to 8-quart pot, add all the ingredients and cook, stirring occasionally, over medium-high heat until the mixture comes to a slight boil.

Reduce the heat to medium low and simmer uncovered for 30 minutes. In a blender, process the soup in batches until all the soup is smooth.

Carrot Squash Soup

Warming ginger is known to improve circulation and digestion, and calm a queasy stomach. Zest from an organic orange peel adds bioflavonoids and pectin.

PREP TIME: 15 MINUTES | **COOK TIME:** 40 MINUTES | **MAKES:** 10 CUPS

  6 large carrots, washed and sliced
  4 cups peeled and diced butternut squash
  8 cups Inside Tract Vegetable Broth (page 287), or commercial
     low-sodium, gluten-free vegetable broth
  2 teaspoons ground ginger
  2 teaspoons orange zest, very finely grated
  Pinch of sea salt (optional)

In a 6- to 8-quart pot, add all the ingredients and cook, stirring occasionally, over medium-high heat until the mixture comes to a slight boil. Reduce the heat to medium low and simmer uncovered for 30 minutes. In a blender, puree the soup in batches until all the soup is smooth. Serve.

Pumpkin Bisque

The sweet winter squash, pumpkin, contains beta-carotene, vitamin C, potassium, and dietary fiber. Nutmeg, a known carminative, may reduce flatulence and bloating.

PREP TIME: 5 MINUTES | **COOK TIME:** 30 MINUTES | **MAKES:** 8½ CUPS

  3½ cups pumpkin (29-ounce can organic)
  5 cups Inside Tract Vegetable Broth (page 287), or commercial
     low-sodium, gluten-free vegetable broth
  1 teaspoon nutmeg
  Pinch of sea salt (optional)

In a 6- to 8-quart pot, add all the ingredients and cook, stirring occasionally, over medium-high heat until the mixture comes to a slight boil. Reduce the heat to medium low and simmer for 20 minutes. Serve.

Cucumber Avocado Mint Soup

Naturally hydrating, the cooling mint and cucumber contain vitamin C, potassium, and dietary fiber. Select organic varieties to avoid wax-coated cucumbers and to enjoy the benefits of the mineral-containing skin. Avocado is a rich source of folate and monounsaturated fat in this soothing soup.

PREP TIME: 15 MINUTES | **COOK TIME:** NONE | **MAKES:** 2 CUPS

> 1 cucumber, seeded and quartered
> 1 avocado, peeled and quartered
> 2 tablespoons fresh mint leaves
> 1 tablespoon freshly squeezed lemon juice
> 1 cup Inside Tract Vegetable Broth (page 287), or commercial
>   low-sodium, gluten-free vegetable broth

Place all the ingredients in a blender and puree until smooth. Serve.

Snacks

Baked Sweet Potato

TRACK 1, TRACK 2, & TRACK 3

PREP TIME: 2 MINUTES │ **COOK TIME:** 40 MINUTES │ **MAKES:** 1 SERVING

> 1 medium sweet potato
> Pinch of your favorite spice

Preheat the oven to 375°F. Wrap the sweet potato in aluminum foil and bake for 40 to 50 minutes (test for doneness by pricking a fork in the middle). Season with your favorite spice such as cardamom, curry powder, or cinnamon.

Note: Cut the sweet potato in ¼" slices and wrap in foil for a quicker cooking time of around 25 minutes.

Raw Beet and Walnut Salad

—from www.kripalu.org

TRACK 1 & TRACK 2

PREP TIME: 10 MINUTES │ **COOK TIME:** NONE │ **MAKES:** 4 SERVINGS

For the Dressing:

> ¼ cup extra-virgin olive oil
> 2 tablespoons freshly squeezed lemon juice
> 1 tablespoon chopped fresh dill
> Pinch of sea salt

For the Salad:

> 4 cups grated beets
> ½ cup chopped raw walnuts
> ¼ cup chopped fresh parsley

Whisk together the dressing ingredients in a large mixing bowl. Add the beets, walnuts, and parsley to the dressing and toss together. Serve immediately or refrigerate.

Sunflower Hummus

TRACK 1 & TRACK 2

PREP TIME: 10 MINUTES | **COOK TIME:** NONE | **MAKES:** 1¼ CUPS

> 1 can (15 ounces) organic chickpeas, well-drained
> ¼ cup sunflower seed butter
> 1 clove garlic, finely chopped
> ½ cup freshly squeezed lemon juice
> 1 tablespoon extra-virgin olive oil
> 2 tablespoons water
> Pinch of sea salt
> Freshly ground black pepper (optional)

In a food processor, add the chickpeas, sunflower seed butter, garlic, lemon juice, oil, and water. Puree until thick and creamy. Adjust consistency with additional lemon juice, if desired, and season with salt and pepper, if desired, to taste. Serve on raw vegetables (baby carrots, jicama, red bell pepper, celery, Daikon radish).

Bean Flour Crepes

TRACK 1 & TRACK 2

PREP TIME: 5 MINUTES | **COOK TIME:** 20 MINUTES | **MAKES:** 7–8 CREPES

> 1 cup bean flour (chickpea or black bean)
> ½ teaspoon favorite spice (cumin, curry powder, rosemary, sage, thyme, turmeric), see note
> 1 cup water
> Extra-virgin olive oil

In a medium bowl, mix together the flour, spice, and water. Oil a small, heavy skillet and heat over medium-high heat. Drop ¼ cup of the batter into the hot skillet and immediately rotate it to spread the batter evenly and make a thin round. Cook until the crepe begins to brown on the bottom. Carefully turn it over and cook the other side. Repeat until all the batter is used up, re-oiling the pan between each crepe.

Note: Add your favorite finely chopped herbs in the batter while cooking. These wraps can be used at any meal and filled with vegetables, tofu, organic poultry, or fish, and can also be used as a thin, gluten-free pizza crust.

Antipasto

TRACK 1 & TRACK 2

PREP TIME: 5 MINUTES | **COOK TIME:** NONE | **MAKES:** 1 SERVING

> 6–8 black or green olives
> ½ cup roasted red bell peppers, drained
> 2 artichoke hearts, drained
> 4 hearts of palm, drained

Arrange the vegetables on a plate and serve.

Yogurt Parfait

TRACK 1 & TRACK 2 (USE SOY YOGURT)

PREP TIME: 5 MINUTES | **COOK TIME:** NONE | **MAKES:** 1 SERVING

> 8 ounces plain yogurt
> 1 cup favorite fruit, fresh or frozen
> 2 teaspoons coconut flakes
> ¼ cup oats or granola, gluten-free
> 1 tablespoon nuts or seeds

Layer the ingredients in a small bowl or parfait glass and enjoy.

Erica's Sweet and Sour Comfort

TRACK 1

PREP TIME: 10 MINUTES | **COOK TIME:** 10 MINUTES | **MAKES:** 1 SERVING

> 2 organic chicken sausages
> ½ cup sauerkraut
> ½ cup unsweetened organic applesauce
> ¼ teaspoon caraway seeds

In a small skillet over medium-high heat, cook the sausages until browned. Combine the sauerkraut, applesauce, and seeds. Place on top of the cooked sausages.

RECOMMENDED SNACKS

Crackers
Foods Alive: www.foodsalive.com
Mary's Gone Crackers: www.marysgonecrackers.com

Bars
Organic Food Bar: www.organicfoodbar.com
Larabar: www.larabar.com
Pure Organic: www.thepurebar.com
Rawma Bar: www.gopalshealthfoods.com
Kind Healthy Snacks: www.kindsnacks.com

Fresh fruit with a handful of nuts or seeds or a dollup of nut or seed butters
Rotate for variety: almond butter; hazelnut butter; walnut butter; pumpkin seed butter; cashew butter; macadamia nut butter; sunflower seed butter

Natural Nut and Seed Butters
Artisana: www.premierorganics.org
MaraNatha: www.maranathafoods.com
Arrowhead Mills: www.arrowheadmills.com
Omega Nutrition: www.omeganutrition.com

Track 1 Spring/Summer Shopping List

NONPERISHABLES

WHOLE GRAINS

- [ ] Almond meal/flour
- [ ] Brown rice tortillas
- [ ] Buckwheat
- [ ] Quinoa, red
- [ ] Rice, black
- [ ] Rice, brown basmati
- [ ] Rolled oats
- [ ] Teff
- [ ] Whole grain bread
- [ ] Whole grain pasta
- [ ] Whole or sprouted grain tortillas
- [ ] •Whole wheat pastry flour

BEANS

- [ ] Black beans, canned
- [ ] Chickpeas, canned
- [ ] Lentils, red
- [ ] White cannellini beans, canned

PANTRY PICKS

- [ ] Apple cider vinegar
- [ ] Artichoke hearts, canned
- [ ] Baking powder
- [ ] Baking soda
- [ ] Cocoa powder
- [ ] Coconut, shredded
- [ ] Creamed coconut
- [ ] Diced tomatoes, canned
- [ ] Dijon mustard, organic
- [ ] Extra-virgin olive oil
- [ ] Grape seed oil
- [ ] Honey
- [ ] Kalamata olives
- [ ] Miso
- [ ] Olive tapenade
- [ ] Red wine vinegar
- [ ] Tamari, gluten-free
- [ ] Vegetable or tomato juice, low sodium
- [ ] 100% maple syrup, organic

PERISHABLES

FRUITS

- [ ] Apples (green and red)
- [ ] Avocados
- [ ] Bananas
- [ ] Frozen juice concentrate
- [ ] Honeydew or cantaloupe melon
- [ ] Lemons
- [ ] Limes
- [ ] Mangoes
- [ ] Mixed berries
- [ ] Oranges
- [ ] Pears
- [ ] Pineapple
- [ ] Tart cherry juice

VEGETABLES

- [ ] Arugula
- [ ] Beets
- [ ] Bok choy
- [ ] Broccoli rabe

PROTEINS

- [ ] Chicken, breasts
- [ ] Cod, wild
- [ ] Eggs, organic, free-range
- [ ] Lamb or beef, lean, cubed
- [ ] Lox, wild, nitrate-free
- [ ] Salmon, wild, canned
- [ ] Salmon, wild, fillets
- [ ] Sardines, canned
- [ ] Shrimp, large
- [ ] Tilapia, fillets
- [ ] Tofu
- [ ] Turkey, breasts
- [ ] Turkey, ground, 94% lean

FRESH HERBS

- [ ] Basil
- [ ] Chives
- [ ] Cilantro
- [ ] Dill
- [ ] Ginger

NUTS

- ☐ Almonds
- ☐ Cashews
- ☐ Macadamia nuts
- ☐ Pecans
- ☐ Walnuts

SEEDS

- ☐ Chia seeds, ground
- ☐ Crunchy flax cereal
- ☐ Pumpkin seeds
- ☐ Sunflower seeds

NATURAL BUTTERS

- ☐ Almond butter
- ☐ Cashew nut butter
- ☐ Macadamia nut butter
- ☐ Tahini

DRIED FRUITS

- ☐ Apricots
- ☐ Dates
- ☐ Prunes
- ☐ Raisins

OTHER

- ☐ Whey protein powder

DRIED HERBS & SPICES

- ☐ Caraway seeds
- ☐ Chinese five-spice powder
- ☐ Cinnamon
- ☐ Cumin
- ☐ Curry powder
- ☐ Dry mustard powder
- ☐ Garam masala
- ☐ Ginger
- ☐ Ground pepper, black
- ☐ Nutmeg
- ☐ Oregano
- ☐ Red-pepper flakes
- ☐ Sage
- ☐ Sea salt
- ☐ Turmeric

VEGETABLES (cont.)

- ☐ Carrots
- ☐ Celery
- ☐ Chinese or Napa green cabbage
- ☐ Cucumber, English
- ☐ Garlic
- ☐ Green beans
- ☐ Green bell peppers
- ☐ Mesclun greens
- ☐ Red bell peppers
- ☐ Red cabbage
- ☐ Red leaf lettuce
- ☐ Red onions
- ☐ Red potatoes
- ☐ Romaine lettuce
- ☐ Scallions
- ☐ Shallots
- ☐ Spinach
- ☐ Sunflower sprouts
- ☐ Sweet potatoes
- ☐ Tomatoes, cherry
- ☐ Tomatoes, plum
- ☐ Yellow bell peppers
- ☐ Yellow summer squash
- ☐ Zucchini

FRESH HERBS (cont.)

- ☐ Mint
- ☐ Oregano
- ☐ Parsley
- ☐ Thai basil

DAIRY/ DAIRY SUBSTITUTES

- ☐ Almond beverage, unsweetened
- ☐ Butter
- ☐ Coconut milk
- ☐ Feta cheese
- ☐ Goat or sheep cheese
- ☐ Hazelnut beverage
- ☐ Yogurt, plain
- ☐ 2% cottage cheese, small curd

Track 1 Fall/Winter Shopping List

NONPERISHABLES

WHOLE GRAINS
- [ ] Almond meal/flour
- [ ] Amaranth
- [ ] Barley
- [ ] Brown rice flour
- [ ] Buckwheat
- [ ] Muesli or granola
- [ ] Quinoa, red
- [ ] Rice, brown basmati
- [ ] Rice, wild
- [ ] Rolled oats
- [ ] Sprouted corn tortillas
- [ ] Steel-cut oats
- [ ] Teff
- [ ] Whole grain pasta
- [ ] Whole or sprouted grain tortilla
- [ ] ~~Whole wheat bulgur~~

BEANS
- [ ] Adzuki beans

DRIED FRUITS
- [ ] Apricots
- [ ] Dates
- [ ] Prunes
- [ ] Raisins

PANTRY PICKS
- [ ] Baking soda
- [ ] Cocoa powder
- [ ] Coconut, shredded
- [ ] Coconut oil
- [ ] Creamed coconut
- [ ] Diced tomatoes, canned
- [ ] Extra-virgin olive oil
- [ ] Grape seed oil
- [ ] Kalamata olives
- [ ] Marinara or tomato sauce
- [ ] Pumpkin puree, canned, organic
- [ ] Red wine
- [ ] Salsa

PERISHABLES

FRUITS
- [ ] Apples
- [ ] Avocados
- [ ] Bananas
- [ ] Frozen juice concentrate
- [ ] Lemons
- [ ] Limes
- [ ] Mixed berries, fresh or frozen
- [ ] Oranges
- [ ] Pears
- [ ] Tart cherry juice

VEGETABLES
- [ ] Arugula
- [ ] Baby portobello mushrooms
- [ ] Beets
- [ ] Broccoli
- [ ] Carrots
- [ ] Cauliflower

PROTEINS
- [ ] Chicken, breasts
- [ ] Chicken, whole
- [ ] Cod, wild or sole; fillets
- [ ] Edamame
- [ ] Eggs, organic, free-range
- [ ] Hummus
- [ ] Lamb or beef, lean
- [ ] Salmon, wild, canned
- [ ] Salmon, wild, fillets
- [ ] Sardines, canned
- [ ] Shrimp, large
- [ ] Turkey, breasts
- [ ] Turkey, ground, 94% lean

FRESH HERBS
- [ ] Basil
- [ ] Cilantro
- [ ] Dill
- [ ] Ginger
- [ ] Mint

FRESH HERBS *(cont.)*

- [ ] Oregano
- [ ] Parsley
- [ ] Sage
- [ ] Tarragon

DAIRY/ DAIRY SUBSTITUTES

- [ ] Butter
- [ ] Goat or sheep cheese
- [ ] Hazelnut beverage
- [ ] Rice beverage
- [ ] Yogurt, plain

VEGETABLES *(cont.)*

- [ ] Celery
- [ ] Collard greens
- [ ] Cucumbers
- [ ] Escarole
- [ ] Fennel bulb
- [ ] Garlic
- [ ] Mesclun greens
- [ ] Onions
- [ ] Parsnips
- [ ] Red bell peppers
- [ ] Red potatoes
- [ ] Scallions
- [ ] Shiitake mushrooms
- [ ] Spinach
- [ ] Sunflower sprouts
- [ ] Sweet potatoes
- [ ] Swiss chard
- [ ] Tomatoes
- [ ] Tomatoes, cherry
- [ ] Turnips
- [ ] Yellow bell peppers
- [ ] Zucchini

BEANS *(cont.)*

- [ ] Black beans, canned
- [ ] Cannellini beans, canned
- [ ] Chickpeas, canned
- [ ] Lentils, red

NUTS

- [ ] Almonds
- [ ] Cashews
- [ ] Pecans
- [ ] Walnuts

SEEDS

- [ ] Chia seeds, ground
- [ ] Crunchy flax cereal
- [ ] Flaxseed, ground
- [ ] Pumpkin seeds
- [ ] Sunflower seeds

NATURAL BUTTERS

- [ ] Cashew nut butter
- [ ] Peanut butter
- [ ] Sunflower seed butter
- [ ] Tahini

OTHER

- [ ] Hempseed protein powder

PANTRY PICKS *(cont.)*

- [ ] Tomato paste
- [ ] Vegetable broth, low-sodium, gluten-free
- [ ] 100% maple syrup, organic

DRIED HERBS & SPICES

- [ ] Allspice
- [ ] Basil
- [ ] Bay leaf
- [ ] Cayenne pepper
- [ ] Chili powder
- [ ] Cinnamon
- [ ] Cloves
- [ ] Cumin
- [ ] Curry powder
- [ ] Dry mustard powder
- [ ] Garam masala
- [ ] Ginger
- [ ] Ground pepper, black
- [ ] Pumpkin pie spice
- [ ] Red-pepper flakes
- [ ] Rosemary
- [ ] Sea salt
- [ ] Turmeric

Track 2 Spring/Summer Shopping List

NONPERISHABLES

WHOLE GRAINS

- [ ] Almond meal/flour
- [ ] Brown rice tortillas
- [ ] Pasta, gluten-free
- [ ] Quinoa
- [ ] Quinoa, red
- [ ] Rice, black
- [ ] Rice, brown basmati
- [ ] Steel-cut oats, gluten-free

BEANS

- [ ] Black beans, canned
- [ ] Chickpeas, canned
- [ ] Lentils, red
- [ ] White beans

NUTS

- [ ] Almonds
- [ ] Cashews
- [ ] Macadamia nuts
- [ ] Walnuts

PANTRY PICKS

- [ ] Artichoke hearts, canned
- [ ] Baking soda
- [ ] Coconut, shredded
- [ ] Diced tomatoes, canned
- [ ] Dijon mustard, organic
- [ ] Extra-virgin olive oil
- [ ] Grape seed oil
- [ ] Kalamata olives
- [ ] Marinara or tomato sauce
- [ ] Miso
- [ ] Olive tapenade
- [ ] Red wine vinegar
- [ ] Tamari, gluten-free
- [ ] Tomato paste
- [ ] Vegetable broth, low sodium, gluten-free
- [ ] 100% maple syrup, organic

PERISHABLES

FRUITS

- [ ] Avocados
- [ ] Blueberries
- [ ] Kiwifruit
- [ ] Lemons
- [ ] Limes
- [ ] Oranges
- [ ] Pineapple
- [ ] Raspberries
- [ ] Strawberries

VEGETABLES

- [ ] Arugula
- [ ] Beets
- [ ] Bok choy
- [ ] Boston lettuce or Savoy cabbage
- [ ] Carrots
- [ ] Celery
- [ ] Cucumber, English
- [ ] Escarole

PROTEINS

- [ ] Chicken, breasts
- [ ] Chicken, whole
- [ ] Cod, wild, fillets
- [ ] Lox or smoked salmon, wild, nitrate free
- [ ] Salmon, wild, canned
- [ ] Salmon, wild, fillets
- [ ] Sardines, canned
- [ ] Tilapia, fillets
- [ ] Tofu
- [ ] Turkey, breasts
- [ ] Turkey, ground, 94% lean

FRESH HERBS

- [ ] Basil
- [ ] Chives
- [ ] Cilantro
- [ ] Dill
- [ ] Ginger
- [ ] Mint

SEEDS

- ☐ Flaxseeds, ground
- ☐ Pumpkin seeds
- ☐ Sunflower seeds

NATURAL BUTTERS

- ☐ Cashew nut butter
- ☐ Pecan nut butter
- ☐ Tahini

OTHER

- ☐ Brown rice protein powder, organic
- ☐ Hempseed protein powder

DRIED HERBS & SPICES

- ☐ Allspice
- ☐ Bay leaf
- ☐ Chinese five-spice powder
- ☐ Cinnamon
- ☐ Cloves
- ☐ Cumin
- ☐ Curry powder
- ☐ Dry mustard powder
- ☐ Garam masala
- ☐ Ginger
- ☐ Ground pepper, black
- ☐ Nutmeg
- ☐ Rosemary
- ☐ Sage
- ☐ Sea salt
- ☐ Turmeric

VEGETABLES (cont.)

- ☐ Fennel bulb
- ☐ Garlic
- ☐ Green beans
- ☐ Parsnips
- ☐ Red bell peppers
- ☐ Red leaf lettuce
- ☐ Red potatoes
- ☐ Romaine lettuce
- ☐ Scallions
- ☐ Spinach
- ☐ Sunflower sprouts
- ☐ Sweet potatoes
- ☐ Tomatoes, plum
- ☐ Turnips
- ☐ Watercress
- ☐ Yellow summer squash
- ☐ Zucchini

FRESH HERBS (cont.)

- ☐ Oregano
- ☐ Parsley
- ☐ Tarragon
- ☐ Thai basil

DAIRY/ DAIRY SUBSTITUTES

- ☐ Almond beverage, unsweetened
- ☐ Soy beverage, plain unsweetened
- ☐ Yogurt, soy

Track 2 Fall/Winter Shopping List

NONPERISHABLES

WHOLE GRAINS

- ☐ Almond meal/flour
- ☐ Amaranth
- ☐ Brown rice tortillas
- ☐ Buckwheat
- ☐ Millet
- ☐ Muesli or granola, gluten-free
- ☐ Pasta, gluten-free
- ☐ Quinoa
- ☐ Quinoa, red
- ☐ Rice, black
- ☐ Rice, brown basmati

BEANS

- ☐ Adzuki beans
- ☐ Black beans, canned
- ☐ Cannellini beans, canned
- ☐ Chickpeas, canned
- ☐ Lentils, red

PANTRY PICKS

- ☐ Baking soda
- ☐ Coconut, shredded
- ☐ Coconut oil
- ☐ Diced tomatoes, canned
- ☐ Dijon mustard, organic
- ☐ Extra-virgin olive oil
- ☐ Grape seed oil
- ☐ Kalamata olives
- ☐ Kombu strips
- ☐ Marinara or tomato sauce
- ☐ Pumpkin puree, canned, organic
- ☐ Red wine vinegar
- ☐ Tamari, gluten-free
- ☐ Tomato paste
- ☐ Vegetable broth, low sodium, gluten-free
- ☐ 100% maple syrup, organic

PERISHABLES

FRUITS

- ☐ Avocados
- ☐ Bananas
- ☐ Lemons
- ☐ Limes
- ☐ Mixed berries
- ☐ Oranges
- ☐ Pineapple
- ☐ Pink grapefruit
- ☐ Strawberries

VEGETABLES

- ☐ Arugula
- ☐ Baby portobello mushrooms
- ☐ Beets
- ☐ Bok choy
- ☐ Broccoli
- ☐ Carrots
- ☐ Celery
- ☐ Cucumber, English

PROTEINS

- ☐ Chicken, breasts
- ☐ Chicken, whole
- ☐ Cod, wild, fillets
- ☐ Edamame
- ☐ Hummus
- ☐ Lamb or beef, lean
- ☐ Lox or smoked salmon, wild, nitrate free
- ☐ Salmon, wild, canned
- ☐ Salmon, wild, fillets
- ☐ Sardines, canned
- ☐ Tilapia, fillets
- ☐ Turkey, breasts
- ☐ Turkey, ground, 94% lean

FRESH HERBS

- ☐ Basil
- ☐ Chives
- ☐ Cilantro
- ☐ Dill

NUTS

- Almonds
- Macadamia nuts

SEEDS

- Flaxseeds, ground
- Pumpkin seeds
- Sunflower seeds

NATURAL BUTTERS

- Almond butter
- Walnut butter

OTHER

- Brown rice protein powder, organic
- Vegetable and fruit powder, organic

DRIED HERBS & SPICES

- Allspice
- Basil
- Bay leaf
- Chinese five-spice powder
- Cinnamon
- Cloves
- Cumin
- Curry powder
- Dry mustard powder
- Garam masala
- Ginger
- Ground pepper, black
- Pumpkin pie spice
- Red-pepper flakes
- Rosemary
- Sage
- Sea salt
- Turmeric

VEGETABLES (cont.)

- Escarole
- Fennel bulb
- Garlic
- Green beans
- Kale
- Onions
- Parsnips
- Scallions
- Shiitake mushrooms
- Sunflower sprouts
- Sweet potatoes
- Swiss chard
- Tomatoes, cherry
- Tomatoes, plum
- Turnips
- Yellow bell peppers
- Yellow summer squash
- Zucchini

FRESH HERBS (cont.)

- Ginger
- Mint
- Oregano
- Parsley
- Tarragon

DAIRY/ DAIRY SUBSTITUTES

- Hempseed beverage, unsweetened
- Yogurt, soy

Track 3 Shopping List

NONPERISHABLES

PANTRY PICKS

☐ Extra-virgin olive oil
☐ Kombu strips
☐ Pumpkin puree, organic, canned
☐ Vegetable broth, low sodium, gluten-free
☐ 100% maple syrup, organic

DRIED HERBS & SPICES

☐ Bay leaf
☐ Cinnamon
☐ Curry powder
☐ Dry mustard powder
☐ Ginger
☐ Ground pepper, black
☐ Nutmeg
☐ Sage
☐ Sea salt
☐ Turmeric

OTHER

☐ Balanced 3-6-9 liquid oil

PERISHABLES

PROTEINS

☐ Chicken, breasts
☐ Cod, wild, or sole; fillets
☐ Salmon, wild, canned
☐ Salmon, wild, fillets
☐ Sardines, canned
☐ Skipjack tuna, canned
☐ Turkey, breast
☐ Turkey, ground, 94% lean

FRESH HERBS

☐ Basil
☐ Burdock root
☐ Chives
☐ Cilantro
☐ Dill
☐ Ginger
☐ Mint
☐ Parsley

FRUITS

☐ Avocados
☐ Bananas
☐ Lemons
☐ Oranges

VEGETABLES

☐ Bok choy
☐ Carrots
☐ Celeriac (celery root)
☐ Collard greens
☐ Cucumber, English
☐ Green beans
☐ Kale
☐ Parsnip
☐ Red potatoes
☐ Shiitake mushrooms
☐ Spinach
☐ Sweet potatoes
☐ Swiss chard
☐ Turnips

VEGETABLES *(cont.)*

☐ Yellow summer squash
☐ Zucchini

OTHER *(cont.)*

☐ Brown rice protein powder, organic
☐ Vegetable and fruit powder, organic

Resources

Cooking

MyFoodMyHealth
www.myfoodmyhealth.com

My Foundation Diet
www.myfoundationdiet.com

The World's Healthiest Foods
www.whfoods.com

Environmental

Eat Well Guide
www.eatwellguide.org

Environmental Defense Fund
www.edf.org/page.cfm?tagID=17694 *(safe seafood list)*

Environmental Working Group
www.ewg.org and www.foodnews.org

Local Harvest: Community Supported Agriculture
www.localharvest.org/csa

Monterey Bay Aquarium
www.montereybayaquarium.org/cr/cr_seafoodwatch/
    sfw_recommendations.aspx *(safe seafood list)*

The Organic Center
www.organic-center.org

Rodale Institute: Farm Locator
www.rodaleinstitute.org/farm_locator

Favorite Food Brands

Bob's Red Mill
www.bobsredmill.com *(whole grains and gluten-free grains)*

Hodgson Mill
www.hodgsonmill.com *(whole grains and gluten-free grains)*

Edward & Sons
www.edwardandsons.com *(variety of products)*

Ducktrap River of Maine
www.ducktrap.com *(naturally smoked, nitrate-free lox)*

Vital Choice Wild Seafood and Organics
www.vitalchoice.com *(wild cold-water fish and seafood)*

Running Food
www.runningfood.com *(chia seed products)*

Enjoy Life Foods
www.perkysnaturalfoods.com *(low-allergy and gluten-free products)*

Frontier Natural Products Co-op
www.frontiercoop.com *(organic spices and seasonings)*

Food for Life
www.foodforlife.com *(gluten-free breads and wraps)*

The Gluten-Free Mall
www.glutenfreemall.com *(variety of gluten-free products)*

Glutenfree.com
www.glutenfree.com *(variety of gluten-free products)*

Eden Organic
www.edenfoods.com *(beans, soups, and sauces)*

Lotus Foods
www.lotusfoods.com *(rice varieties and stainless steel rice cooker)*

South River Miso
www.southrivermiso.com *(misos)*

Pulmuone Wildwood Organics
www.pulmuonewildwood.com *(organic soy foods)*

Maine Coast Sea Vegetables
www.seaveg.com *(seaweed products)*

MaraNatha
www.maranathafoods.com *(natural nut and seed butters)*

Organic Sunshine Burgers
www.sunshineburger.com *(gluten-free veggie burgers)*

Food Allergy and Gluten Sensitivity

Celiac.com
www.celiac.com

Gluten-Free Certification Organization
www.gfco.org

Corn Allergens
www.cornallergens.com

Celiac Disease Foundation
www.celiac.org

The Food Allergy and Anaphylaxis Network
www.foodallergy.org

Gluten Intolerance Group of North America
www.gluten.net

The Gluten Syndrome
www.theglutensyndrome.net

National Foundation for Celiac Awareness
www.celiaccentral.org

Gastrointestinal Disease

American College of Gastroenterology
www.acg.gi.org

American Dietetic Association
www.eatright.org

American Gastroenterological Association
www.gastro.org

American Liver Foundation
www.liverfoundation.org

International Foundation for Functional Gastrointestinal Disorders
www.iffgd.org

American Academy of Allergy, Asthma and Immunology
www.aaaai.org

Crohn's and Colitis Foundation of America
www.ccfa.org

National Eczema Association
www.nationaleczema.org

National Digestive Diseases Information Clearinghouse
www.digestive.niddk.nih.gov

National Center for Complementary and Alternative Medicine
http://nccam.nih.gov

Integrative and Functional Medicine Practitioners

Dietitians in Integrative and Functional Medicine
www.integrativeRD.org

The Institute for Functional Medicine
www.functionalmedicine.org

Continuum Center for Health and Healing
www.healthandhealing.org

University of Arizona Center for Integrative Medicine
www.integrativemedicine.arizona.edu

Supplements

Extensive line of professional formulations that support digestive wellness
www.MnMvites.com
www.swiftnutrition.com

Acknowledgments

From Gerard E. Mullin, MD: I would like to first acknowledge my creator who has guided me during some very difficult times in my life. It was my faith in Him that gave me the strength to overcome the many dark nights that I encountered while I was incapacitated, homebound, and jobless. In retrospect, it was a blessing since now I can serve as a guidepost to help others to restore their health and transform their lives.

I had the love and support of many whose energies and spirits formed the backbone of my strength during challenging times. My parents when they were alive were, first and foremost, my lifeline. They sacrificed so much to ensure that I was well educated. My mother, in essence, also served as my first mentor for learning how to overcome a chronic illness with food as medicine. My brothers, Patrick and Tim, have been impeccable advisors and outstanding role models. There were many decision points along the way and they both provided invaluable counsel. I cannot imagine where I would be today without the both of them. To my sisters and their children who provided invaluable assistance as caregivers when I became disabled in 2004.

To my many close, personal friends who sustained me during difficult times. In particular, Dr. Loren Marks, for his insight and generosity over the years. To Dr. Christopher Houlihan and his wife, Debbie, for their unwavering support for more than 30 years. To Jose Negrin and Ms. Maria Valdez, who were always there for me in times of trouble. Mrs. Maria Keena, for her spiritual guidance through the years, in particular since the passing of my mother. We are all connected in spirit and are family.

To Drs. Roseanne Russo and Lisa Lih-Brody. I would have passed on if it were not for their heroic efforts while hospitalized in 2004. To Dr. Lisa Conway and Bernarto Vargas for their compassionate care. To Fanny Cruz, a lifesaver, who came to my rescue in times of trouble, and Wanda, a fountain of wisdom, energy, and light for the ages. To Donna Jackson Nakazawa, for featuring my reversal of fortune in her book, *The Autoimmune Epidemic*. Deborah Hocutt, for introducing me to Larry Kirshbaum and Meghan Thompson, my literary agents.

Over the years, I was mentored by outstanding individuals. Dr. Louis Rivela was my college chemistry professor who remains one of the most outstanding educators and role models of my life. Dr. Tony Kalloo from Johns Hopkins who has mentored me since I began my fellowship there in 1988.

Alternative healthcare providers who have passed on: Dr. John Gerrath, Dr. Bill Timmins, Dr. Jeffrey Berg, and Dr. Shari Lieberman. Bill revolutionized laboratory testing and adrenal physiology. Dr. Shari Lieberman was a national expert in complementary nutrition and my mentor during my master's program in human nutrition. Drs. Frederick Smith and Daniel Sulmasy OFM, who blended compassion, spirituality, and ethical principles in the practice of medicine. Mr. Richard Baxter, for his professional guidance and friendship over the years.

In the field of integrative medicine, there were some key individuals who fostered my growth. Dr. Adrian Dobs from Johns Hopkins, Dr. James Gordon from the Center for Mind-Body Medicine, Drs. Jeffrey Bland and David Jones from the Institute for Functional Medicine, Drs. Tieraona Low Dog and Victoria Maizes, who guided me during my fellowship in integrative medicine at the University of Arizona, and most of all, Dr. Andrew Weil, for his continued mentorship and support.

I also had the privilege of working with accomplished nutritionists in more recent times that I would like to acknowledge. Dr. Judith Porcari and Sylvia McAdoo who collaborated with me to make important policy changes regarding the delivery of nutrition in the hospital setting. Dr. Loren Marks, Kathie Swift, Kasia Kines, Amy Fischer, and Ashley Koff for providing outstanding nutrition care to my patients. Dr. Carol Irenton-Jones and Dr. Mark DeLegge from the American Society for Enteral and Parenteral Nutrition. I would also like to acknowledge the many journal editors I have worked with over the years, in particular, Dr. Jeanette Hasse from Nutrition in Clinical Practice. To the American Dietetic Association for bestowing upon me an honorary membership. To an outstanding dietitian and human being, Dr. Laura Matarese, who coedited two nutrition books with me. Most of all, to my coauthor, Kathie Swift, who has been a guiding light over the years.

I would also like to acknowledge Dr. Sajida Chaudry and Ms. Annette Bourne for helping me deliver integrative care to the patients at Johns Hopkins Community Physicians at Odenton, Maryland.

A special thank you to Laura Turnbull, RN, for friendship, support, and assistance. To Julie McKenna, my senior level medical office assistant. In my 20 years of practice, no one lights a candle to you for lending a helping hand to patients with your heart.

To my patients, for their trust, patience, and mentorship through the many years.

From Kathie Madonna Swift: I am deeply grateful to the following individuals and groups for their support.

To my treasured family, Dan, Kadan, Michael, Katie, Marty, and our sweet little Lauren Madonna, for your constant love and laughs.

To my nutrition interns, Emily Mohar and Erica Kasuli, who helped me in more ways than I can mention.

To my dear friend Sheila Dean, who is always there to enlighten me in nutritional medicine; to Mary Alice Gettings, for her constant encouragement and support; and to Amy Jarck, who helped me for endless hours in the kitchen, at the table, and the computer.

To Dr. Susan Lord, gifted healer and friend, visionary and mind body pioneer and to Noushin Bayat, spiritual guide and sister friend.

To my long-time colleagues at the Food As Medicine program, the remarkable Jo Cooper, Dr. James Gordon, Dr. John Bagnulo, Dr. Cindy Geyer, Dr. Patrick Hanaway, Dr. Joel Evans, our incredible Chef Rebecca Katz, and all the heart-centered faculty and friends at the Center for Mind-Body Medicine.

To my wonderful colleagues at the UltraWellness Center, including the amazing Dr. Mark Hyman, Dr. Elizabeth Boham, Dr. Todd Lepine, Maggie Wad, Deb Phillips, and the entire dedicated healthcare team.

To my brilliant partners at the Optimal Health and Prevention Research Foundation, Colleen Fogarty Draper, Dr. Paula Nenn, and founder Gene Vaisberg.

To my treasured associates at Kripalu Center for Yoga and Health, Annie B. Kay, Jennifer Young and Jim Conzo . . . what a joy it is to work with you and all the others in healthy living!

To my delicious recipe contributors, Caroline Nation, MyFoodMyHealth.com founder; Myra Kornfeld; Leslie Cerier; and the Kripalu kitchen. To Dr. Janice Vickerstaff Joneja, my food allergy mentor, for her expertise and contributions.

To the professional medical and nutrition organizations for their leadership in health care, including Dietitians in Integrative and Functional Medicine Dietetic Practice Group and the Institute for Functional Medicine and my functional medicine teacher and mentor for decades, the brilliant Dr. Jeffrey Bland.

To my coauthor, Dr. Gerard Mullin, who brings his heart to healing.

From Kathie and Gerry: The authors would like to thank Spencer Smith for editorial guidance, as well as Larry Kirshbaum and Meghan Thompson from LJK Literary Management LLC, and Gena Smith, our book editor from Rodale Inc.

Endnotes

Introduction

1. Special Report of the US Census Bureau, 2007.
2. http://www.sciencedaily.com/releases/2008/01/080108082944.htm

Chapter 1

1. Michael Gershon, *The Second Brain* (New York: Harper Collins, 1999).
2. An English translation of the *Sushruta samhita*, based on original Sanskrit text. Edited and published by Kaviraj Kunja Lal Bhishagratna. Vol. 1. (Introduction)—Sutrastharam. Calcutta: no. 10. Kasni Ghose's Lane 1907.
3. http://digestive.niddk.nih.gov/statistics/statistics.htm#all.
4. American Gastroenterological Association, The Burden of Chronic Gastrointestinal Diseases Study, 2001.
5. Gerard Mullin, *Integrative Gastroenterology* (Oxford: Oxford University Press, 2011).

Chapter 2

1. T. Just et al., "Cephalic phase insulin release in healthy humans after taste stimulation?" *Appetite* 51, no. 3 (Nov 2008): 622–27.
2. M. Sanaka, T. Yamamoto, and Y. Kuyama, "Effects of proton pump inhibitors on gastric emptying: a systematic review," *Dig Dis Sci* 55, no. 9 (2010 Sep): 2431–40.
3. U. Nöthlings et al., "Sugary sodas related to increase risk of pancreatic cancer," *Am J Clin Nutr* 86, no. 5 (2007 Nov): 1495–1501; N. T. Mueller et al., "Cancer Epidemiol Biomarkers," *Prev* 19, no. 2 (2010 Feb): 447–55; F. Bravi et al., "Folate intake may decrease pancreatic risk," *Ann Oncol* 22, no.1 (2011 Jan.): 202–6.
4. A. M. O'Hara and F. Shanahan, "The gut flora as a forgotten organ," *EMBO* (July 2006): Rep. 7 (7): 688–93. PMID 16819463.
5. "Gut bacteria can manufacture defenses against cancer and inflammatory bowel disease," Feb. 9, 2009, *Science Daily*, www.sciencedaily.com/releases/2009/02/090205214418.htm.

Chapter 3

1   P. Green, *Celiac Disease: The Hidden Epidemic* (New York: William Morrow, 2010).
2   L. Weinstock et al., "Restless leg syndrome is associated with celiac disease," *Dig Dis Sci* 55 (2010): 1667–73.
3   P. Boyle and J. Ferlay, "Cancer incidence and mortality in Europe," 2005. *Ann Oncol* 16, no. 3 2005: 481–88.
4   G. Rennert, "Prevention and early detection of colorectal cancer—new horizons," *Recent results in cancer research [Fortschritte der Krebsforschung]* 174 (2007): 179–87.
5   E. J. Coups et al., "Multiple behavioral risk factors for colorectal cancer and colorectal cancer screening status," *Cancer Epidemiol Biomarkers Prev* 16, no. 3 (2007): 510–16.
6   C. L. Thompson et al., "Short duration of sleep increases risk of colorectal adenoma," *Cancer* 117, no. 4 (2011): 841–47.
7   Neurologic manifestations reportedly associated with celiac or gluten sensitivity: peripheral neuropathy, 49%; headache, 46%; depression/anxiety, 31%; ataxia, 5.4%; migraines, 4.4%; epilepsy, 3.3–5.5%. L. Hernandez and P. H. Green, "Extraintestinal manifestations of celiac disease," *Current Gastroenterology Reports* 8, no. 5 (2006): 383–89.
8   L. Weinstock et al., "Restless leg syndrome is associated with celiac disease," *Dig Dis Sci* 55 (2010): 1667–73.
9   L. Weinstock et al., "Crohn's disease is associated with restless leg syndrome," *Journal of Inflammatory Bowel Disease* 16, no. 2 (2010 Feb): 275–79.
10 R. P. Allen et al., "Restless leg syndrome prevalence and impact: REST general population study," *Arch Intern Med* 165 (2005): 1286–92.
11 E. D. Harris et al., *Kelley's Textbook of Rheumatology,* 7th ed. (St. Louis, MO: W. B. Saunders, 2005), 525.
12 S. A. Buechner, "Rosacea: an update," *Dermatology* 210 (2005): 100–108.
13 S. Larsen, K. Bendtzen, and O. H. Nielsen, "Extraintestinal manifestations in inflammatory bowel disease: epidemiology, diagnosis, and management," *Ann Med* 42, no. 2 (2010 Mar): 97–114 (review).
14 M. Aloi and S. Cucchiara, "Extradigestive manifestations of IBD in pediatrics," *Eur Rev Med Pharmacol Sci* 13, suppl. 1 (2009 Mar): 23–32.
15 A. Alkhalifah et al., "Alopecia areata update: part I. Clinical picture, histopathology, and pathogenesis," *J Am Acad Dermatol* 62, no. 2 (2010 Feb): 177–88.
16 M. Sárdy and J. Tietze, "Dermatitis herpetiformis. An update of the pathogenesis," *Hautarzt* 60, no. 8 (2009 Aug): 627–30, 632 (review).

[17] A. Jalel, G. S. Soumaya, and M. H. Hamdaoui, "Vitiligo treatment with vitamins, minerals, and polyphenol supplementation," *Indian J Dermatol* 54, no. 4 (2009): 357–60.

Chapter 4

[1] jn.nutrition.org/content/early/2010/08/11/jn.110.124826.short.
[2] www.mypyramid.gov/pyramid/index.html.
[3] http://goodreads.com/author/quotes/61107.MargaretMead.
[4] A. Wilde, "Gluten Intolerance Symptoms—How Do You Know If Gluten Is Making You Sick?" March 11, 2007, retrieved April 6, 2009 from www.gluten freenetwork.com/faqs/symptoms-treatments/gluten-intolerance-symptoms-how-do-you-know-if-gluten-is-making-you-sick/
[5] E. Lionetti et al., "Headache in pediatric patients with celiac disease and its prevalence as a diagnostic clue," *J Pediatr Gastroenterol Nutr* 49, no. 2 (2009): 202–7.
[6] C. Efe et al., "Silent celiac disease presenting with polyarthritis," *J Clin Rheumatol* 16, no. 4 (2010): 195–96.
[7] W. Hauser et al., "Anxiety and depression in adult patients with celiac disease on a gluten-free diet," *World J Gastroenterolo* 16, no. 22 (2010): 2780–87.
[8] J. Yamahara et al., "The anti-ulcer effect in rats of ginger constituents," *J Ethnopharmacol* 23, nos. 2–3 (1988 Jul–Aug): 299–304.
[9] T. M. Moraes et al., "Effects of limonene and essential oil from *Citrus aurantium* on gastric mucosa: role of prostaglandins and gastric mucus secretion," *Chem Biol Interact* 180, no. 3 (2009 Aug 14): 499–505.
[10] K. Eamlamnam et al., "Effects of aloe vera and sucralfate on gastric microcirculatory changes, cytokine levels, and gastric ulcer healing in rats," *World J Gastroenterol* 12, no. 3 (2006 Apr 7): 2034–39.
[11] P. Khosla, R. S. Karan, and V. K. Bhargava, "Effect of garlic oil on ethanol induced gastric ulcers in rats," *Phytother Res* 18, no. 1 (2004 Jan): 87–91; S. Y. Lee, Y. W. Shin, and K. B. Hahm, "Phytoceuticals: mighty but ignored weapons against *Helicobacter pylori* infection," *J Dig Dis* 9, no. 3 (2008 Aug): 129–39.
[12] www.brainyquote.com/words/so/soil221344.html. http://en.wikiquote.org/wiki/Franklin_D_Roosevelt
[13] H. Marlow et al., "Diet and the environment: Does what you eat matter?" *The American Journal of Clinical Nutrition* 89, no. 5 (2009): 1699S–1703S.
[14] www.cnpp.usda.gov/dietaryguidelines.gov
[15] jn.nutrition.org/content/early/2010/08/11/jn.110.124826.short

[16] M. Chiba et al., "Lifestyle-related disease in Crohn's disease: relapse prevention by a semi-vegetarian diet," *World J Gastroenterol* 16, no. 20 (2010): 2484–95.

[17] A. Strohle, A. Hahn, and A. Sebastian, "Estimation of the diet-dependent net acid load in 229 worldwide historically studied hunter-gatherer societies," *Am J Clin Nutr* 91 (2010): 406–12.

[18] S. Berkemeyer, "Acid-base balance and weight gain: are there crucial links via protein and organic acids in understanding obesity?" *Med Hypothesis* 73 (2009): 347–56.

[19] N. R. Cook et al., "Joint effects of sodium and potassium intake on subsequent cardiovascular disease: the Trials of Hypertension Prevention follow-up study," *Arch Intern Med* 169, no. 1 (2009): 32–40.

[20] www.genengnews.com/gen-news-highlights/interleukin-genetics-introduces-weight-management-genetic-test/55899549.

[21] http://www.diabetes.org/diabetes-basics/diabetes-statistics/

[22] Ibid.

[23] I. Glemziene et al., "Enteropathies and oxidative stress," *Acta Medicat Lituanica* 13, no. 4 (2006): 232–35.

[24] J. Ko and L. Mayer, "Oral tolerance: lessons on treatment of food allergy," *Eur J Gastroenterol Hepatol* 17, no. 12 (2005 Dec): 1299–1303.

[25] Yu, L. C. "The epithelial gatekeeper against food allergy." *Pediatrics & Neonatology* 50, no. 6 (December 2009): 247–54.

[26] V. Rosenfeldt et al., "Effect of probiotics on gastrointestinal symptoms and intestinal permeability in children with atopic dermatitis," *J Pediatr* 145, no. 5 (2004): 612–16.

[27] A. Fassano and T. Shea-Donohue, "Mechanisms of disease: the fold of intestinal barrier function in the pathogenesis of gastrointestinal autoimmune diseases," *Nat Clin Gastroenterol Hepatol* 2, no. 9 (2005): 416–22.

[28] P. Collin et al., "Endocrinological disorders and celiac disease," *Endocr Rev* 23 (2002): 464–83.

[29] www.foodallergy.org/allergens/index.html; Guidelines for the Diagnosis and Management of Food Allergy in the United States: Report of the NIAID-Sponsored Expert Panel, www.jacionline.org/article/S0091-6749 (10)01566-6/fulltext.

[30] B. J. Cowart, "Taste, our body's gustatory gatekeeper," *Cerebrum* 7 (2005): 7–22.

[31] http://bami.us/Diet/ArtificialSweeteners.html.

[32] N. Sakamoto et al., "Dietary risk factors for inflammatory bowel disease: a multi-center case control study in Japan," *Inflamm Bowel Dis* 11, no. 2 (2005): 154–63.

[33] www.tcme.org/.

Chapter 5

1. http://www.medscape.com/viewarticle/727323?sssdmh=dm1.633691&src=nldne&uac=6824HR
2. Weil, A. *Health and Healing.* Houghton Mifflin. New York. 1998: 62.
3. http://www.drweil.com/drw/u/ART00521/three-breathing-exercises.html
4. Brumett, B. H., M. J. Helms, W. G. Dahlstrom, I. C. Sieger. Prediction of all-cause mortality by the Minnesota Multiphasic Inventory Optimism-Pessimism Scale Scores: Study of a college sample during a 40-year follow-up period. Mayo Clinic Proceedings. 2006; 81; 12: 1541–44.
5. Drossman, D. A., L. Chang, S. Schneck, C. Blackman, W. F. Norton, N. J. Norton. *Dig Dis Sci.* 2009 Jul; 54 (7): 1532–41. A focus group assessment of patient perspectives on irritable bowel syndrome and illness severity.
6. Drossman, D. A. *Aliment Pharmacol Ther.* 1999 May; 13 Suppl 2: 3–14. Review. Review article: an integrated approach to the irritable bowel syndrome.
7. De La Fuente Mochales, M. B., and M. E. González Cascante. *Rev Enferm.* 2010 Jun; 33 (6): 43–44.
8. Vlachopoulos, C., P. Xaplanteris, N. Alexopoulos, K. Aznaouridis, C. Vasiliadou, K. Baou, E. Stefanadi, C. Stefanadis. *Psychosom Med.* 2009 May; 71 (4): 446–53. Divergent effects of laughter and mental stress on arterial stiffness and central hemodynamics.
9. Levy, R. L., J. A. Linde, K. A. Feld, M. D. Crowell, R. W. Jeffery. *Clin Gastroenterol Hepatol.* 2005 Oct; 3 (10): 992–6 The association of gastrointestinal symptoms with weight, diet, and exercise in weight-loss program participants.
10. Heitkemper, M. M., M. E. Jarrett, R. L. Levy, K. C. Cain, R. L. Burr, A. Feld, P. Barney, P Weisman. *Clin Gastroenterol Hepatol.* 2004 Jul; 2 (7): 585–96 Self-management for women with irritable bowel syndrome.
11. Cohen, D. C., A. Winstanley, A. Engledow, A. C. Windsor, J. R. Skipworth. Marathon-induced ischemic colitis: why running is not always good for you. *Am J Emerg Med.* 2009 Feb; 27 (2): 255.
12. Izakson, Z. A. *Vopr Kurortol Fizioter Lech Fiz Kult.* 1971; 36 (1): 79–80. Observations on strengthening abdominal press and reinforcing the abdominal wall by exercise therapy in digestive organ diseases.
13. Zhang, S. X., Guo H. Z., Jing B. S., Liu S. F.. *Aviat Space Environ Med.* 1992 Sep; 63 (9): 795–801 The characteristics and significance of intrathoracic and abdominal pressures during Qigong (Q-G) maneuvering.
14. Yang Yang. Taijiquan. Zhenwn Publications. Champaign, Illinois. 2005.
15. Sullivan, S. N. *N Engl J Med* 304 (1981), p. 915. The gastrointestinal symptoms of running.
16. Fischer, L. R., L. F. MacMahon, Jr, M. J. Ryan et al., *Dig Dis Sci* 31 (1986), p. 1226. Gastrointestinal bleeding in competitive runners.

[17] van Nieuwenhoven, M. A., F. Brouns, R. J. Brummer. *Eur J Appl Physiol.* 2004 Apr; 91 (4): 42–34. Gastrointestinal profile of symptomatic athletes at rest and during physical exercise.

[18] www.sleepfoundation.org.

[19] Cremonini, F., M. Camilleri, A. R. Zinsmeister, L. M. Herrick, T. Beebe, N. J. Talley. Sleep disturbances are linked to both upper and lower gastrointestinal symptoms in the general population. *Neurogastroenterol Motil.* 2009 Feb; 21(2): 128–35.

[20] Baccari, B. C. Orexins and gastrointestinal functions. *Curr Protein Pept Sci.* 2010 Mar; 11 (2): 148–55.

[21] Stein, E., Katz P. O.. GERD: GERD and insomnia-first degree relatives or distant cousins? *Nat Rev Gastroenterol Hepatol.* 2010 Jan; 7 (1): 8–10. Review.

[22] Chopra, D. *Seven Spiritual Laws of Success: A Practical Guide to the Fulfillment of Your Dreams.* Amber-Allen Publishing, San Rafael, CA. November, 1994. Pg 4.

[23] Harris, W., M. Gowda, J. W. Kolb. et al. A randomized controlled trial of the effects of remote intercessory prayer in patients admitted to the coronary care unit. *Arch Intern Med* 1999; 159: 2273–78.

[24] Evans, J. Meditation for Digestive Health. In *"Integrative Gastroenterology."* 1st Edition. Mullin GE Editor. Oxford University Press, New York. Publication date. April 27, 2011.

[25] Mokdad, A. H., J. S. Marks, D. F. Stroup, J. L. Gerberding. *JAMA.* 2004; 291: 1238–45.

[26] James, S. Gordon, M. D.: connecting mind, body, and beyond, Interview by Karolyn A. Gazella and Suzanne Snyder. *Altern Ther Health Med.* 2006 Mar-Apr; 12 (2): 69–74.

[27] Loucks, E. B., L. M. Sullivan, R. B. D'Agostino Sr, et al. Social networks and inflammatory markers in the Framingham Heart Study. *J Biosoc Sci* 2006; 38: 835–842.

[28] House, J. S., K. R. Landis, D. Umberson. Social relationships and health. *Science* 1988; 241: 540–45.

[29] Frasure-Smith et al. Social support, depression, and mortality during the first year after myocardial infarction. *Circulation.* 2000 Apr 25; 101 (16): 1919–24.

[30] Seeman, T. E., S. L. Syme. Social Networks and CAD: A comparison of the structure and function of social relations as predictors of disease. *Psychosomatic Medicine.* 1987; 49 (4): 341–54.

[31] Cohen, S., W. J. Doyle, D. P. Skoner, B. S. Rabin, J. M. Gwaltney Jr. Social ties and susceptibility to the common cold *JAMA.* 1997 Jun 25; 277 (24): 1940–44.

[32] Westaway, M. S.; J. R. Seager; P. Rheeder; DG Van Zyl. *Ethn Health* 2005 10 (1): 73–89.

[33] Kaplan, G. A., T. E. Seeman, R. D. Cohen, L. P. Knudsen, J. Guralnik. Mortality among the elderly in the Alameda County Study: behavioral and demographic

risk factors. *Am J Public Health* 1987; 77 (3): 307–12. & *Am J Public Health* 1987; 77 (7): 818.

[34] Spiegel, D., J. R. Bloom, H. C. Kraemer, E. Gottheil. The effect of psychosocial treatment on survival of patients with metastatic breast cancer. *Lancet.* 1989, ii: 888–91.

[35] Muscatello, M. R., A. Bruno, G. Pandolfo, U. Micò, S. Stilo, M. Scaffidi, P. Consolo, A. Tortora, S. Pallio, G. Giacobbe, L. Familiari, R. Zoccali. Depression, Anxiety and Anger in Subtypes of Irritable Bowel Syndrome Patients *J Clin Psychol Med Settings.* 2010 Mar; 17 (1): 64–70.

[36] Denollet, J., Y. Gidron, C. J. Vrints, V. M. Conraads. Anger, suppressed anger, and risk of adverse events in patients with coronary artery disease *Am J Cardiol.* 2010 Jun 1; 105 (11): 1555–60.

[37] Bennett, E. J., P. Evans, A. M. Scott, C. A. Badcock, B. Shuter, R. Höschl, C. C. Tennant, J. E. Kellow. Psychological and sex features of delayed gut transit in functional gastrointestinal disorders *Gut.* 2000 Jan; 46 (1): 83–87.

[38] Blomhoff, S., S. Spetalen, M. B. Jacobsen, M. Vatn, U. F. Malt. Intestinal reactivity to words with emotional content and brain information processing in irritable bowel syndrome *Dig Dis Sci.* 2000 Jun; 45 (6): 1160–65.

[39] Ornish, Dean. *Love & Survival: 8 Pathways to Intimacy and Health.* Harper Collins. New York, New York. 1998.

[40] Oz, Lisa. *US.* Free Press, a Division of Simon & Schuster, Inc. New York, New York. 2010.

[41] Nakazawa, D. *The Autoimmune Epidemic.* Simon and Schuster. New York, New Work. 2008.

[42] Kang, J. H., F. Kondo. Bisphenol A migration from cans containing coffee and caffeine *Food Addit Contam.* 2002 Sep; 19 (9): 886–90.

[43] Matsumoto, A., N. Kunugita, K. Kitagawa, T. Isse, T. Oyama, G. L. Foureman, M. Morita, T. Kawamoto. Bisphenol A levels in human urine *Environ Health Perspect.* 2003 Jan; 111 (1): 101–4.

[44] Bray, G. A. J. Fructose: pure, white, and deadly? Fructose, by any other name, is a health hazard *Diabetes Sci Technol.* 2010 Jul 1; 4 (4): 1003–07.

[45] Nseir, W., F. Nassar, N. Assy. Soft drinks consumption and nonalcoholic fatty liver disease *World J Gastroenterol.* 2010 Jun 7; 16 (21): 2579–88.

[46] Hayward, D., J. Wong, A.J. Krynitsky. Polybrominated diphenyl ethers and polychlorinated biphenyls in commercially wild caught and farm-raised fish fillets in the United States *Environ Res.* 2007 Jan; 103 (1): 46–54.

[47] Pall, M. L. Do sauna therapy and exercise act by raising the availability of tetrahydrobiopterin? *Med Hypotheses.* 2009 Oct; 73 (4): 610–130.

[48] http://www.realage.com/tips/skirt-ulcers-with-this-salad-topper?eid=7214& memberid=13730500

Chapter 6

1 Marakis, G., A. F. Walker, R. W. Middleton et al. Artichoke leaf extract reduces mild dyspepsia in an open study *Phytomedicine*. 2002; 9: 694–99.

2 Holtmann, G., B. Adam, S. Haag. et al. Efficacy of artichoke leaf extract in the treatment of patients with functional dyspepsia: a six-week placebo-controlled, double-blind, multicentre trial *Aliment Pharmacol Ther*. 2003; 18: 1099–1105.

3 Brett, 1998.

4 Misharina, T. A., M.B. Terenina, N. I. Krikunova. Antioxidant properties of essential oil *Prikl Biokhim Mikrobiol*. 2009 Nov-Dec; 45 (6): 710–16.

5 Perveen, T., S. Haider, S. Kanwal, D. J. Haleem.Pak Repeated administration of Nigella sativa decreases 5-HT turnover and produces anxiolytic effects in rats. *J Pharm Sci*. 2009 Apr; 22 (2): 139–44.

6 Mullin, G. E., J. O. Clarke. Role of complementary and alternative medicine in managing gastrointestinal motility disorders *Nutr Clin Pract*. 2010 Feb; 25 (1): 85–87.

7 Nadkarni, A. K. 1976. *Indian Materia Medica* (3 ed. Vol. 1). Bombay: Popular Prakashan.

8 Deitelhoff, P., O. Petrowicz, and B. Müller. 2000. *Phytomedicine* 7S2: 92.

9 WHO, 1999.

10 Igimi, H., R. Tamura, K. Toraishi et al. Medical dissolution of gallstones. *Dig Dis Sci* 1991; 36: 200–208.

11 Igimi, H., T. Hisatsugu, M. Nishimura. The use of D-limonene preparation as a dissolving agent of gallstones *Am J Dig Dis* 1976; 21: 926–39.

12 Wilkins, J. Jr. Method for treating gastrointestinal disorder. U.S. Patent (642045). 2002.

13 Sweetman, S. C 2005. Martindale: *The Complete Drug Reference*. Pharmaceutical Press: London, 1254–55, 1264.

14 Kassir, Z. A. 1985. Endoscopic controlled trial of four drug regimens in the treatment of chronic duodenal ulceration *Ir Med J* 78: 153–56.

15 Aly, A. M, L. Al-Alousi, H. A. Salem. 2005. Licorice: a possible anti-inflammatory and anti-ulcer drug *AAPS Pharm Sci Tech* 6: E74–E82.

16 Bradley, P. R. (ed). 1992b. Slippery Elm Bark in British Herbal Compendium Vol. 1 British Herbal Medicine Association, Bournemouth, Dorset, 204.

17 Suarez, F., M. D. Levitt, J. Adshead, et al. Pancreatic supplements reduce symptomatic response of healthy subjects to a high fat meal *Dig Dis Sci*. 1999; 44: 1317–21.

18 Borrelli, F., R. Capasso, G. Aviello, et al. Effectiveness and safety of ginger in the treatment of pregnancy-induced nausea and vomiting *Obstetrics & Gynecology* 2005; 105 (4): 849–56.

[19] Chaiyakunapruk, N., N. Kitikannakorn, S. Nathisuwan et al. The efficacy of ginger for the prevention of postoperative nausea and vomiting: a meta-analysis. American journal of obstetrics and gynecology 2006; 194 (1): 95–99.

[20] Gonlachanvit, S., Y. H. Chen, W. L. Hasler et al. 2003. Ginger reduces hyperglycemia-evoked gastric dysrhythmias in healthy humans: possible role of endogenous prostaglandins. *Journal of pharmacology and experimental therapeutics* 307 (3): 1098–1103.

[21] El-Abha, H. S., L. N. Hammad, H. S. Gawad. Modulating effect of ginger extract on rats with ulcerative colitis *J Ethnopharmacol.* 2008 Aug 13; 118 (3): 367–72.

[22] Soh, N. L., Walter G. Complementary medicine for psychiatric disorders in children and adolescents *Curr Opin Psychiatry.* 2008 Jul; 21 (4): 350–5.

[23] Dabos, K. J., E. Sfika, L. J. Vlatta, D. Frantzi, G. I. Amygdalos, G. Giannikopoulos. Is Chios mastic gum effective in the treatment of functional dyspepsia? A prospective randomized double-blind placebo controlled trial. *J Ethnopharmacol.* 2010 Feb 3; 127 (2): 205–9.

[24] Paraschos, S., P. Magiatis, S. Mitakou, K. Petraki, A. Kalliaropoulos, P. Maragkoudakis, A. Mentis, D. Sgouras, A.L. Skaltsounis. In vitro and in vivo activities of Chios mastic gum extracts and constituents against Helicobacter pylori. *Antimicrob Agents Chemother.* 2007 Feb; 51 (2): 551–59.

[25] Werbach, M. R. Melatonin for the treatment of gastroesophageal reflux disease. *Altern Ther Health Med.* 2008 Jul-Aug;14 (4): 54–58.

[26] Kandil, T.S., A. A. Mousa, A. A. El-Gendy, A. M. Abbas. The potential therapeutic effect of melatonin in Gastro-Esophageal Reflux Disease. *BMC Gastroenterol.* 2010 Jan; 10:7.

[27] Bundy, R., A. F. Walker, R. W. Middleton, G Marakis, and J C. Booth. 2004. Zinc L-carnosine protects colonic mucosal injury through induction of heat shock protein 72 and suppression of NF-kappaB activation. *Journal of Alternatie and Complementary Medicine* 10: 667–9.

[28] Walker, A. F., R. W. Middleton, and O. Petrowicz. 2001. Artichoke leaf extract reduces symptoms of irritable bowel syndrome in a post marketing surveillance study *Phytotherapy Research* 15: 58–61.

[29] Bundy, R., A. F. Walker, A. F. Middleton R. W. et al. Artichoke leaf extract reduces symptoms of irritable bowel syndrome and improves quality of life in otherwise healthy volunteers suffering from concomitant dyspepsia: a subset analysis. *J Altern Complement Med.* 2004; 10: 667–69.

[30] De la Motte, S., S. Bose-O'Reilly, M. Heinisch, and F. Harrison. 1997. Double-blind comparison of an apple pectin-chamomile extract preparation with placebo in children with diarrhea *Arzneimittelforschung* 47: 1247–49.

[31] Becker, B., U. Kuhn. and B. Hardewig-Budny. Double-blind, randomized evaluation of clinical efficacy and tolerability of an apple pectin-chamomile extract in children with unspecific diarrhea 2006. *Arzneimittelforschung* 56: 387–93.

32 Savino, F., F. Cresi, E. Castagno, L. Silvestro, and R. Oggero. 2005. A random-ized double-blind placebo-controlled trial of a standardized extract of Matri-cariae recutita, Foeniculum vulgare and Melissa officinalis (ColiMil) in the treatment of breastfed colicky infants *Phytotherapy Research* 19:335–40.

33 Weizman, Z., Alkrinawi, S., D. Goldfarb, and C. Bitran. Efficacy of herbal tea preparation in infantile colic 1993. *Journal of Pediatrics*. 122: 650–52.

34 von Arnim, U., U. Peitz, B. Vinson, K. J. Gundermann, P. Malfertheiner. STW 5, a phytopharmacon for patients with functional dyspepsia: results of a multi-center, placebo-controlled double-blind study *Am J Gastroenterol*. 2007 Jun; 102(6): 1268–75.

35 Rösch, W., T. Liebregts, K. J. Gundermann, B. Vinson, G. Holtmann. Phyto-therapy for functional dyspepsia: a review of the clinical evidence for the herbal preparation STW 5. *Phytomedicine*. 2006; 13 Suppl 5: 114–21.

36 Leng, P. H, K. A. Gwee, S. M. Moochhala, K. Y. Ho. Melatonin improves abdominal pain in irritable bowel syndrome patients who have sleep distur-bances: a randomized, double blind, placebo controlled study *Gut*. 2005; 54: 1402–7.

37 Lu, W. Z., G. H Song, K. A. Gwee, K. Y Ho. The effects of melatonin on colonic transit time in normal controls and IBS patients. *Dig Dis Sci*. 2008; 54 (5): 1087–93.

38 Pittler, M. H., E. Ernst. Peppermint oil for irritable bowel syndrome: a critical review and metaanalysis. *Am J Gastroenterol* 1998 Jul; 93 (7): 1131–35.

39 Ford, A. C., N. J. Talley, B. M. Spiegel, A. E. Foxx-Orenstein, L. Schiller, E. M. Quigley, P. Moayyedi. Effect of fibre, antispasmodics, and peppermint oil in the treatment of irritable bowel syndrome: systematic review and meta-analysis *BMJ*. 2008 Nov 13; 337: a2313.

40 www.springerlink.com/content/I3677n5733267837/

41 Hoveyda, N., C. Heneghan, K. R. Mahtani et al. A systematic review and meta-analysis: probiotics in the treatment of irritable bowel syndrome. (2009) *BMC Gastroenterol* 9, 15.

42 Chmielewska, A., H. Szajewska. Systematic review of randomised controlled trials: probiotics for functional constipation. *World J Gastroenterol*. 2010 Janu-ary 7; 16 (1): 69–75.

43 Aragon, G., D. B. Graham, M. Borum, D. B. Doman. Probiotic therapy for irri-table bowel syndrome. *Gastroenterol Hepatol* (NY). 2010 Jan; 6(1): 39–44.

44 You, Y., S. Yoo, H. G. Yoon, J. Park, Y. H. Lee, S. Kim, K. T. Oh, J. Lee, H. Y. Cho, W. Jun. In vitro and in vivo hepatoprotective effects of the aqueous extract from Taraxacum officinale (dandelion) root against alcohol-induced oxidative stress *Food Chem Toxicol*. 2010 Jun; 48 (6): 1632–37.

45 Takasaki, M., T. Konoshima, H. Tokuda, K. Masuda, Y. Arai, K. Shiojima, H. Ageta. *Biol Pharm Bull*. 1999 Jun; 22 (6): 602–5.

[46] Rodriguez-Hernandez, H., et al. Hypomagnesemia, insulin resistance, and non-alcoholic steatohepatitis in obese subject *Arch Med Res*, 2005. 36 (4): 362–66.

[47] Koivisto, M., et al., Magnesium depletion in chronic terminal liver cirrhosis. *Clin Transplant*, 2002. 16 (5): p. 325–28.

[48] Cani, P. D., et al. Selective increases of bifidobacteria in gut microflora improve high-fat-diet-induced diabetes in mice through a mechanism associated with *endotoxaemiaDiabetologia*, 2007. 50 (11): p. 2374–83.

[49] Daubioul, C. A., et al., Dietary oligofructose lessens hepatic steatosis, but does not prevent hypertriglyceridemia in obese zucker rats. *J Nutr*, 2000. 130 (5): p. 1314–19.

[50] Carithers, R. L. and C. M. McClain, Alcoholic Liver Disease, in Sleisenger and Fordtran's Gastrointestinal and Liver Disease *Pathophysiology/Diagnosis/Management*, M. Feldman, L. Friedman, and L. Brandt, Editors. 2006, Saunders Elsevier: Canada. 1771–92.

[51] McClain, C. J., et al., Cytokines in alcoholic liver disease *Semin Liver Dis*, 1999. 19 (2): p. 205–19.

[52] Gazak, R., D. Walterova, V. Kren. *Gastroenterology*. 2008 Nov;135 (5): 1561–67.

[53] Saller, R., R. Brignoli, J. Melzer, R. Meier. An updated systematic review with meta-analysis for the clinical evidence of silymarin *Forsch Komplementmed*. 2008 Feb; 15 (1): 9–20.

[54] Sanyal, A. J., et al., Pioglitazone, vitamin E, or placebo for nonalcoholic steatohepatitis. *N Engl J Med*. 362 (18): p. 1675–85.

[55] Stamoulis, I., G. Kouraklis, and S. Theocharis. Zinc and the liver: an active interaction *Dig Dis Sci*, 2007. 52 (7): p. 1595–1612.

[56] Shea-Budgell, M. et al. Marginal zinc deficiency increased the susceptibility to acute lipopolysaccharide-induced liver injury in rats. *Exp Biol Med* (Maywood), 2006. 231 (5): p. 553–58.

[57] Keyhanian, S., E. Stahl-Biskup. Phenolic constituents in dried flowers of aloe vera (Aloe barbadensis) and their in vitro antioxidative capacity *Planta Med*. 2007 Jun; 73 (6): 599–602.

[58] Bautista-Pérez, R., D. Segura-Cobos, B. Vázquez-Cruz. *J Ethnopharmacol*. 2004 Jul; 93 (1): 89–92.

[59] Pogribna, M., Freeman J. P., D. Paine, M. D. Boudreau. *Lett Appl Microbiol*. 2008 May; 46 (5): 575–80.

[60] Korkina, L., M. Suprun, A. Petrova, E. Mikhal'chik, A. Luci, C. De Luca. The protective and healing effects of a natural antioxidant formulation based on ubiquinol and Aloe vera against dextran sulfate-induced ulcerative colitis in rats *Biofactors*. 2003; 18 (1–4): 255–64.

[61] Langmead, L., R. J. Makins, D. S. Rampton. Randomized, double-blind, placebo-controlled trial of oral aloe vera gel for active ulcerative colitis. *Aliment Pharmacol Ther.* 2004 Mar 1; 19 (5): 521–27.

[62] Eamlamnam, K., S. Patumraj, N. Visedopas, D. Thong-Ngam. Effects of Aloe vera and sucralfate on gastric microcirculatory changes, cytokine levels and gastric ulcer healing in rats *World J Gastroenterol.* 2006 Apr 7; 12 (13): 2034–39.

[63] Sotnikova, E. P. Therapeutic use of aloe in experimental stomach ulcers *Vrach Delo.* 1984 Jun; (6): 71–74.

[64] Gawron-Gzella, A., E. Witkowska-Banaszczak, M. Dudek. Herbs and herbal preparations applied in the treatment of gastric hyperacidity, gastric and duodenal ulcer in cigarette smokers *Przegl Lek.* 2005; 62 (10): 1185–87.

[65] Blitz, J. J., J. W. Smith, J. R. Gerard. Aloe vera gel in peptic ulcer therapy: preliminary report *J Am Osteopath Assoc.* 1963 Apr; 62: 731–35.

[66] Ammon, H. P. Boswellic acids in chronic inflammatory diseases. Boswellic acids in chronic inflammatory diseases. *Planta Med* 2006; 72 (12): 1100–16.

[67] Gupta, I., A. Parihar, P. Malhotra, et al. Effects of Boswellia serrata gum resin in patients with ulcerative colitis *Eur J Med Res* 1997; 2 (1): 37–43.

[68] ———. Effects of gum resin of Boswellia serrata in patients with chronic colitis *Planta Med* 2001; 67 (5): 391–5.

[69] Gerhardt, H., F. Seifert, P. Buvari, H. Vogelsang, R. Repges. Therapy of active Crohn disease with Boswellia serrata extract H 15 Z *Gastroenterol* 2001; 39(1): 11–7.

[70] Madisch, A., S. Miehlke, O. Eichele, J. Mrwa, B. Bethke, E. Kuhlisch, E. Bästlein, G. Wilhelms, A. Morgner, B. Wigginghaus, M. Stolte. Boswellia serrata extract for the treatment of collagenous colitis. A double-blind, randomized, placebo-controlled, multicenter trialInt *J Colorectal Dis.* 2007 Dec; 22(12): 1445–51.

[71] Holt, P. R., S. Katz and R. Kirshoff. Curcumin therapy in inflammatory bowel disease: a pilot study 2005. *Dig Dis Sci.* 50: 2191–93.

[72] Hanai, H., T. Iida, et al. Curcumin maintenance therapy for ulcerative colitis: randomized, multicenter, double-blind, placebo-controlled trial 2006. *Clinical Gastroenterology and Hepatology* 4: 1502–6.

[73] Amasheh, M., S. Andres, S. Amasheh, M. Fromm, J. D. Schulzke. Barrier effects of nutritional factors *Ann N Y Acad Sci.* 2009 May; 1165: 267–73.

[74] Crowther, M. *Proc Nutr Soc.* Hot topics in parenteral nutrition. A review of the use of glutamine supplementation in the nutritional support of patients undergoing bone-marrow transplantation and traditional cancer therapy 2009 Aug; 68(3): 269–73.

[75] Coëffier, M., R. Marion-Letellier, P. Déchelotte. Potential for amino acids supplementation during inflammatory bowel diseases *Inflamm Bowel Dis.* 2010 Mar; 16(3): 518–24.

[76] Lecleire, S., A. Hassan, R. Marion-Letellier, M. Antonietti, G. Savoye, C. Bôle-Feysot, E. Lerebours, P. Ducrotté, P. Déchelotte, M. Coëffier. Combined glutamine and arginine decrease proinflammatory cytokine production by biopsies from Crohn's patients in association with changes in nuclear factor-kappaB and p38 mitogen-activated protein kinase pathways. *J Nutr.* 2008 Dec; 138(12): 2481–86.

[77] Siguel, E. N., R. H. Lerman. Prevalence of essential fatty acid deficiency in patients with chronic gastrointestinal disorders *Metabolism* 1996, vol 45, pp 12–23.

[78] Ruggiero, C., F. Lattanzio, F. Lauretani, B. Gasperini, C. Andres-Lacueva, A. Cherubini. Omega-3 polyunsaturated fatty acids and immune-mediated diseases: inflammatory bowel disease and rheumatoid arthritis *Curr Pharm Des.* 2009; 15 (36): 4135–48.

[79] Turner, D., S. H. Zlotkin, P. S. Shah, A. M. Griffiths. Omega 3 fatty acids (fish oil) for maintenance of remission in ulcerative colitis Cochrane Database Syst Rev, 2007 Apr 18; (2): CD006320.

[80] Turner, D., P. S. Shah, A. H. Steinhart, S. Zlotkin, A. M. Griffiths. Maintenance of remission in inflammatory bowel disease using omega-3 fatty acids (fish oil): a systematic review and meta-analyses. *Inflamm Bowel Dis.* 2011 Jan; 17 (1): 336–45. doi: 10.1002/ibd.21374.

[81] Turner, D., S. H. Zlotkin, P. S. Shah, A. M. Griffiths. Omega 3 fatty acids (fish oil) for maintenance of remission in Crohn's disease Cochrane Database Syst Rev. 2009 Jan 21; (1): CD006320.

[82] Feagan, B. G., W. J. Sandborn, U. Mittmann, S. Bar-Meir, G. D'Haens, M. Bradette, A. Cohen, C. Dallaire, T. P. Ponich, J. W. McDonald, X. Hébuterne, P. Paré, P. Klvana, Y. Niv, S. Ardizzone, O. Alexeeva, A. Rostom, G. Kiudelis, J. Spleiss, D. Gilgen, M. K. Vandervoort, C. J. Wong, G. Y. Zou, A. Donner, P. Rutgeerts. Omega-3 free fatty acids for the maintenance of remission in Crohn disease: the EPIC Randomized Controlled Trials. *JAMA,* 2008 Apr 9; 299 (14): 1690–97.

[83] Seidner, D. L., B. A. Lashner, A. Brezzinski and The Enteral Nutrition in Ulcerative Colitis Study. An oral supplement enriched with fish oil, soluble fiber, and antioxidants for corticosteroid sparing in ulcerative colitis: a randomized, controlled trial *Clinical Gastroenterology and Hepatology* Volume 3, Issue 4, April 2005, 358–69.

[84] Hallert, C., I. Bjorck, M. Nyman, A. Pousette, C. Granno, H. Svensson. Increasing fecal butyrate in ulcerative colitis patients by diet: controlled pilot study. *Inflamm Bowel Dis,* 2003 Mar; 9 (2): 116–21.

[85] Bamba, T., O. Kanauchi, A. Andoh, Y. Fujiyama. A new prebiotic from germinated barley for nutraceutical treatment of ulcerative colitis. *J Gastroenterol Hepatol,* 2002 Aug; 17 (8): 818–24.

[86] Kanauchi, O. H., K. H. Mitsuyama, T. H. Homma, et al. Treatment of ulcerative colitis patients by long-term administration of germinated barley foodstuff: multi-center open trial *Int J Mol Med,* 2003 Nov; 12 (5): 701–4.

[87] Hanai, H., O. Kanauchi, K. Mitsuyama, et al. Germinated barley foodstuff prolongs remission in patients with ulcerative colitis. Germinated barley foodstuff prolongs remission in patients with ulcerative colitis *Int J Mol Med,* 2004 May; 13 (5): 643.

[88] Williams, N. T. Probiotics *Am J Health Syst Pharm.* 2010 Mar 15; 67 (6): 449–58.

[89] Clarke, J. O., G. E. Mullin. A review of complementary and alternative approaches to immunomodulation *Nutr Clin Pract.* 2008 Feb; 23 (1): 49–62.

[90] Sang, L. X., B. Chang, W. L. Zhang, X. M. Wu, X. H. Li, M. Jiang. Remission induction and maintenance effect of probiotics on ulcerative colitis: a meta-analysis.*World J Gastroenterol* 2010 April; 16 (15): 1908–15.

[91] Scheppach, W., H. Sommer, T. Kirchner, et al. Effect of butyrate enemas on the colonic mucosa in distal ulcerative colitis *Gastroenterology.* 1992; 103 (1): 51–56.

[92] Breuer, R. I., S. K. Buto, M. L. Christ, et al. Rectal irrigation with short-chain fatty acids for distal ulcerative colitis. Preliminary report. *Dig Dis Sci.* 1991; 36 (2): 185–87.

[93] Steinhart, A. H., A. Brzezinski, J. P. Baker. Treatment of refractory ulcerative proctosigmoiditis with butyrate enemas 1994; 89 (2): 179–183.

[94] Patz, J., W. Z. Jacobsohn, S. Gottschalk-Sabag, S. Zeides, D. Z. Braverman. Treatment of refractory distal ulcerative colitis with short chain fatty acid enemas *Am J Gastroenterol.* 1996; 91 (4): 731–34.

[95] Vernia, P., M. Cittadini, R. Caprilli, A. Torsoli. Topical treatment of refractory distal ulcerative colitis with 5-ASA and sodium butyrate *Dig Dis Sci.* 1995; 40 (2): 305–7.

[96] Mullin, G. E., L. Turnbull, K. Kines. Vitamin D: a D-lightful health supplement *Nutr Clin Pract.* 2009 Oct-Nov; 24 (5): 642–4.

[97] Harries, A. D., R. Brown, R. V. Heatley, et al. Vitamin D status in Crohn's disease: association with nutrition and disease activity *Gut.* 1985; 26: 1197–203.

[98] Cantorna, M. T. Vitamin D and its role in immunology: multiple sclerosis, and inflammatory bowel disease. *Prog Biophys Mol Biol.* 2006; 92: 60–64.

[99] Mullin, G. E., L. K. Turnbull, K. Kines. Vitamin D: a D-lightful health supplement: part II *Nutr Clin Pract.* 2009 Dec; 24 (6): 738–40.

[100] Froicu, M., Y. Zhu, M. T. Cantorna. Vitamin D receptor is required to control gastrointestinal immunity in IL-10 knockout mice *Immunology.* 2006; 117: 310–318.

[101] Jørgensen, S. P., J. Agnholt, H. Glerup, S. Lyhne, G. E. Villadsen, C. L. Hvas et al. Clinical trial: vitamin D_3 treatment in Crohn's disease—a randomized double-blind placebo-controlled study *Aliment Pharmacol Ther.* 2010; 32: 377–83.

[102] Sturniolo, G. C., V. Di Leo, A. Ferronato, A. D'Odorico, R. D'Inca. Zinc supplementation tightens "leaky gut" in Crohn's disease *Inflamm Bowel Dis.* 2001 May; 7 (2): 94–98.

[103] Hendricks, K. M., W. A. Walker. Zinc deficiency in inflammatory bowel disease *Nutrition Reviews.* 1988, vol 46, pp 401–8.

[104] Watanabe, T., M. Ishihara, K. Matsuura, K. Mizuta, Y. Itoh. Polaprezinc prevents oral mucositis associated with radiochemotherapy in patients with head and neck cancer. *Int J Cancer.* 2010 Oct 15; 127 (8): 1984–90.

[105] Odashima, M., M. Otaka, M. Jin, I. Wada, Y. Horikawa, T. Matsuhashi, R. Ohba, N. Hatakeyama, J. Oyake, S. Watanabe. *Life Sci.* 2006 Nov 10; 79 (24): 2245–50.

Chapter 7

[1] B. Spiegel et al., "Measuring irritable bowel syndrome patient-reported outcomes with an abdominal pain numeric rating scale," *Aliment Pharmacol Ther* 30, no. 11–12 (2009 Dec 1): 1159–70.

[2] S. Vermeire et al., "Correlation Between the Crohn's Disease Activity and Harvey-Bradshaw Indices In Assessing Crohn's Disease Severity," *Clin Gastroenterol Hepatol* 8, no. 4 (2010): 357–63.

[3] I. Clara et al., "The Manitoba IBD Index: Evidence for a new and simple indicator of IBD activity," *Am J Gastroenterol* 104, no. 7 (2009 Jul): 1754–63.

[4] S. L. Oyer, L. C. Anderson, and S. L. Halum, "Influence of anxiety and depression on the predictive value of the Reflux Symptom Index," *Ann Otol Rhinol Laryngol* 118, no. 10 (2009 Oct): 687–92.

Chapter 8

[1] Center for Science in the Public Interest, www.cspinet.org/reports/chemcuisine.htm

[2] Deanna M. Minich, *An A-Z Guide to Food Additives: Never Eat What You Can't Pronounce* (San Francisco: Conari Press, 2009).

[3] W. D. Heizer, S. Southern, and S. McGovern, "The role of diet in symptoms of irritable bowel syndrome in adults: a narrative review," *J Am Diet Assoc* 109 (2009): 1204–14.

Chapter 9

[1] National Institute of Allergy and Infectious Diseases, National Institutes of Health, "Guidelines for Diagnosis and Management of Food Allergy in the United States," Washington DC, 2010.

[2] Peter Farb and Geoge J. Armelagos, *Consuming Passions: An Anthropology of Eating.* Houghton-Mifflin, New York. 1980.

[3] W. D. Heizer, S. Southern, and S. McGovern, "The role of diet in symptoms of irritable bowel syndrome in adults: a narrative review," *J Am Diet Assoc* 109 (2009): 1204–14.

[4] P. R. Gibson and S. J. Shephard, "Evidence-based dietary management of functional gastrointestinal symptoms: the FODMAP approach," *J Gasto and Hepatology* 25 (2009): 252–58.

[5] Kate Scarlata, "The FODMAPs approach: minimize consumption of fermentable carbs to manage functional gut disorder symptoms," *Today's Dietitian,* 12, no. 8 (2010 August): 30–34.

[6] J. Mathieu, "What is orthorexia?" *J Am Diet Assoc* 105, no. 10 (2005): 1510–12.

[7] C. Fargo Ware, "Morsels, nibbles, and bites," *Tastings* (Newsletter of the Food and Culinary Professionals, American Dietetic Association) 15, no. 1 (2010): 4.

[8] Adapted from *Dealing with Food Allergies* by Janice Vickerstaff Joneja, PhD, RDN (Boulder, Colorado: Bull Publishing Company, 2003).

Chapter 11

[1] B. M. Sun et al., "Acupuncture versus metoclopramide in treatment of postoperative gastroparesis syndrome in abdominal surgical patients: a randomized controlled trial," *Zhong Xi Yi Jie He Xue Bao.* 2010 Jul; 8(7): 641–44.

[2] A. Sugumar, A. Singh, and P. J. Pasricha, "A systematic review of the efficacy of domperidone for the treatment of diabetic gastroparesis," *Clin Gastroenterol Hepatol* 6, no. 7 (2008): 726–33.

Index

Underscored page references indicate boxed text and tables. **Boldface** references indicate illustrations.